I invite you to come with me on a voyage of discovery. It will take you a few hours, yet it took me four years. The journey began with the publication of my first book, Understanding Chronic Pain, and ends, or at least pauses—for there is much yet to learn—with this work.

Curing Chronic Pain is a bold, even audacious title, but I think it is appropriate. Admittedly, neither I nor anyone else can cure everyone with chronic pain, but that goal is nearly within reach, and I believe my optimism is warranted.

In my first book, I explored the relationship of pain to depression, childhood trauma, and substance abuse. I explored also, however tentatively, its relationship to bipolar disease. This work moves many steps forward, for in it I examine the relationship of pain to delusions, hallucinations, phobias, obsessive-compulsiveness, dementia, narcolepsy, cravings, and anger. All of these offer incredible clues for successful treatment, and I will describe many cases in which miraculous cures have been achieved. Many of these have occurred with the usage of opiates, a group of drugs I disdained in my first book because of their potential for addiction. My thinking on this matter has turned 180 degrees, for I have learned to weigh the potential for addiction against the probability of cure. The balance tips strongly to the latter, and I now employ opiates regularly and with great success, for I know that their therapeutic spectrum extends far beyond the mere relief of pain.

Those of you who have read Understanding Chronic Pain will find that this work follows almost seamlessly. Although Curing Chronic Pain will stand on its own, I encourage those unfamiliar with my first book to take a look at it. I believe you will marvel, as constantly I do now, at just how much a doctor can learn in four years.

Robert T. Cochran Jr., MD

CURING
CHRONIC
PAIN

Stories of Hope
and Healing

ROBERT T. COCHRAN JR., MD

Providence House Publishers
WWW.PROVIDENCEHOUSE.COM
FRANKLIN, TENNESSEE

Printed in the United States of America

13   12   11   10   09   1   2   3   4   5

Library of Congress Control Number: 2008937367

ISBN: 978-1-57736-412-2

Cover and page design by LeAnna Massingille

PROVIDENCE HOUSE PUBLISHERS
238 Seaboard Lane • Franklin, Tennessee 37067
www.providencehouse.com
800-321-5692

To Donna, Elma, and Bob

*It is much more important to know
what sort of patient has a disease
than what sort of a disease a patient has.*

—Sir William Osler

Contents

PREFACE AND ACKNOWLEDGMENTS   ix

1. How Did You Know What to Do?   1
2. Pharmacy for Pain   17
3. Pain in the Jaw   35
4. Depression and Pain   49
5. Demons and Ghosts   73
6. Remembered Pain   91
7. The Damaged Brain   113
8. Pain Behavior   129
9. Drugs of Abuse   145
10. Why I Fail   163
11. Analgesic Rebound   183
12. Childhood Abuse   205
13. The Bipolar Spectrum   229
14. The Opiate Cure   249
15. Anger and Pain   279
16. Dreams and Pain   299

EPILOGUE   323
INDEX   331
ABOUT THE AUTHOR   338

Preface and Acknowledgments

I want to tell you a little about myself, and in doing so, explain how this book came to be. I was cradle gifted with a B+ intelligence and an A+ imagination (I am glad it was not the reverse). This is to say ideas, not always necessarily good ones, come easily to me. I was also gifted with an even disposition, and that, I assure you, is an important attribute in one who spends his life listening to others talk about how much they hurt.

After I completed my formal academic studies, I entered internship and residency in the field of internal medicine—certainly a happy career choice. Also a happy choice was my decision to spend a year as a resident in neurology. During their subspecialty year, most of my classmates entered the sexy and rapidly developing fields of infectious disease, rheumatology, and above all, cardiology, where great things were being done. The field of neurology was much less seductive because little was being done, but I did feel the brain, although little understood, was not an unimportant part of the body.

I entered practice and did what internists do: treat heart attacks, strokes, bladder infections, and all the rest. I did see my share, however, maybe more than my share, of painful people—those with migraine and a disorder then known as fibrositis, but now described more eloquently as fibromyalgia (which means quite literally, pain in the muscles and the connective tissue that attaches to them). I began prescribing psychiatric drugs, chiefly antidepressants, for the treatment of those disorders, with some success. Intrigued by this, I elected to attend a psychopharmacology (drugs for the mind) conference—an enterprise about as far removed from my daily professional life as one could imagine. I enjoyed it enormously, and from that point on some thirty years ago, most of my obligatory continuing medical education credits have been in the field of psychiatry and psychopharmacy.

Perhaps it was my simultaneous interest in several different medical fields that led me to be invited to join a new pain clinic that was opening at Centennial Hospital in Nashville, Tennessee. There I met and had daily conversation with anesthesiologists, psychiatrists, neurologists, physical therapists, and psychologists. Our clinic was multi-disciplinary, that is, many different minds were working to solve very difficult problems. And problems they were—the sickest people I have ever seen in my life, suffering badly, sleepless, frustrated, and depressed.

Although I respected my colleagues greatly, I found the multi-disciplinary approach fragmented and without direction. I resolved that if I was ever going to make any sense out of the pain thing, I would have to do it with my own brain, not somebody else's. I left the clinic to pursue my study with my own agenda. Gradually it started coming to me. I realized that there was great commonality in people who suffered pain. Whether it was due to migraine, neuritis, lumbar spine disease, irritable bowels, or whatever, I kept hearing the same story. Disordered sleep. Disordered mood. Disordered memory. Disordered appetite. I began to realize that chronic pain was not many diseases, it was a single, core illness with many different expressions. As my experience grew, and as the new psychopharmaceuticals came on the scene in great variety, I found that my patients' recovery rates were improving substantially, up to as much as 50 percent.

Some ten years into my study of chronic pain, my ideas had crystallized enough for me to at least begin writing a book. It was an exercise that was to take nearly five years. I discovered that by putting ideas to paper, I was better able to organize them and make them coherent. I was beginning to see a pattern.

Understanding Chronic Pain: A Doctor Talks to His Patients was published in January 2004. Although published by a smaller, regional press and having little marketing effort other than my willingness to go anywhere for a book signing, it achieved national distribution and has been a top-rated book on the subject on Internet sources from early on. It is now in its second edition.

Understanding Chronic Pain has had a favorable impact on many lives. I know this from conversations with readers and from letters and e-mails received from near and far. I have been deeply touched by these communications, and I have included a number of them in this text. They are eloquent, describing in the first person the plight of the painful, and I am sure that they will resonate with many readers who suffer and who sometimes feel they are alone. They are not.

Following the publication of my book, I continued my work and the learning curve gradually ascended with my outcomes ever improving. Pleased with my success, I decided to write another book, but for some reason it went slowly. Then, about a year before this writing, I began to see things more clearly. I found my imagination sometimes running away with me. There were good ideas, lots of them, and also good luck. There were remarkable observations and experiences and cures so dramatic that they seemed almost providentially directed. That which had begun at a glacial pace had become meteoric in velocity. To put that in some perspective for you, a third of the content of this book consists of material that I did not even know existed when I began writing it one year ago. Indeed, I have found it difficult to conclude this book because it seems weekly, and sometimes daily, a patient offers me a new insight.

Curing Chronic Pain, like its predecessor and companion, consists of the stories of people who suffer pain and who have entered my life seeking help. Some of the stories evolve in such a melodramatic manner that they may appear contrived. I assure you they are not. They are true stories of real people. The changes I have made are to disguise identities and some-times to simplify the story so my reader does not have to go down as many blind alleys as I have had to do. I will admit that I have condensed two stories (that is, people) into one. This has been done in the interest of making an important point with economy of space. I have exercised it only on a few occasions and in no instance have I deviated from the funda-mental truth. I write only what I see and hear.

I believe I have some remarkable things to tell you. I will write about wonderful people, wonderful new drugs, and most incredibly, wonderful old drugs. I will describe cures that I could not have imagined a year ago.

In *Understanding Chronic Pain*, I admonished that I was not writing a book that offered the quick and easy answer. I was writing a book that offered understanding, for I believed that it would be through understanding that we would find the answers. I still believe that, and I believe that we are rapidly gaining ever more under-standing. Nonetheless—and I don't want to give you false hope—there may be some incredibly quick and easy answers out there. We will have to disobey convention and change some of our thinking, but they are out there.

I want to express my gratitude to many people who have assisted me with my work. Donna, my wife of fifty years, has once again given me time and space, and for that simple act of courtesy and love, I am profoundly grateful. My office staff—Janet Epstein, Pat Lovell, Linda Harris, Sandy Cooper, Jan Diehl, Sherry Jolly, and Jennifer Hargrove—has helped me enormously, and I am appreciative. I am indebted to Andrew Miller and the staff at Providence House Publishers for their support and energy in seeing this book to publication.

I am deeply indebted to my colleagues, who have paid me great tribute by referring their most difficult patients to me. My referrals come from across the medical spectrum, encompassing the fields of neurosurgery, orthopedics, urology, gynecology, gastroenterology, rheumatology, and neurology. Thus, I am able to see patients with a great variety of painful states, and I am grateful for that opportunity.

Lastly, my greatest debt is to those people who have come to me for care and submitted to my therapies. I have been able to help most of them, and I am thankful for that because my respect for them and my affection knows virtually no bounds.

Each of the human beings I describe in this book, and many others also, brought me a gift—that of knowledge. Some gave me but little, others quite a lot. But the way they were so conveniently layered one upon another in time and complexity has allowed me to construct something that may turn out to be important. The manner in which they appeared, each teaching me something, sometimes almost more than I could handle, was not, I believe, the product of chance. I believe it was the product of design. This is to say that I did not create this book alone. I write these words on Christmas Day 2007.

CURING
CHRONIC
PAIN

CHAPTER ONE

How Did You Know What to Do?

Ann's pain bothered her only at night. She would go to bed and sleep well for a couple of hours and then awaken with pain in the neck, and as time went by, in the back of the head also. She would move to a reclining chair, place a heating pad behind her neck, and after a while the pain would diminish sufficiently to allow her to sleep—at least until she would again awaken with pain.

X-rays showed changes of degenerative arthritis in the cervical spine, a finding not unexpected in an elderly woman. Her physician prescribed Naproxen, an anti-inflammatory drug commonly used for the treatment of arthritis. It was without effect. He then prescribed Ultram, an analgesic. He instructed her to take it every four hours as needed for pain or, if she chose, to take it at bedtime in order to prevent painful awakenings. Neither exercise worked. Suspecting his patient's pain derived from pressure on the nerve roots by bone spurs or a ruptured disc, he referred her to a neurosurgeon. An MRI showed some narrowing of the neural foramina, the gaps in the vertebral column through which the cervical nerves pass. None of the several constrictions were severe enough, however, to warrant surgery, and even if they had been, I doubt the surgeon would have elected to operate on an eighty-four-year-old whose pain went away with an hour on a heating pad.

She was referred to an anesthesiologist for a procedure known as epidural steroid injection. A hypodermic needle was inserted through the muscles of the back of the neck and cortisone was injected adjacent to the spine to bathe the inflamed nerve roots. Pain abated for a week or so, but then returned full force each night. Nevertheless, she submitted to a second injection a month later, but that was of even less benefit. The thoughtful anesthesiologist told Ann there was no need for any more steroid injections. He suggested another procedure, the occipital nerve block. Anesthetic was injected into the area of the occipital nerves, those which carry sensation from the back of the skull and the upper neck. Following the procedure, Ann slept well for one night only. Her pain then returned, again full force.

Such is the unfortunate lot of the painful. They typically see many doctors, and they are subject to many treatment forms that sometimes don't work very well at all.

The persistent anesthesiologist, unable to relieve pain by the application of cortisone or anesthetic to inflamed nerves, opted for another form of therapy, known as Botox injection. Botox is a trademarked, proprietary drug, its name a contraction of botulinum toxin. Botulism is the most virulent form of bacterial food poisoning. The organism releases a paralyzing toxin which in severe cases can lead to death. However, the localized placement of small quantities of the toxin can be helpful in preventing unwanted muscular spasm. The anesthesiologist hoped the injections would diminish the force of muscle contractions, which, he surmised, were causing the strange nocturnal pain. They helped not at all. The anesthesiologist, thrice burned, referred her to me.

Ann, over the course of several months, had seen three different doctors. She had undergone x-rays and an MRI. She had received anti-inflammatory drugs and analgesics. She had been subjected to injections, first cortisone, then an anesthetic, and then Botox. Such is the unfortunate lot of the painful. They typically see many doctors, and they are subject to many treatment forms that sometimes don't work very well at all.

She was a handsome and vivacious woman with gold-rimmed glasses and bright, blue eyes. She was accompanied by a friend who was equally charming. They obviously enjoyed each other's company, and their conversation was quick and clever. Ann was certainly exhibiting no angst.

Her past medical history was, for an eighty-four-year-old, quite unremarkable. She had required a few operations, but her recovery from each was prompt and complete. Her emotional health had also been quite good. She denied any history of depression and, until the onset of her pain, she slept well. I inquired about her personal history because chronic pain often appears according to the dictates of destructive personal events. She had her share. What eighty-four-year-old has not? She was twice a widow. Her first marriage lasted happily for fifty years. Her second, to her husband's cousin, lasted for seven. Following his death, she returned to her ancestral home in Kentucky where she enjoyed the companionship of good friends and her church and garden club.

As we shall see in the case studies which follow, only occasionally does chronic pain strike out of the blue. It usually appears under the persuasion of forces such as depression, drug abuse, or emotional trauma. Ann, it seemed, was an exception. Until the onset of pain, her life had been of one of social, emotional, and physical comfort.

The examination was unremarkable. She described no pain as she rotated her neck to the left and to the right, and even the extremes of extension (looking up at the ceiling) and flexion (looking to the floor) produced no discomfort at all. Her arthritic neck was certainly not bothering her at the time of my examination.

"Ann, I am very taken with the fact that your pain seems to appear only at night. Does it ever occur during the day? Are there certain activities that seem to bring it on?"

"No, I never have pain during the day. My activities are not limited at all. I am able to garden, and just a couple of weeks ago I painted my kitchen."

"Did you have more pain that night?"

"No, no more than usual."

One does not comfortably paint a kitchen with a badly arthritic neck nor does such a neck flare up exactly at midnight. I will suggest to the reader that I was not treating a person who suffered from cervical arthritis, pinched nerves, or spastic muscles. I was treating a person who suffered chronic pain. There is a difference.

"Ann, I am going to give you a couple of medicines that I believe may be helpful. One of them is known as Nortriptyline and the other Clonazepam. I want you to take a single pill every night. I'm not sure they will work, but it is certainly worth a try. I would like to see you again in two weeks."

On her return, she took my hand and said, "This really has been remarkable. From the first night I had no more pain, and I have slept quite well."

"That's wonderful. I thought I might be able to help you, but as you say, this is truly remarkable."

"I feel like I have been cured."

"Well, perhaps you are. I will write you a long-term supply of medicines, enough to last six months. I will have you come back at the end of that time to see how you are doing. In the meantime, if there are problems, I want you to call me."

"That's fine with me. I promise you, I will keep taking the medicine. I look forward to seeing you again. I am very grateful for what you have done." Then she squeezed my hand, looked me in the eye, and said, "Young man, how did you know what to do? I've seen several doctors, and I have had all kind of injections in my head and neck, and none of them worked. And then you gave me some pills and immediately my pain went away. I want you to tell me how you knew what to do."

Pat was tall and blond and attired in a loose-fitting, beltless cotton dress. She was not unhandsome, but her face suggested desperation. I would have put her age at sixty-five had I not known that she was forty-eight. She began the conversation by saying, "You are my last resort. If you can't help me, my life is over."

I hear this kind of declaration a lot. It is a testament to the destructiveness of chronic pain, and it holds enormous implications for treatment. The physician must always be guided by the dictum *primum non nocere*, that is—first, do no harm. Thus, whether administering pharmaceuticals, performing an operation, or engaging in psychotherapy, the doctor must, at the very least, avoid making the patient worse. Unfortunately—or perhaps fortunately—this is hard to do in those who truly suffer chronic pain. Many of them are at the absolute end of their tether, and that offers an opportunity for imagination and creativity that would not be employed in those who suffer less destructive illnesses. This is what makes the treatment of the painful patient so exciting—and challenging. If the doctor is not excited and challenged by hearing his patient say, "You are my last resort," that doctor has no fire in the belly at all.

Only within the past few years has come the recognition that chronic pain may be a unique disorder, a thing unto itself.

I reviewed the notes of the referring physicians, an internist and a gastroenterologist. Both recorded her lifelong history of abdominal pain and increasingly frequent attacks of explosive diarrhea. They listed the various medications she had taken and noted that none had been particularly helpful except for the opiate Hydrocodone, which she was using in suspiciously large quantity. They reviewed the diagnostic studies which had been performed, and reported that all had been quite normal. Both described the physical examination as unremarkable, save for some abdominal distention and tenderness. They concluded that Pat suffered from irritable bowel syndrome.

The internist, in his summation, observed that she was sleepless and chronically depressed and also that she was having difficulty with some of her personal relationships. He suggested consultation with a psychiatrist. The gastroenterologist offered the terse judgment that *this patient suffers more of a pain problem than an intestinal problem*. Had he seen her ten years before, I doubt he would have written that. Only within the past few years has come the recognition that chronic pain may be a unique disorder, a thing unto itself.

Being a pain doctor is arduous work, but there is one advantage that comes with it. He or she does not have to reinvent the wheel. My patient's medical history and physical and laboratory examinations had been recorded in elegant detail by physicians of competence at least equal and probably exceeding my own. I was able—indeed I was invited—to spend my time on other matters. These, as we shall see time and time again, include the exploration of the patient's personal, social, and emotional history as well as their medical, for only by doing so can we understand the true meaning of chronic pain.

"Your doctors have told me that you have irritable bowel syndrome and a lot of pain in your abdomen. Tell me about it."

"I hurt all the time. I have a lot of constipation, and sometimes I have diarrhea. It swings from one to the other. I have a lot of gas, and that is embarrassing."

"You have taken lots of different medicines. I see you are taking Hydrocodone now. That is a pretty strong pain killer."

"Yes, I have taken all the medicines, and I have taken so much Metamucil that I get sick when I even think about it. The drugs have never helped me very much. The Hydrocodone does help a bit, but I don't like the way it makes me feel. Sometimes, though, I have to take it—lots of it."

"Your doctors have some concerns that you are using too much of it. What is your take on that?"

"Yes, I do take more than I should. They will only give me a little bit at a time. I use it up in just a few days, then I suffer for weeks."

"How long has your stomach trouble been going on?"

"As long as I can remember. I used to be able to put up with it, but now it is really interfering. I am not sure I can keep working."

"Why is that?"

"The pain is getting worse and worse, and I am getting to where I soil myself. I can't control my bowels." She then placed her hands on her abdomen, pulled the dress tightly about it, and said, "Look at my stomach. It's huge. People think I am pregnant. I have to wear clothes like this to hide it. You may not believe this, but I can't even wear panties. The elastic hurts my stomach."

"I assure you, I have heard that kind of complaint before."

"You have?"

"Yes, many times, but let's move on to another subject. I understand that you are having trouble sleeping."

"Yes, I have a terrible problem with sleep. Sometimes I lose control of my bowels during the night, and I have to change the bed."

"How long have you had insomnia?"

"Most of my life. I have never been a very good sleeper."

"How do you feel when you wake up in the morning?"

"Terrible. I wake up exhausted."

"Your internist made reference to some difficulties you are having in your personal life. I would like to explore that a little bit, if you don't mind."

"Go ahead. I will tell you when I want you to stop."

"Are you married? Do you have children?"

"No to both."

"Have you ever been married?"

"No, never. I would like to be married, and I have certainly had plenty of opportunities. I have been engaged nine times."

"Nine times! Why so many?"

"I don't know, really. I guess it has just been my bad luck to not find the right man."

I will suggest to the reader that *nine* unsuccessful engagements do not happen just by bad luck. Nor does irritable bowel syndrome happen just by bad luck.

"Pat, do you ever suffer periods of depression?"

"Oh, yes. I have been depressed many times in my life. I have taken Wellbutrin and Prozac, but they never worked very well. Most of the time the depression goes away on its own."

"Have you ever thought of suicide?"

"Yes, I have thought about it a lot, but I don't believe I could ever do it. Let's just say it is against my religion."

"I want to ask you a strange question. Are you a spender? Do you sometimes go out and buy things that you don't need? Are you irresponsible with money?"

"Actually, I am rather good with money. I have worked hard and made a very good living. It's been easy for me. I've always had a lot of energy, at least until a few years ago when my stomach pain got so bad. I will admit that I do have a vice. I get a big kick out of gambling. I travel a lot, and whenever I am in a river town, I will go to a casino. I lose a lot of money that way, sometimes $1,000 a pop."

"Does that bother you?"

"Not really. Sometimes it makes me feel good."

"Did you have a happy childhood?"

"Yes, my father was very well-to-do. I went to private schools. My parents, both of them, treated me very well."

"There were no destructive events when you were young?"

"Why in the world do you ask that?"

"Because it may be important. It may help me understand your illness."

She hesitated and then said, "Well, yes, something did happen to me when I was twenty years old, but I don't want to talk about it."

"Was it a bad thing that happened to you?"

"Yes, it was really bad."

"So bad that you sometimes dream about it or flashback to it? Do you sometimes relive it?"

"Yes, I do, but I am not going to tell you what it was. I'll just say it was something that was against my religion."

"Did you see a psychologist or psychiatrist about it?"

"Yes, I've seen many of them, at least a half dozen."

"Why so many?"

"Well to tell you the truth, I didn't like most of them. One was really nice, though. I spent a couple of months with her."

"What did you talk about?"

"Mostly about my feelings about what happened. She said I had a disease called traumatic stress or something like that. I can't remember exactly."

"Post-traumatic stress disorder?"

"Yes, that is what she said it was."

"Did she give you medicine?"

"Yes, she was the one who gave me Prozac. It didn't do me any good, so I decided to quit seeing her."

"Do you think that was a pretty hasty decision?"

"Yes, I suppose so."

"I imagine you have seen lots of different doctors for your bowel problem."

"Indeed I have. I have seen three or four internists and a lot of gastroenterologists. I have been scoped four or five times altogether, some from above and some from below, and I am scheduled for another one pretty soon."

"Pat, I am going to make an observation here, and I hope I don't offend you. It seems like your relationships with your lovers, your therapists, and your physicians are about as irregular as the workings of your bowels. Do you suppose there could be some kind of connection?"

She hesitated and then said, "I never thought about it quite that way, but you may be right. You know, you are pretty good. I like talking to you."

Pat suffered chronic pain in the form of irritable bowel syndrome. She also suffered post-traumatic stress disorder, a common legacy of severe emotional trauma. She also, quite possibly, had

An aggressive, energized lifestyle with periodic depression and periodic disinhibition (gambling) certainly suggests bipolar disease.

bipolar (manic-depressive) disease. An aggressive, energized lifestyle with periodic depression and periodic disinhibition (gambling) certainly suggests bipolar disease. Nine unsuccessful engagements are virtually diagnostic of it. This is the way it usually plays out in chronic pain. Co-existent psychiatric diseases are the rule, not the exception. Unfortunate though this may seem to be, it offers an incredible variety of treatment options. As I began my therapy, I chose, unlike the physicians who had seen her before, to treat her mind rather than her bowels.

"I am giving you two prescriptions. One is for Nortriptyline and the other for Clonazepam. I want you to start on a low dosage and, if you tolerate them, to gradually increase the amount according to my instructions. I expect the first good thing that will happen to you is that you will begin to sleep. I will see you back in two weeks."

"I like you. I want to talk to you some more."

"I will talk with you as much as time allows, but you must understand I am not a psychologist or psychiatrist. I am not trained to address the issues that I suspect you may want to talk about. What I will be doing mostly is to administer medication that I think has a real prospect of helping you."

My enthusiasm for the use of pharmacy in the treatment of chronic pain is so great that in *Understanding Chronic Pain* I wrote that it is the drugs that cure pain, not the doctor. In that judgment, I believe now I was at least partially wrong. The drugs can be enormously helpful—of that there is absolutely no doubt—but they must be administered by a physician who connects with the patient. And that connection begins with understanding their illness. This invites trust and confidence, and it is in this environment that the drugs really work best.

Pat returned at the appointed time and began the conversation in a manner that surprised me—to show me her new engagement ring. She said, "This time I am really in love. He's a wonderful man. He's a machinist, and he doesn't have a lot of money, but that doesn't matter. He insists on a prenuptial agreement before we get married. He doesn't want to inherit any of my father's money. Isn't that wonderful? Do you think I ought to marry him?"

"I wouldn't dare offer you advice on a matter like that."

"I thought you would probably say that."

"How is your pain—and your sleep? Have the drugs made any difference?"

"Yes, I am sleeping a lot better. My stomach doesn't bother me as much. I think the medicines may be doing some good, but the real reason for my improvement, I am sure, is that I am finally in love."

Medication, the right medication, can certainly relieve chronic pain. So can falling in love. That experience is probably the best non-pharmacologic treatment there is for chronic pain. I suspected, though, that this woman's love experience would be a short one, and in the long run it would be the drugs that would see her through. I congratulated her on her good fortune, but suggested she increase the dose of Nortriptyline.

She appeared two weeks later exactly as scheduled. She spoke excitedly and rapidly about her plans for marriage, and then getting back to work.

"I have a lot more energy now. I feel better in every way. I will let you in on a little secret. Sex is better."

"How so?"

"I used to poop in the bed when I had sex. I don't do that anymore." She was in my face.

"I am not using any protection. I am forty-eight years old. Do you think I will get pregnant?"

Pat was exhibiting two of the major features of bipolar mania, disinhibition and flight of ideas. I followed up with an important question.

"How are you sleeping now?"

"It's strange, I don't seem to need sleep. I have a lot of energy, and I am staying awake a lot. My mind is full of ideas. I really feel good."

"Pat, have you ever had experiences like this before where you got wound up and energized?"

"Yes, I have had lots of them."

"How long do they usually last?"

"A few days usually."

"And then?"

"Then I get down."

The employ of pharmacy entails inherent risk because unwanted side effects certainly do occur. Victims of bipolar disease seem to be particularly disposed to a very strange one. Sometimes the administration of antidepressants incites mania in the form of grandiosity, disinhibition, and mind-busy hyperactivity. Chief among the drugs which do this (and there are many) are the tricyclic antidepressants, of which Nortriptyline is an example. Unfortunately, the tricyclics are among the very best drugs for the treatment of pain. They must be used with caution, however, for many victims of chronic pain are bipolar. So the risk must be accepted, but the physician must remain vigilant.

"I am going to give you a new medicine. It's called Seroquel. I want you to add it to the other drugs."

"What is it supposed to do?"

"It has many uses, but I'm employing it as a mood stabilizer."

"Do you think I'm bipolar?"

It is astonishing how often I am asked that question. Many victims of chronic pain, I have learned, suspect that they are bipolar, but they usually hesitate to address the issue with their physicians.

"Why do you ask that? I have never mentioned that word before, have I?"

"No, you never did, but I have thought for a long time that I was manic-depressive."

"Did you ever mention that to any of your other doctors?"

"Only to the psychiatrist. She said I wasn't. She said I had post-traumatic stress disorder."

"Well, you probably have both and chronic pain as well. They all seem to run together."

"I really like talking to you."

"I like talking to you, too."

Chronic pain is the most complex of diseases. It cohabits with many disorders of the mind, be this stress disorder, depression, bipolarity, drug addiction, and host of others. Recognition of this, which I consider an unassailable truth, offers the beginning of understanding into the true nature of the disease. I instructed Pat to continue her Nortriptyline and Clonazepam. They had been quite helpful in tempering her bowels. She needed, however, another drug, one which would temper her moods.

On her return visit, she greeted me by saying, "Thanks for giving me the Seroquel. It is a wonder drug. For the first time in my life, I feel like I am even! I'm actually in control of my emotions. I have never felt that way before."

"How is your pain?"

"So much better. My BM's are regular, and I don't soil myself. My stomach still swells up some, but my clothes don't hurt me the way they used to. Are you going to ask me about my engagement?"

"Well, I figured we would get around to that sooner or later."

"It's off." She held up her left hand and said, "Look, no ring."

"Are you happy with that decision?"

"Very happy. Let me ask you something. I have been thinking about this bipolar thing, and I have been reading about it a lot. Do you think it is possible that my engagements took place when I was manic and my separations when I was depressed? It seems bizarre, but I am beginning to think that is what was going on."

"You may be correct, but it could be the other way around."

"And the thing I was involved in so many years ago—could that have happened when I was manic?"

"It certainly could have."

"Then I am not a bad person, after all."

"No, you are a good person with a very bad disease."

"There is a lot more to it than irritable bowels, isn't there?"

"Yes, a whole lot more."

She looked at me with her brown eyes full of tears and said, "I've seen lots of doctors, some of the best. None of them helped me like you have, and I want to know why. This is important to me. Why has it taken me twenty-five years to understand what was wrong with me? Tell me, how did you know what to do?"

> *Medication, the right medication, can certainly relieve chronic pain.*

The answer to that question is, I believe, at the very core of understanding chronic pain. It is certainly not because I am more intelligent than other physicians or that I am better trained (I am forty-five years removed from my formal academic studies, and the field of pain medicine did not even exist at that time). My success rate certainly does not derive, as some have suggested, from my great compassion for those who suffer chronic pain. The notion that I am more compassionate than other physicians is patently absurd. And besides, we will not cure chronic pain with compassion, we will cure it, and understand it, by clinical observation.

I suggest that I know what to do because I recognize, as do few other physicians, *that chronic pain is a mental illness.*

It is not that others are not trying. Pat's gastroenterologist, competent and knowledgeable, recorded that she suffered more of a pain problem than an intestinal problem. He was getting close, and so was the internist who tried to explore her relationships and the pattern of her life in an effort to understand her pain. Their efforts were noble.

Ann and Pat were very different people. Ann's life was one of well being and comfort. Only late into it did she experience pain, this in the head and neck. Pat's life was chaotic and disturbed, and her abdominal pain began when she was quite young. The two women hurt at different times in their lives and at different places in their bodies, and the patterns of their fundamental existence were remarkably unalike. And yet, their pains responded to the very same drugs (admittedly, in Pat, whose disease was much more complex, an add-on drug was necessary).

> *I suggest that I know what to do because I recognize, as do few other physicians, that chronic pain is a mental illness.*

Readers may be surprised to learn that I find Ann's illness much harder to understand than Pat's. She had none of the common antecedents or risk factors for the development of chronic pain and very few of the symptoms of the disease. I chose to treat her as I did only because her pain occurred exclusively at night and regularly at the same hour of the night. These features are quite common in those who suffer chronic pain. They were enough to invite me to make a least a tentative diagnosis of that disease and to initiate therapy that, fortunately, worked quite well and continues to work well three years later.

Pat practically wrote the book on chronic pain. She suffered a common antecedent in the form of trauma in her youth. We don't know what it was, but it was enough to make her flashback to the experience and enough for her psychiatrist to make a diagnosis of post-traumatic stress disorder. She almost certainly suffered another psychiatric disorder—bipolar disease. She had many of the symptoms of chronic pain, sleeplessness among them. Another was the experience of *allodynia*, which means perception of pain in response to a trivial sensory stimulus. The elastic waistband of her panties hurt her.

Pat, four years later, has done less well than Ann. She is the victim of a cruel disease characterized by erratic mood swings with pain along for the ride. She is better than when we started, but by no means has her recovery been complete.

In this book I will describe many people who suffer chronic pain. I will illustrate the commonalties among them and will suggest that chronic pain, like all diseases, has discernible origins. It has a complex, but nonetheless predictable, pattern of clinical behavior, and it has a somewhat predictable response to drug therapy. I will suggest chronic pain can best be understood as a disease of the mind, and I will emphasize that we have many drugs, hundreds of them, which can alter the conduct of that organ and diminish pain.

CHAPTER TWO

Pharmacy for Pain

All of us suffer painful injuries and illnesses throughout the course of our lives. The experience can be quite bitter, but in the majority of cases pain goes away in time. This happens not only because the wound heals but also because the brain has the resources to diminish pain that no longer serves a useful purpose, that is, to protect us from further injury by telling us that something is amiss and remedial action is necessary.

This book is about those whose pain is not self-limited, those who do not recover from illness or injury and as a result suffer incessant chronic pain. Some examples: The migraine headache does not go away in the anticipated hours or days, and that form of chronic pain, formerly known as tension headache but better described as transformed migraine, afflicts the sufferer with a constant, unremitting headache. The muscle sprain or overuse injury does not go away in the anticipated days or weeks, and that form of chronic muscular pain known as fibromyalgia evolves. The surgical operation for the removal of a painfully ruptured spinal disc is performed successfully, but the victim continues, unaccountably, to have pain in the back that may persist for a lifetime. There are countless other examples of the evolution of acute into chronic pain, and many will be explored in this book.

Now let's look at what happens when we move from the pain of the acute injury or illness into chronic pain. The timeline on this can be measured in days or weeks, and it is during that interval, I suggest, that the pain is leaving the body and entering the mind. Sleep becomes disordered, and pain often worsens at night. It may, as we have already seen, occur exclusively at night. Tremors in the form of large muscle jerkings (myoclonus) occur throughout the night, and attempts to sleep are hindered by restless movements of the lower (or even upper) extremities, the disorder known as restless legs (or arms—or both). In some with chronic pain, sleep is impaired by an inability to turn off the mind, and victims suffer thought racing and thought scatter. Hope for recovery gives way to despair and depression—usually an apathetic, listless despondency but occasionally a state of restless, purposeless hyperactivity. Energy—physical, mental, and sexual—is diminished, and victims experience fatigue, want of memory and mental focus, and

This book is about those whose pain is not self-limited, those who do not recover from illness or injury and as a result suffer incessant chronic pain.

diminished libido and sexual response. The perception of pain changes, and even lightly touching the area of pain evokes discomfort (allodynia again). Blood flow changes and the skin over the painful area becomes cool to touch. Pain spreads beyond the bounds of the original injury and may actually extend to the opposite side of the body in the fashion of a mirror image. It may even spread to encompass the entire body. Appetite diminishes with weight loss in some, but more often appetite is increased with sweet cravings and weight gain—sometime enormous weight gain. Disposition changes with fractiousness and irritability. Thought is sometimes bent into obsessive ruminations about pain and also impulse to suicide.

Many readers will find themselves in this book. Indeed, I suspect that many have already found themselves in the above paragraph. Standing back and looking at all this, it is truly remarkable that so many brain systems—those that control appetite, mood, memory, sleep, energy, and thought—are disordered in the painful. Remarkable also is the uniformity of these symptoms. The great majority of pain sufferers experience most of them.

Let's examine this a little bit more. Why do those with chronic pain all experience virtually the same symptoms? If those symptoms were merely a reflection of our emotional reaction to pain, why should we expect them to occur with such uniformity? Think about it and consider the diversity of human beings and their emotional behaviors. Considering this diversity, we would reasonably expect great variation in the way people react to pain. And this is exactly what happens with acute pain. Some react stoically, others demonstratively and excitably. Some exhibit their emotions, and others hide them. However, when chronic pain evolves, there is much less variation in the victims' behaviors. They become rather stereotyped, even predictable. This tells us, I believe, that the disease we call chronic pain is actually also a disorder of sleep, appetite, mood, memory, and even thought. It is the biggest disease there is and the most complicated. As I have written before, there are more things going wrong in the brain and body in those who suffer chronic pain than in any other disease.

Now let's look at the complex clinical array that is chronic pain and introduce another observation, one that I believe is of uncontestable validity. Many of the symptoms that we logically ascribe to the effects of chronic pain are actually operative long before pain appears. Thus, many people who develop chronic pain have experienced intervals of depression *before* they became painful. Eating disorders, including anorexia-bulimia and obesity, often appear *before* the advent of pain. Insomnia—and even restless legs—frequently appear *before* pain. Intervals of unaccountable fatigue are by no means uncommon experiences *before* pain appears, nor are intervals of mind-racing hyperactivity.

I suggested in my first book that the frequency of these disorders in those who become painful is sufficient to consider them risk factors for the development of the disease. Just as there are risk factors for lung cancer, heart disease, diabetes, and osteoporosis, there are risk factors for the development of chronic pain. I believe that chronic pain is not a chance and random occurrence. It is not bad luck. It is the product of biologic design, and it can best be understood, as I have written before, within the context of the totality of the victim's life.

I will introduce a few more extremely important risk factors. One is drug dependency and abuse. It is a sad fact that many people who enter recovery from drugs of abuse become painful, some in short order, others years later. I will, in this book, offer some examples of the phenomenon and offer explanations as to why it happens. Another risk factor, and one sadly of prime importance, is the experience of childhood abuse, particu-

Few of us are unblemished, and that is why chronic pain can happen to any of us.

larly sexual abuse. This is the mother of all risk factors. Childhood trauma deforms a developing mind and invites a host of illnesses that generally make their appearance in adolescence or early adulthood. These include obesity, drug addiction, chronic pain, and a variety of psychiatric diseases, certainly including post-traumatic stress disorder. Yet another risk factor, and this is quite understandable if we accept that chronic pain is a disease of the mind, is the presence of underlying neurologic diseases such as stroke, Parkinson's disease, and Alzheimer's.

Let's pause now and let the reader note that chronic pain is a disease that comes to abused, obese, sleepless, drug-addicted, mentally ill, or brain-damaged people. It reads badly, but it is really not. We must accept that the majority of us have, along the way, suffered some form of neuropsychiatric illness. Few of us are unblemished, and that is why chronic pain can happen to any of us. Nonetheless, we have to recognize that through good fortune and perhaps God's grace, some of us are more favorably endowed than others and, therefore, are perhaps less suscep-tible to chronic pain. With that said, a disclaimer: Even the most resolute and emotionally integrated of us could, under the provocation of over-whelming life events, come to suffer chronic pain, and I have made a special effort to write about that particular subject.

In the pages that follow, I will tell the stories of people who have been cured or at least marvelously helped by the administration of pharmacy. I will report failures also, but the prospect of success with the use of drug therapy is, at least in my own experience, increasing rapidly. In *Understanding Chronic Pain*, I wrote that when I began to focus my prac-tice almost exclusively on the treatment of chronic pain, some twenty years ago, I was actually able to help about 25 percent of my patients. When my book was published in 2004, I was helping about 60 percent.

Now, four years later, I am closer to 80 percent, and importantly, when I fail, I now usually know why.

I hope you are as eager to get into the case histories as I am, but first we must talk a little about pharmacy. This will of necessity entail some technical material. I will try to keep it as simple as possible. I know that you, reader with chronic pain, have taken and are familiar with many of the drugs that I describe. I believe I can offer some interesting insights into how and why they actually work.

Nerve cells communicate with one another by the release of a chemical known as a neurotransmitter from one nerve cell, and the reception of that chemical by an adjacent one. The receiving cell becomes energized and transmits down its length an electrical message through the lining of the cell known as the membrane. At the end of that journey, the message is relayed to another cell, again by the mechanism of neurotransmitter release and reception. There are four basic ways in which pharmacy can modify this system. One is to increase the release of the neurotransmitter (this is an agonist effect); another is to block the reception of that neurotransmitter (an antagonistic effect); another is by changing the nerve cell membrane's ability to conduct the electrical message; and lastly, by the administration of the neurotransmitter itself.

There are a great number of neurotransmitter systems in the brain. This book will reference half a dozen major ones. Their names are serotonin, noradrenaline, gamma-aminobutyric acid (GABA), dopamine, glutamine, and endorphin or opioid. These different systems constitute a majority of the brain's neurotransmitter activity and, integrated together, they constitute the brain's infrastructure

Be advised, when I refer to a neurotransmitter system, I am referring to a cluster of nerve cells and their attached filaments (axons), which employ a certain neurotransmitter in their function. Be advised also that there are subtypes of the different neurotransmitters, and these subtypes may be located in many different areas within the brain to serve quite different functions.

As I discuss the different neurotransmitter systems, I will briefly describe those drugs or families of drugs that act on those systems. You will see that many of the drugs act on multiple neurotransmitter systems. At the end of this chapter, the various drugs will be listed in tabular form.

Serotonin and Noradrenaline

Serotonin and noradrenaline systems are interdependent and kindred in their function. They are located predominantly in the brain base, and they serve the control of sleep-wakefulness, appetite, energy, attention (or perhaps better, vigilance), sexual response, mood, and the perception of pain. We can conceptualize that most of these are neurovegetative functions, that is, they are essential for sustaining life.

We have several groups of drugs that are agonists (enhancing) to either serotonin, noradrenaline, or both. The most well known of these is the group identified as selective serotonin reuptake inhibitors (SSRI) of which Prozac is an example. They are selective agonists to serotonin and have little influence on noradrenaline. They are preeminent in the treatment of depression, but seemingly because of their lack of effect on noradrenaline, have rather little usefulness as analgesic (pain-relieving) drugs. Conversely, a group of antidepressant drugs identified in this text as tricyclic-like are agonist to noradrenaline but antagonist to serotonin. They have modest analgesic effect presumably because of their antagonism to serotonin.

Most psychiatrists believe that mania and panic represent a kind of glutamine storm. I will suggest that pain . . . also represents a glutamine storm.

Many readers certainly have taken an SSRI drug and know of its sex-inhibiting effect. This is because serotonin itself is a sex-inhibiting system. Curious that a neurotransmitter system that is necessary for emotional wellness should diminish sexual response. This is a good time to remind the reader that the brain is a system of checks and balances, and just as there is a sex-inhibiting system, there is a sex-enhancing system—that of noradrenaline. In the same sense that serotonin is sex-inhibiting, serotonin and noradrenaline taken together may be considered pain-inhibiting. And drugs that are agonists to both do have the property of analgesia, and they are well established in the treatment of chronic pain. They fall into two groupings—the tricyclic antidepressants (TCA), which have been around for more than fifty years, and the more recently derived serotonin and noradrenaline reuptake inhibitors (SNRI). There are two of them, and they are known as Effexor and Cymbalta. They are both useful not only for the treatment of pain but also depression.

Glutamine, GABA, Dopamine, and Opioid

We now move into more complex neurotransmitters, those which control not only our pain and mood but also to a remarkable degree our personal and social behaviors. These systems are located in the mid-brain and forebrain (the behavior controlling frontal lobes).

Glutamine is the brain's excitatory transmitter. It functions by allowing an increase in the amount of calcium and other ions that enter the cell. This destabilizes the cell, and it becomes irritable and hyper-excitable. It is this irritability that leads to a bunch of very bad things including convulsive seizures, delirium, panic, and the hyperactive mania of bipolar disease. The subject of bipolar disease (and its relationship to pain) will come up repeatedly throughout this book, so I will introduce you to some of the emotions, thoughts, and behaviors that attend the bipolar state. They are sleep-needless hyperactivity, impulse and disinhibition (social, financial, and sexual), unprovoked anger, mind-racing, mood shifts, and suicidality and homicidality. There are a lot more, but at least I have introduced you to the subject.

Most psychiatrists believe that mania and panic represent a kind of glutamine storm. I will suggest that pain, particularly that which recurs either randomly or predictably through time—in the manner of mania and panic—also represents a glutamine storm. I doubt that few authorities would really disagree with that.

We have only a few drugs that actually antagonize the glutamine receptors, but we have a great number that can combat its effect by closing up the cell membrane and diminishing the entry of calcium. They are known collectively as anticonvulsants. Virtually all of them were released for the treatment of epilepsy but were found in short order to also be effective in the treatment of bipolar mania, migraine, and chronic pain!

Before leaving glutamine and assigning it the role as the brain's bad guy, we have to recognize that a little cellular hyperactivity is not a bad thing at all. Many great works of art, literature, and music were created under the influence of glutamine-driven bipolar mania.

Now let's look at the good guys, all of which, in their own way, oppose the effect of glutamine. They are GABA, opioid, and dopamine.

GABA is the brain's inhibiting or calming neurotransmitter, and drugs that are GABA agonists are recognized as anxiolytic or, in lay terms, tranquilizers. Almost all of them belong to a chemical class known as benzodiazepine, that word derived from their chemical structure. Three of them, Diazepam, Lorazepam, and Clonazepam, are also anticonvulsant and perhaps for that reason are especially useful in the treatment of chronic pain.

The opioid neurotransmitter system is, of course, the brain's endogenous (within the brain) agency for the relief of pain. Its effect can be magnified, obviously, by the administration exogenously (from outside the brain) of morphine and other opioids.

Dopamine is certainly one of the brain's more complex neurotransmitter systems. It is involved in multiple activities, including the maintenance of posture and muscle tone, and a deficiency of this subtype of dopamine causes Parkinson's disease. Another dopamine function is the maintenance of the integrity of thought, and an excess of this subtype is responsible for the hallucinations of schizophrenia. Lastly, dopamine is the neurotransmitter system responsible for the feeling states and emotions of gratification, reward, and joy. The power of these emotions to control our behavior is remarkable.

It is possible to place electrodes into dopamine-rich areas of an experimental animal's brain and connect them to a pedal in the animal's cage so that depressing the pedal will stimulate dopamine. The animal quickly learns that depressing the pedal will give it what we presume is ineffable joy. The creature will no longer eat, drink, sleep, or procreate. It will only continue to depress the pedal until the system is mercifully turned off.

Virtually all drugs of abuse, those that give us well-being and joy, do so by stimulating dopamine. Some (cocaine) do this directly and others indirectly through intermediary neurotransmitters; opiates, of course, to opioid receptors; alcohol and tranquilizers to GABA; and marijuana through receptors known as cannaboid—yes, if there is any drug that alters our mood and behavior, it is because we have receptors to receive it!

Let's reflect on all this. Glutamine is the bad guy, and it does bad things. Against the bad guy are GABA, which calms; opioid, which gives comfort (relief of pain); and dopamine, which gives pleasure. A theme that will reappear through this book is the role of drugs that are agonists to GABA, opioid, and dopamine in the treatment of bipolar disease—and also chronic pain.

Before leaving this subject, which I assure you has been addressed in an extremely simplistic manner, I need to inform you that just as a little extra glutamine can be a very good thing for the agency of imagination and creativity, a little extra GABA, opioid, and dopamine can be a very bad thing. Repeated gratification, reward, and pleasure lead to cravings, and that is addiction.

Drugs Useful for the Treatment of Pain

There is, regrettably, no really coherent way to classify and organize the various drugs discussed in this book. Collectively they can be identified as *neuropsychiatric* drugs, which means that they are employed in the treatment of either neurologic or psychiatric disease (and quite commonly both). Some of them are identified by their chemical structure (tricyclic, benzodiazepine), and others by their mechanism of action (selective serotonin reuptake inhibitors). These terms are quite cumbersome for the lay reader, and so I will follow the convention of identifying drugs by their clinical indication—that is, which drug for which disease. The reader must be reminded, however, that this classification is archaic because none of the drugs listed below, absolutely none, have a single clinical indication. Each of them is used for a variety of disorders.

Antidepressants

Selective Serotonin Reuptake Inhibitors (SSRI)

The SSRIs are the most widely used antidepressants. They are serotonin agonists, and they are both antidepressant and anti-anxiety. They are only marginally effective, however, as analgesic drugs.

Proprietary	Generic
Celexa	Citalopram
Lexapro	Escitalopram
Luvox	Fluvoxamine
Paxil	Paroxetine
Prozac	Fluoxetine
Zoloft	Sertraline

Tricyclic Antidepressants (TCA)

The TCAs were among the first antidepressant drugs, and for some twenty years they held center stage. They are serotonin and noradrenaline agonists, and they were discovered early on to be analgesic. This is not in the sense that the opiates are analgesic. Administering a tricyclic will not diminish pain immediately. It often takes days or even weeks for them to exert their effect. Many readers are certainly aware of the side effects of the tricyclics. They are, among others, weight gain, sexual dysfunction, and impaired memory. These effects relate to the fact that the tricyclics are "dirty" drugs, that is, they influence multiple neurotransmitter systems. They are agonists to serotonin, which accounts for sexual dysfunction, and they are antagonists to both histamine, which accounts for the weight gain, and acetylcholine, which accounts for memory impairment. It is these side effects that have been an obstacle, understandably, to their more frequent administration. They remain, however, among the preeminent drugs in the treatment of chronic pain.

Proprietary	Generic
Anafranil	Clomipramine

Norpramine	Desipramine
Elavil	Amitriptyline
Pamelor	Nortriptyline
Sinequan	Doxepin
Trofranil	Imipramine

Selective Noradrenaline and Serotonin Reuptake Inhibitors (SNRI)

These drugs are selective agonists to both serotonin and noradrenaline. Unlike the tricyclics, they influence no other transmitters and on that account, have fewer side effects. They can be very effective in the treatment of chronic pain, perhaps comparable to the tricyclics.

Proprietary	Generic
Cymbalta	Duloxetine
Effexor	Venlafaxine

Tricyclic-Like Antidepressants

These drugs, which are chemically different from the tricyclics, are noradrenaline agonists and serotonin antagonists. They have antidepressant effects, and they found great favor when they were introduced some thirty years ago because they lacked some of the disturbing side effects of the tricyclics. They do have some analgesic effect but currently are employed chiefly as sleeping aids.

Proprietary	Generic
Desyrel	Trazadone
Serzone	Nefazodone

Dopamine Antidepressants

We currently have very few drugs that selectively target the dopamine system for the treatment of depression, but the search for such is being aggressively conducted. One of the drugs listed below, Emsam, actually first appeared, and is still used, for the treatment of

Parkinsonism. The other, Wellbutrin, in addition to being antidepressant, is employed for smoking cessation.

Proprietary	Generic
Wellbutrin	Bupropion
Emsam	Selegiline

Opioid Analgesics

These drugs all are opioid agonists, and they virtually all stimulate the same subtype of opioid receptor. They are unrivaled in the treatment of the acutely painful illness or injury. They can also be helpful in the treatment of chronic pain, but in some instances discussed in this text, they can be quite ineffective. They can, perhaps surprisingly, be quite helpful in the treatment of depression and bipolar disease. The reader is advised that I have not included in this list the well-known non-steroidal anti-inflammatory drugs (NSAID). These are useful in the treatment of everyday pains but of marginal benefit in those people that I write about in this book.

Importantly, we have a single opioid antagonist. It is known as Naltrexone, and it is available in every emergency room for the treatment of opiate overdosage.

Proprietary	Generic
Darvon	Propoxyphene
Demerol	Meperidine
Dilaudid	Hydromorphone
Duragesic, Actiq, Fentora	Fentanyl
Lortab, Vicodin	Hydrocodone
Methadose	Methadone (Dolophine)
MS Contin, Kadian	Morphine
Nubain	Nalbuphine
Percodan, Tylox, Oxycontin	Oxycodone
Stadol	Butorphanol
Subutex	Buphrenorphine
Ultram	Tramadol

Many of the opiates are formulated in combination with the non-opiate analgesic Tylenol, generically acetaminophen. The suffix, "cet," identifies this formulation. Thus, we have names such as Darvocet, Lorcet, Percocet, and Ultracet.

Anxiolytics/Tranquilizers

These drugs share a common chemical structure known as benzodiazepine. They are GABA agonists and useful as sleep aids and as anti-anxiety drugs. A few of them, asterisked below, are also anti-convulsant and as such can be extremely helpful in the treatment of pain.

Proprietary	Generic
Ativan*	Lorazepam
Klonopin*	Clonazepam
Restoril	Temazepam
Serax	Oxazepam
Tranxene	Clorazepate
Valium*	Diazepam
Xanax	Alprazolam

Antipsychotic

A recently discovered group of drugs are widely employed in the treatment of schizophrenia. They are antagonist to both dopamine and serotonin. They can be useful as mood stabilizing drugs in the person with bipolar disease. One of them, Seroquel, is widely employed as a sleeping pill.

Proprietary	Generic
Abilify	Aripiprazole
Geodon	Ziprasidone
Risperdal	Riseridone
Seroquel	Quetiapine
Zyprexa	Olanzapine

Anti-Migraine

A group of drugs with a common chemical structure identified as triptan are serotonin agonists with activity predominantly in the arteries and not within the brain. Their usage is somewhat peripheral to the main theme of this book, but several of them will be referenced in the text. They are splendid drugs for the immediate relief of the pain of migraine headache.

Proprietary	Generic
Amerge	Naratriptan
Frova	Frovatriptan
Imitrex	Sumatriptan
Maxalt	Rizatriptan
Relpax	Eletriptan
Zomig	Zolmitriptan

Anticonvulsant

The anticonvulsants constitute a variety of drugs of dissimilar chemical configuration. They were thought, early in their development, to be GABA agonists. On this account, one of them, Neurontin, was identified generically as Gabapentin because of its presumed effect on GABA. Its derivative, Lyrica, was identified as Pregabaline for the same reason. That has all gone by the board, and we now believe that the anticonvulsant drugs inhibit the influx of excitatory calcium ions through the cell membrane. They are, in a physiologic sense, membrane stabilizers. In a clinical sense they are mood stabilizers, useful in the treatment of bipolar disease and, as I have mentioned before, for the prevention of migraine and the treatment of all sorts of chronic pain.

I have included in this group a single drug that is not anticonvulsant.* It was, however, the first mood stabilizer discovered, and it remains useful in the treatment of bipolar disease and occasionally in the treatment of migraine. It is known as Lithium.

Proprietary	Generic
Depakote	Valproate

Dilantin	Phenytoin
Keppra	Levetiracetam
Lamictal	Lamotrigine
Lithonate*, Eskalith*	Lithium*
Lyrica	Pregabaline
Neurontin	Gabapentin
Tegretol	Carbamazepine
Topamax	Topiramate
Zonegran	Zonisamide

Psychostimulants

These drugs, all derived from the stimulant amphetamine, are of similar chemical configuration. They have proven useful in the treatment of attention deficit disorder, narcolepsy, fatigue, and daytime sleepfulness. They can be helpful in the treatment of bipolar disease, although they are little used for that purpose, perhaps on account of their addictive properties. Perhaps surprisingly, they can be analgesic. They, like the recreational drug cocaine, are all dopamine agonists. Some are prepared in an extended release formulation.*

Proprietary	Generic
Adderall, Adderall XR*	Amphetamine
Dexedrine	Dextroamphetamine
Ritalin, Concerta*	Methylphenidate
Focalin XR*	Dexmethylphenidate

There are two psychostimulants that are not amphetamine derived and are not dopamine agonists. Rather, they are agonists to noradrenaline, and they are useful in the treatment of excessive sleepiness and attention deficit disorder.

Proprietary	Generic
Provigil	Modafinil
Strattera	Atomoxetine

Drugs That Influence Glutamine

A small group of drugs of quite different chemical configurations have their antagonism to glutamine in common. One, Ketalar, is an analgesic comparable to the opiates. However, it has no influence at all on opioid receptors. It is little used now because of side effects, but conceptually it was a breakthrough drug because it demonstrated the importance of the glutamine system in the perception of pain. A true opiate, Methadone, in addition to being an opioid agonist, is also a glutamine antagonist. It is an excellent analgesic and may turn out to be incredibly effective in the treatment of bipolar disease. Namenda, an anti-Alzheimer's drug, is also a glutamine antagonist and may have analgesic properties.

Proprietary	Generic
Ketalar	Ketamine
Methadose	Methadone (Dolophine)
Namenda	Memantine

I have listed in this chapter more than fifty drugs useful for the treatment of chronic pain. The list is representative but by no means inclusive. There are hundreds of other drugs with potential utility. Listing all of them would be an exercise in tedium, both for the author and the reader. Suffice it to say that I have included most of the important ones.

Be advised that most of the drugs discussed in this book are identified by their trademarked, proprietary names. A few, those whose usage extends over several decades, are identified by their generic. I have chosen the form that I find most recognizable by my patients. I have placed those drug names of universal recognition, such as morphine and alcohol, in the lower case and all others in capitals. This avoids the thought-interrupting alteration of the upper case for proprietary and lower case for generic drugs.

Virtually every patient that I am currently attending for the treatment of pain is on several of the drugs listed on these pages, a practice known as polypharmacy. You will soon recognize that I have certain favorites. Among the tricyclics, I favor Nortriptyline and Imipramine, and among the benzodiazepines, I favor Clonazepam. The reasons for this are, in the main, quite unscientific. Doctors, like everyone else, are creatures of habit. I do not attest that Imipramine and Nortriptyline are better than the other tricyclics, only that I am more familiar with them and, therefore, use them preferentially.

I want now to introduce you to the term genetic pleomorphism (pleo—many; morph—shape). This recognizes that there is great variation in human beings and their neurotransmitters, and it explains why there is such variation in patient response to drugs. For example, Imipramine is an excellent analgesic, soporific, and antidepressant in most people. In a minority, however, and this effect is not rare, Imipramine induces (often quite suddenly) a weeping, suicidal despair and occasionally manic hyperexcitability. Lamictal, the mood-stabilizing anticonvulsant, can be a good drug for

We must prepare not only for the unexpected adverse effect, but also the unexpected beneficial effect.

evening out the bipolar, but it can, rarely, induce either mania or depression. The examples are endless, and we will encounter many of them in this book. There is not a drug listed on these pages that has not in someone induced adverse mood and behavioral changes. This is not to say that we should fear the drugs—only to say that we must respect them and be vigilant to their capacity for harm.

Now let's reverse the coin and look at how genetic pleomorphism can work in our favor. We must prepare not only for the unexpected adverse effect, but also the unexpected beneficial effect. I will present many case studies in this book in which the administration of a drug, even counterintuitively, was very advantageous—thus, the employ of the therapeutic trial. It is a reasonable and proper exercise done in the anticipation that the chosen drug just *might* be helpful.

The reader is reminded that many of the usages of the drugs I have discussed have not been officially approved by the Federal Drug Administration (FDA). Knowledge of their usefulness has not derived from formal drug testing but rather from lessons learned by experience, a process known as empiricism. The prescription of drugs for purposes other than that for which they have been approved, known as off-label prescribing, is a widely accepted activity. Were it to be otherwise, the practice of pain medicine and also of psychiatry would be set back not by years, but by decades.

CHAPTER THREE

Pain in the Jaw

B ill's pain began with a trip to the dentist. He had cracked a molar on a kernel of popcorn and an extraction was necessary. The dentist injected an anesthetic at the back of the jawbone to block the lingual nerve, which serves sensation on one side of the jaw and tongue. Within moments Bill experienced a pain like none he had ever known, a deep, searing, burning pain into the right side of his jaw and tongue. Tears welled up in his eyes and profuse sweating drenched his body. He gagged a few times and then vomited his morning coffee. He screamed and clamored out of the dental chair and paced down the hallway pounding his jaw with his fist in an effort to somehow override the pain.

"I was totally out of control. I was almost insane. I'd never had a pain like that."

"How long did it last?"

"Only a few minutes, but it seemed like forever. After a while, when my jaw started getting numb, it went away, and I was able to get back in the chair and let the dentist pull the tooth. It was really strange. Once the pain went away, I felt real good. It was almost like an elation."

The object of local anesthesia, that is, the blocking of the action of a certain nerve, is to place the anesthetic in proximity to the nerve, bathing it with an agent that temporarily disrupts its function. The lingual nerve is not much bigger than the lead of a mechanical pencil, but by dumb unluck, the dentist actually penetrated the nerve and distended it with the injection of anesthesia. One can easily imagine the pain generated by such an injury to a nerve of sensation. As the anesthetic began to take effect, however, the pain dissipated.

Bill's violent reaction to his pain is certainly understandable, and it brings up a curious paradox about the way we behave when we perceive pain. Most people with migraine prefer to remain quite still. Movement worsens the pain. However, those with a variant of migraine known as cluster headaches can't sit still. They have to pace until the pain goes away. The same kind of paradox occurs with pains induced by severe corporal injury. A person with a fractured bone obviously doesn't want to move. A person with a kidney stone, however, cannot stay still. Nor could Bill.

The extraction was completed uneventfully. Bill accepted the dentist's apology and explanation and returned to work at the bank. After the anesthetic wore off, his jaw and tongue numbness disappeared, or nearly so. The tip of his tongue on the right side remained numb and very painful. Although not nearly so severe as the first pain, it was bad enough to keep him awake through the night. He returned to the dentist the following day, and x-rays were done to ensure that his violent maneuvers had not broken off a tip of the hypodermic needle. The dentist explained that the nerve had indeed been injured, but only slightly. The numbness and pain were confined to but a tiny part of the lingual nerve distribution. The lesion in the nerve was certainly quite small, perhaps even microscopic in dimension. The dentist told him he would be better in a few days. He prescribed Hydrocodone every four hours as needed for pain.

There is more to chronic pain than nerve injury, and there is more to recovery from chronic pain than the regeneration of nerves.

Bill's pain did not go away. The tip of his tongue remained numb on the right side. It would periodically burn, almost exclusively at night, awakening him from his sleep. After a couple of weeks, he was referred to an oral surgeon who concurred with the dentist's diagnosis, damage to the lingual nerve by an anesthetic needle. Recovery, probably in a short time, was to be expected.

"And then?"

"I continued to hurt. I would awaken at night with pain on the tip of my tongue and sometimes in my jaw on the right side. Occasionally, I would wake up and feel the pain on both sides of my tongue."

"Both sides?"

"Yes, both sides."

"And then?"

"I was referred to a neurologist who was expert in peripheral nerve injuries. He told me the same thing that everybody else had—an injury to the lingual nerve. He told me that he anticipated the pain would go away in about forty-five days."

"Forty-five days? Do you mind telling me how he knew that with such certainty?"

"He told me that nerves regenerate at a very slow but measurable rate. By dividing that rate into the distance between the back of the jaw where I was injected and the tip of my tongue where I was hurting, he was able to calculate how many days it would take to recover."

I offered no judgment on that calculation, but I did think it represented a perhaps unwarranted confidence. There is more to chronic pain than nerve injury, and there is more to recovery from chronic pain than the regeneration of nerves. I kept that particular thought to myself and asked only if the neurologist had prescribed any medicines.

"Yes, he gave me Neurontin."

"That is certainly an appropriate choice. Did it help?"

"Yes, the Neurontin helped quite a lot, but I had to take a pretty big dose to get any real effect, and I found it very sedating. I was unable to concentrate, and I was very forgetful."

"The treatment was worse than the disease."

"Yes, it surely was. I went back to the neurologist, and he told me to discard the Neurontin. He prescribed Amitriptyline, and I am taking that now. My dose is 75 mg. every night."

"Has it helped?"

"Yes, I am not as sedated now, and I am doing fairly well with it."

"Do you still have pain?"

"Oh yes, especially at night. There were a couple of times when it was really bad, not just in my mouth but also in my face. My chin and my nose hurt, and sometimes—this is really strange—I would have sneezing attacks."

"You would have pain on both sides of your mouth and your face?"

"Yes, both sides."

"That's interesting. The nerve that was damaged supplied only the right side of the jaw and tongue, and yet you are hurting on both sides of your mouth and even into your face. Did you mention that to the neurologist?"

"Yes, I told him about it, but he was dismissive. I guess he thought it was my imagination."

"Well, it seems that we are past the time when he told you you would recover."

"That's quite correct. We are at least a month past that date."

"But the Amitriptyline is helping you?"

"Quite a lot, but I have a problem, and that is why I am here. Since I have been on Amitriptyline my diabetes has gotten a lot worse. My internist was perplexed about it and wanted your opinion."

"Well, it can happen. I think I have seen it once or twice before. Let's check it out."

I reached for the *Physician's Desk Reference* and searched the index for a reference to Amitriptyline.

"You don't have to do that. I have already looked it up. Amitriptyline can raise the blood sugar."

"Did you mention that to the neurologist?"

"Yes. He said it couldn't happen."

I will offer to the reader a judgment that I did not express to Bill. The more one, physician or otherwise, knows about a certain subject, the less he seems to know about other subjects. This is understandable and quite forgivable, but it introduces a queer mindset—that which the expert knows is quite important, and that which he or she doesn't know is unimportant. The neurologist treated Bill's pain, it would seem, effectively and for that deserves credit. For the overconfident calculation of the date of recovery, the discounting of the strange migration of pain *away* from the path of the damaged lingual nerve, ignoring the effect of Amitriptyline on the blood sugar, and perhaps not really exploring the true origins of Bill's pain, I must give him low marks.

"Tell me about your diabetes."

"I have had it four years, and I am taking pills for it, Glucotrol and Actos."

"Have they kept it under control?"

"Yes, my blood sugars were in good order until I started on Amitriptyline. Since then, I have had to double the dose of both medicines, and my blood sugar is still running too high."

"The treatment is worse than the disease?"

"Yes, and there is another problem. I am a little reluctant to bring it up but it is important to me."

"I can guess. Sexual dysfunction?"

"How did you know that?"

"It is very common with drugs like Amitriptyline. Are you impotent?"

"Well, let's just say I am impaired, and it bothers me a lot. I am in a new relationship. I am very fond of her, and we are both frustrated."

"You are not married?"

"No, I lost my wife about nine months ago. I have found a companion. Her husband died a couple of years ago. We go to the same church, and we really have connected."

"Bill, we have a problem here, but I think it is solvable. Before we get into that, though, I'd like to talk a little bit more about your wife's death with you. I suspect that may have some bearing on why you became so painful."

"I am happy to talk with you about it because I think you are right. You must know after my wife's death, I was grieving enormously."

"When did your wife die?"

"In July of last year."

"When did you break the tooth?"

"In August."

"How long had you been married?"

"Almost twenty-five years."

"Children?"

"Two, away at college."

"The cause of your wife's death?"

"Cancer, breast cancer. It was very aggressive, and she died about two years after her mastectomy. It was a real ordeal. I did the best I could for her, and when she left, the house was really lonely."

"You were depressed?"

"No, I don't think so. I could still work at the bank and really do it rather effectively. In fact, work was my release. I wasn't depressed, but I did have occasional spells when I thought about her and cried, but I could still function. I felt it was something I just had to work my way through. Finding Rachel really helped me. She is a wonderful person."

"Bill, I will offer my opinion that your loss and your grief had quite as much to do with your pain as did the damage to your nerve. I don't see how it could be otherwise."

"I agree with you 100 percent."

"Did you tell the neurologist about your wife's death?"

"Yes, I did. He said the pain was due to damage to the nerve, and it probably would have happened whether I was grieving or not."

I prescribed the drug Cymbalta. It is a new drug, and it has a unique chemical structure, different from that of the tricyclics, but its clinical effect, particularly for the treatment of pain, is similar. It certainly has its own set of problems, but raising the blood sugar and sexual dysfunction do not seem to be among them. I advised a slow taper of his Amitriptyline rather than a sudden cessation. Whether with opiates, tranquilizers, or antidepressants, sudden withdrawal can produce some disturbing effects. I told Bill that I could by no means guarantee that we would improve things by this change of therapy. I only told him, and I truly believe this, that there is a drug or combination of drugs that will relieve pain in nearly everybody, most of the time without major side effects. I told him also, certainly without giving a specific date, that in time he would probably get better. I doubted, however, that the pain would ever go entirely away. The onset of his pain and the death of his wife appeared almost simultaneously, within but a month of each other. Their memories were ensconced together in brain place and brain time and were not to be

The onset of his pain and the death of his wife . . . were ensconced together in brain place and brain time and were not to be easily separated.

easily separated. I suspected that just as the memory of his wife would never go away, so would the memory of his pain never go away.

He returned three weeks later to report that he was doing well. He was taking 60 mg. of Cymbalta, and he had been off the Amitriptyline for a week. His blood sugar had fallen with remarkable exactitude. With every 25 mg. reduction in Amitriptyline dosage, he told me, his blood sugar fell about twenty points. He had already reduced the dosage of some of his diabetes medicine. I asked if there had been any improvement in his sexual energy. He only smiled.

"Are you having pain now?"

"Yes, a bit. My lips burn, sometimes during the day, but mostly at night. I will wake up with my lips burning."

"Is it bad?"

"No, it is not really bad at all. They feel kind of tingly. Hard to believe, but it is actually a pleasant sensation."

"Only on the lips, not on the jaw or tongue?"

"Only on the lips, the upper and the lower. They tingle all over— just the lips."

"Bill, you have been through a lot. You are a very intelligent person, and it has been a pleasure to treat you. Let me ask, what do you think really happened to you?"

"I believe my mind was playing tricks on me."

A Nobel neurophysiologist could not have stated it better. Chronic pain is indeed the product of the mind playing tricks. It plays tricks when it makes pain strike only at night, and it plays tricks when it spreads the pain of injury beyond the bounds of its origin.

"Your new relationship, Bill: Is it going well?"

"Yes, and my children adore her. We have something special planned. She and I have both traveled a lot, but we have decided to go somewhere where neither of us has been before. We are going to Santa Fe."

"You won't be disappointed. Are you going to the opera?"

"Yes, we are going to the opera."

Bill's pain began with an injury to the right lingual nerve. At the onset, his pain was appropriate to that injury, the right side of the jaw and the right side of the tongue. As his anesthetic wore off, his pain and numbness disappeared except for the right side of the tip of his tongue. With the passage of time and the evolution of his disease, his discomfort spread to the other side of the tongue, then the lips, and then the lower face, even into the nose. In response to that particular stimulus, he had sneezing attacks—an uncontrollable response to a noxious stimulus, be it pollen or a virus or discomfort within the nose. And then, in part under the sponsorship of treatment and perhaps some other things, the area of his pain became confined to his lips, only the lips, including the lower, which does have some lingual nerve innervation, and the upper, which has absolutely none.

> *Chronic pain is indeed the product of the mind playing tricks. It plays tricks when it makes pain strike only at night, and it plays tricks when it spreads the pain of injury beyond the bounds of its origin.*

I want to offer you now a flight of my imagination, a cerebral event of which I am often victim. I have suggested that Bill's pain would never entirely go away, just as the memory of his wife would never go away. The appearance of his pain was sandwiched in time between the loss of his first love and the discovery of his new one. Bill's brain was simultaneously accommodating to grief, pain, and joy. Processing all this would have been difficult, emotionally, for any of us. Some brain confusion, including the perception of pain, would be expected. In the end, Bill's fundamentally sound emotional integration, his new love, and his pharmacy won out over grief and loss and pain. But why did pain in the jaw and the tongue end up as a pleasurable sensation, nocturnal tingling on the lips? I am not much into symbols, but I will admit they are important in our lives. I will suggest that Bill's pleasurably tingling lips were a memory and a symbol of love, both lost and gained, derived, as it were, from an intensely painful experience. Even chronic pain can have a happy ending!

This may be far-fetched to some readers, but in a later chapter I will explore the importance of memory and pain.

Bogle suffered pain in his jaw. It was due to osteonecrosis, which means, quite literally, dead bone. He was tall, long-limbed, and angular, and he had a great crop of kinky, white hair. He was eighty years old, and he was black. Some of the patients that I describe in this book are black, and some are white. I make no real distinction because I think the issue of race as it relates to pain is highly unimportant, but Bogle was one of the most estimable people I have ever known, and I want to tell you a bit about him. He grew up in the rural South and attended a segregated college. After his studies there were completed, he pursued graduate work at a prestigious Midwestern university. He was awarded a PhD in psychology and returned to his alma mater as a member of the faculty. He became a department head at age thirty. He left that post at age seventy-five and became dean of the college. Shortly after that move, which he described as a happy one, he began to develop pain on the left side of his jaw. He consulted many physicians, but for two years, at least, no cause could be found. In the course of his journeys, he was prescribed many different medicines. Tegretol, an anticonvulsant commonly used for neuritic face pain, was without effect, as was Neurontin. Celexa, the antidepressant, was equally unhelpful. Naproxen, an anti-inflammatory drug, also. Even Hydrocodone gave only modest relief. Some two years into his illness, Bogle consulted an oral surgeon who biopsied the bone of the painful area. The pathologist's report concluded with a diagnosis of osteonecrosis. A portion of Bogle's jawbone had inexplicably died. The oral surgeon gave his unhappy advice. There was no medical or surgical treatment. Bogle would just have to live with the pain. Not wanting to accept this advice, he came to see me.

"Tell me what the pain is like."

He responded slowly and with measured care. "It doesn't hurt all of the time. Most of the time it doesn't hurt at all, but sometimes it can be quite severe."

"Do you see any pattern to the pain? Can you predict when it will start hurting?"

"At night. Sometimes I awaken with a violent pain in the left side of my jaw. When that happens, I take a Hydrocodone and try to go back to sleep. Sometimes it is hard to do, though."

"Does it hurt when you chew?"

"No, and that seems strange to me. Part of my jawbone is dead. You would think it would hurt when I chewed or gritted my teeth, but that doesn't seem to bring it on at all. It is very curious—sometimes I will chew gum, and that seems to make it better. I keep chewing gum by my bed, and I use it a lot."

Curious indeed. Damaged bone should hurt when pressure is applied to it. It should be relieved when it is at rest. Think of a fracture or an arthritic hip.

"Bogle, are you depressed?"

"No, I am really not. Maybe I should be, but I look at myself, and I just don't see depression. My life is very rich, and I wake up every morning hopeful and excited about a new day."

"Tell me about your life. What is it that makes you so hopeful and excited?"

"My granddaughters. They are twins. They have just graduated from high school, and in a few months I will be sending them off to college."

"*You* are sending them to college?"

"Yes, they are my responsibility, and they are the joy of my life."

"Why are they your responsibility?"

"My daughter left her husband a few years back. She wanted to go her own way. She left the girls with me and my wife."

"How do you feel about that? Are you resentful or angry?"

"No, my daughter is doing well. She is having a nice career in real estate. She comes by occasionally, and we have a good relationship. I don't mind taking care of the girls. It has really been a joy. I have been very active in the parent-teacher association, and at the graduation ceremony just a month or so ago, I was recognized as Parent of the Year. Isn't that something?"

"I am impressed, Bogle, very impressed. Let me ask you, though. You said the girls were left with you and your wife. Was she recognized also?"

"Unfortunately, no. My wife is very ill. She has Alzheimer's and is in a nursing home. I visit her every day."

I knew I was in the company of a remarkable man.

"I am very sorry, Bogle, but let me ask you to give me a timeline on all this, your assumption of your granddaughters' care, your wife's illness, and the onset of your pain."

"They all came about the same time—about five years ago."

"Bogle, I am going to give you some medicines that I think may help you. One is called Clonazepam, and the other Imipramine. We will start on a low dose and increase to the limits that are written on the bottles. I am hopeful that you will start sleeping through the night without pain. I will see you back in three weeks, and during that time I want you to think about something. Your biopsy shows osteonecrosis. We cannot be certain, however, that your osteonecrosis began five years ago. We only know that your pain began five years ago. You are a psychologist and knowledgeable in the workings of the mind. I want you to think about whether there might be some connection between your pain, your wife's illness, and the adoption of your granddaughters."

"That I will do."

He returned at the appointed interval and told me that he was sleeping through the night with only occasional breakthroughs of pain. He had used his Hydrocodone only once or twice.

"I am happy that you are better. When we spoke before, I asked you to think about certain things. Do you have any comment?"

"Yes, I have thought quite a lot about it. I am a psychologist, and it is easy for me to look in the minds of others, but, and I suspect you know this, sometimes it is hard to look into one's own mind."

"I know that very well. I think I have spent half of my life in denial."

"I, also. I suppose I have repressed some emotions that perhaps should have come out."

"Well, so be it. I do often see chronic pain such as you have experienced appearing under the provocation of traumas that should, in most of us, lead to depression or at least something like depression, but manifest them-selves instead in chronic pain. What do you think about that?"

"I think you may be correct. I think that may well be what happened to me."

Bogle did well for several months. He continued to have occasional pains, chew on his gum, and take a Hydrocodone, but the frequency and severity of attacks was much diminished. Within a year or so into our treatment, however, he came to me complaining of a sense of fatigue that he thought might be due to his drug therapy. He asked if we might change the medicine.

Traumas that should, in most of us, lead to depression, or at least something like depression . . . manifest themselves instead in chronic pain.

"I am reluctant to do so, Bogle, because the drugs are working so well. However, there is a new drug called Cymbalta that can be very helpful in the treatment of chronic pain. It is much like the Imipramine that you are taking. I suspect that is what is causing your fatigue. Discontinue the Imipramine and take the Cymbalta as directed. I will see you again in a month, and we will reappraise."

On his return, he said, "I have had a lot more pain. The new medicine is not working. I want to go back to the Imipramine, fatigue or not."

I complied with his request, and he returned a month later saying he was quite happy with my treatment. He had decided that his fatigue might be as much a function of his eighty years of age as to the Imipramine.

In later chapters I will tell the stories of many people who suffer chronic pain. I will identify their pain as a disease of the mind, and as such, one that travels in company with mind-bending experiences such as childhood abuse, drug addiction, and psychiatric illness. I have placed the story of Bill and Bogle at the beginning of the book, however, to point out that the most resolute and emotionally well-integrated can suffer pain under the provocation of destructive life events, even in the absence of depression, or for that matter, any other psychiatric illness.

A remarkable attribute of both Bill and Bogle was that they suffered their pain almost exclusively at night. Worsening of pain at night and the appearance of pain only at night are certain indicators—perhaps the most certain indicators—that the victim suffers the disease chronic pain, which responds, predictably, to neuropsychiatric drugs. In both of them, restoration of sleep was associated with diminution of pain. This does not necessarily mean that pain diminished *because* sleep was restored. It only means that pain was diminished *as* sleep was restored.

Both were cured, or nearly cured, by pharmacy. The tricyclic Amitriptyline helped Bill but produced unfortunate side effects. A kindred, Cymbalta, was effective in diminishing pain, correcting diabetes, and restoring sexual function. In Bogle, Cymbalta only made the pain worse. The drugs don't work the same on everybody (genetic pleomorphism again), and we just have to accept that as a fact of life. Bill's pain spread beyond—way beyond—the bounds of his original injury. Bogle's stayed put. And that is the way it goes. There are no hard and fast rules, and we just have to live with it.

Bill and Bogle suffered pain but neither suffered its companion, depression. I do not know why this happened, but I am taken with the commonalities between them. Both, in the throes of their discomfort, almost simultaneously experienced both loss and gain. Bill quite literally lost his wife, and Bogle, quite figuratively, lost his. Bill gained a new love, and Bogle gained his also, his twin granddaughters. Whether this acquisition of new love kept them from depression, I don't know, but it did not keep them from chronic pain.

CHAPTER FOUR

Depression and Pain

R ichard's tongue had been burning for more than a year. He told me that its severity was seven on a pain scale of ten, and that it was there 24/7. I scanned his medical records. He had been seen several times by his primary care doctor and his dentist. He had also consulted a throat specialist, an allergist, and a dermatologist. All the necessary tests, and some unnecessary ones also, had been performed and were unrevealing. Richard had been advised to change his toothpaste and even to change his toothbrush. He had been prescribed a variety of mouthwashes, as well as antihistamines and antibiotics. None helped.

He was fifty-nine years of age and an imposing presence. Handsomely dressed with coat and tie, he had a great head of white hair parted and combed with not a single member out of place. He spoke slowly and with perfect articulation. Each word was uttered as if it represented some sort of small treasure. I sensed that Richard was someone who was used to being looked at and listened to.

"Richard, we will talk about your burning tongue shortly but first, tell me about yourself. Are you married? Do you have children?"

"Yes, I am happily married and have been so for thirty years. I have three children and four grandchildren."

"All doing well?"

"Yes, quite well, thank you."

"What do you do for a living?"

"I am a public speaker, Dr. Cochran. I work for a large publishing house that specializes in inspirational books. I travel all over the world giving speeches."

"What an interesting job!"

"Yes, it is very interesting. I meet many people, and I have been to all of the continents several times."

"Well, I must ask you, does public speaking, an activity in which one uses the tongue a lot, make your pain worse?"

"No, I have often wondered about that myself, but no, speaking has no influence on my pain at all."

"And the travel? You fly across continents, you change time zones and, I would gather, shift from one climate to another. Does all that change have any influence on your pain?"

"Not in the least."

Oh boy. This one is going to be fun, I thought.

"Richard, tell me how your pain began."

"It began right on the tip of my tongue, right in the middle at the very tip."

"Did it hurt badly at first, or did it gradually become more severe?"

"As I recall, it was just a sense of irritation at first, maybe for a matter of a few weeks. And then it started spreading backwards, and when it did, it became more and more painful."

"And now the pain is all over your tongue?"

"Yes, my entire tongue hurts."

"If you place your tongue to the side of your mouth and apply pressure to it by biting down, does your pain increase?"

"No, my pain level does not change at all. My disease, whatever it is, is quite curious, don't you think?"

"Yes, but let me try to comfort you. I am used to treating, and many times curing, the curious disease."

"That is comforting indeed, Dr. Cochran."

"A few more questions. Do you ever feel pain in your gums, your throat, or your lips?"

He raised his hand to his mouth, brushed his index finger across his lips, and said, "Only the lips. Sometimes my lips hurt, although not nearly so bad as my tongue."

"How are you sleeping?"

"Usually I sleep quite well. Sometimes after a long trip, I have to take a sleeping pill, but that is really very infrequent. I think I see where you are taking me with this. My pain tends to worsen as the day goes on, and the pain is quite severe, but it almost never keeps me from sleeping."

"Then it is not 24/7."

He smiled and said, "You are right, it is 16/7."

When my office schedules a new patient appointment, we send that person a request for the usual demographic and insurance information. Included is an intake history form on which the patient is to list current symptoms, medications, prior illnesses, and family history. On the reverse, there is a system review—a questionnaire of perhaps one hundred different symptoms with the request that they be answered yes or no. Richard's system review was extraordinarily negative. Only under the heading of psychiatric symptoms did he acknowledge that he suffered anxiety.

All the necessary tests, and some unnecessary ones also, had been performed and were unrevealing.

Beside it he wrote "slight." His medication list was quite short. He was taking the antacid Protonix and the antidepressant Lexapro. *A good place to start,* I thought.

"Richard, I see that you are taking Lexapro. I suppose you were given that for depression."

"Yes, I have been taking Lexapro for six years now. It has been extremely helpful to me. I really don't have any problem with depression at all now, but my primary care doctor thought it best that I continue taking the drug."

"Tell me what was going on when your depression began."

"I was in a bad automobile accident. I had a concussion and was unconscious for several days. Several of my ribs were broken, and my spleen ruptured. I required surgery and was in the hospital for over two weeks. I was also under a lot of personal stress. I was in sales back then, and it wasn't nearly as pleasant as being a public speaker. I became very anxious and depressed."

"Were you suicidal?"

"No, nothing like that, but I was constantly fatigued, and I had a great deal of trouble sleeping. I have always been an emotional person, but this was something different. I was on a roller coaster. My emotions were running amok."

"Did you see a psychiatrist?"

"No, my primary care doctor prescribed the antidepressant."

"That was the Lexapro?"

"No, the first drug he gave me was Celexa. It helped quite a lot for several months, but then I became listless. Nothing seemed to matter. I didn't care about anything. That is when my doctor changed me to Lexapro. My improvement was dramatic. I have had absolutely no problems with depression since I have been on Lexapro."

Many readers have probably experienced the flattening-out effect of the SSRI antidepressants. They can be very effective in relieving depression, but in its place they sometimes lead to a state of emotional torpor and evenness that deprives the user of the normal experiences of sadness and joy. There is nothing unique about Celexa in this regard, but it is curious that Lexapro, almost an identical drug, had no such effect.

"Richard, I see that you have a slight problem with anxiety. Could you tell me about that?"

"I do become anxious from time to time. Fortunately, it doesn't last very long. I can usually make it go away by doing some sort of exercise. Taking a walk will always relieve it."

"Is there any trigger? Can you identify anything that makes you nervous?"

"I have been quite unable to do that, although I have certainly tried."

"Richard, I do believe that I can relieve your pain and maybe pretty quickly. But I have one more question."

"Sure."

"You have a disease that I recognize as chronic pain. Sometimes it just appears out of the blue, but most of the time, indeed almost all the time, there is some injury to the body from which the victim of chronic pain, for whatever reason, doesn't recover. Can you think of any kind of injury to your tongue when this started? Could you have bitten it or burned it on some hot food?"

"No, I have no memory of anything like that."

"Is it possible that you had some kind of dental work done shortly before this thing came on you?"

He hesitated as he searched his memory. I could sense that he was working hard for me.

"Yes, I do remember now. One of my front teeth was chipped. It was a few weeks before I could arrange a dental appointment to have it repaired, and I do recall that I frequently rubbed the tip of my tongue against the broken tooth. I remember a certain sense of irritation in my tongue then. I think you have hit on something, Dr. Cochran. That is when the pain actually began."

I elected to treat Richard with Clonazepam and Imipramine. The two drugs, or for that matter, the two classes of drugs (benzodiazepines and tricyclics) seem to have a synergistic effect. That is, they work well together, and they create a thing that is greater than the sum of its parts.

Richard was well within a week.

"My pain is almost nonexistent. It is less than a one."

I thought that Richard would respond to my drugs because he carried the legacy of depression and because he experienced the curious phenomena, so common in chronic pain, of the migration of pain beyond the bounds of its origin. Recall Bill from the preceding chapter. His pain began on one side of his tongue and migrated into his lips and lower face.

Sometimes it just appears out of the blue, but most of the time, indeed almost all the time, there is some injury to the body from which the victim of chronic pain, for whatever reason, doesn't recover.

Thoughtful readers may wonder why, if Richard's pain was somehow a derivative of his depression, it appeared at a time when his depression was cured. I am not sure that Richard's depression was totally in control. Recall his tentative response to my questionnaire inquiring about the presence of anxiety. "Yes," he wrote, but "slight." Perhaps his depression was only partially controlled, and his anxiety was a persistent symptom of that disorder. (Yes, anxiety can certainly be a symptom of depression.) Moreover, Richard was on treatment with Lexapro, an SSRI that, although quite helpful in the treatment of depression, is often ineffective in the treatment of pain. His symptoms of sadness were controlled by the drug, and his symptoms of anxiety, nearly so, but his pain was not.

He experienced the curious phenomena, so common in chronic pain, of the migration of pain beyond the bounds of its origin.

Mark's pain began in his right eye. It occurred in the afternoon of a day in which he learned that a close friend had suddenly died. It was severe, and it kept him from sleeping through the night. It continued into the next day, and as he was lifting a suitcase from a shelf in his closet, he experienced an excruciating pain in the back of his head. His vision became doubled and blurred. He was unable to speak, and both his arms and legs felt tingly and weak.

"It was a hemorrhage in the back of my brain. I remember going to the hospital. They did an MRI in the emergency room and then took me up to the operating room. I could hear them talking, but I couldn't respond or move. I remember one of them saying, 'He is a lucky man. He doesn't have an aneurysm, and he is not going to need an operation.'"

"And then?"

"I was in the hospital for a week. My speech gradually returned, and within a few days I was able to walk. My headache went away slowly, but when I left the hospital, I was still seeing double, and glare hurt my eyes. I had to wear sunglasses. It was a month before I could drive a car again, but my recovery from my hemorrhage was complete except for some occasional, pretty severe headaches."

"What were they like?"

"They would strike me in the back of the head and in the right eye, just like before. They were bad but not nearly as bad as when I first got sick."

"How long would they last?"

"Oh, maybe an hour, sometimes longer."

"How often?"

"On the average, a couple of times a week. My hemorrhage was five years ago, and the headaches were a lot more frequent then than now, but I still have them."

"Is there anything that seems to bring them on?"

"Yes, most certainly. I have them when I strain to lift something, and sometimes I have them when I watch a movie or TV show that strikes my emotions."

"That is interesting. Let me ask you, have you ever had a problem with headache before?"

"Yes, sometimes I would have tension headaches and sometimes sinus headaches, but they were never very bad. Ibuprofen would usually take care of them," he chuckled.

"Did you ever think that these might be migraine, or did your doctors suggest they might be migraine?"

"No, I never even went to the doctor about them. They were no big deal."

"Your hemorrhage was five years ago, and that is when your headaches began. You are coming to see me now. Why after so long?"

"Well, I had been under the care of Dr. Jones, the neurologist. I like him a lot, and I think he has done a good job with me, but he has moved to another part of town, and I thought it might be a good idea to let somebody else to take a look. I want you to understand that I am at least 75 percent improved, but I thought another opinion might be helpful."

He laughed when he said this, which struck me as a little inappropriate.

"Dr. Jones is an excellent neurologist. I respect him very much. Could you tell me what medicines he has been giving you?"

"He tried me on Depakote, but I didn't like it. It made me feel unwell and fatigued. Right now I am taking Topamax, and I think it is helping quite a lot. Like I told you, I am really not very sick," he chuckled again.

Mark was exhibiting insouciance, a want of concern. He was, I suspected, lying to himself. He was in denial. If he was unconcerned about his headaches, why did he even bother to come to see me?

"Mark, have you ever had a problem with depression?"

"Yes, actually I have," he said with a smile.

"Tell me about it."

"I had a very successful career in accounting, but I became very stressed. I was working too hard, and I didn't have time for my family. I became depressed, and I went to a psychiatrist. He gave me several different antidepressants, but none of them really worked. Then I had a kind of epiphany. I had enough money to retire, so at age fifty-two, I just walked away from it. The community college was happy to have me on the faculty. I teach there three days a week. On the others I go fishing and hunting."

"What happened to the depression?"

"It lifted. It lifted a lot." Again he chuckled. "I threw away the anti-depressant pills."

"When did all this happen?"

"Just shortly before my brain hemorrhage."

"So no problem with depression now?"

"No, not really."

"You are no longer seeing a psychiatrist?"

"Well yes, I still see him. Mostly we talk about stress management. That is still a little bother for me." Once again he chuckled.

"How are you sleeping?"

He smiled and said, "That is a problem for me."

"Are you taking any medicine for sleep?"

"No."

"Mark, have you ever had a problem with drugs or alcohol?"

"Absolutely not."

"Do you have a family history of depression?"

"Yes, my mother and two brothers have chronic depression."

"Okay, Mark. I want to prescribe a couple of medicines for you, and you need to be advised they are useful for sleep, and they are also useful for pain. I think there is real prospect for improvement."

"Well," he laughed, "if they will make me better I will take them, but I want you to know I am really not very sick. I am 75 percent improved from where I was five years ago."

I wrote him a prescription for Imipramine and Clonazepam and in short order dictated my consultation note to his primary care physician with a copy to his psychiatrist and neurosurgeon. I called the latter right away to find out just what had happened to Mark.

"Yes, I remember Mark quite well. He had a mesencephalic subarachnoid hemorrhage."

Mesencephalic refers to the mid-brain. Subarachnoid refers to the space within the lining of the brain and hemorrhage, of course, to the rupture of a blood vessel. Subarachnoid hemorrhage is almost always due to rupture of an artery weakened and ballooned out in the form of an aneurysm, but it almost never occurs in the mid-brain. Aneurysms are usually found in the arteries of the upper brain, the big cauliflower-shaped portion of that organ. The stalk of the cauliflower corresponds to the mid-brain.

Mark was exhibiting insouciance, a want of concern. He was, I suspected, lying to himself. He was in denial.

"Mid-brain hemorrhages are very rare. They seem to occur almost always in people with migraine, and sometimes they occur after sexual intercourse. We do arteriograms, but we never find an aneurysm. We really don't understand why this thing happens."

I thanked my colleague for the information and didn't let on that I had never heard about this—and I thought I knew something about migraine. It did fit. Mark's occasional sinus and tension headaches were almost certainly migraine, and the intense eye pain he experienced the day preceding his stroke was definitely a migraine. The sudden pain in the back of the head was the hemorrhage.

I was about to close up the chart and give it to my transcriptionist when something caught my eye. It was a piece of notepaper on which Mark had written the following:

Bending over gives me a headache
Picking up things, straining, makes my head hurt
My future—what can I expect?
Hollow feeling in my temples
Emotional—temples feel pressed in,

throbbing in the head, pressure
Stress—vacuum chamber feeling—outer space

The act of clue-giving is a theme that will recur throughout this book. I am repeatedly astonished (and delighted) when my patient offers me hints about his illness. This happens with such frequency and to such benefit that it seems almost providential. Sometimes in the spoken word and sometimes in the written, my patient will tell me something that he thinks I ought to know, but is reluctant or perhaps fearful of expressing. Did Mark leave his notes by accident? I don't know, and I suppose if I had asked him, he would say it was. But deep in my heart, and I suspect Mark's also, we know that it was not. Mark was trying to tell me that he was very depressed.

At the time of Mark's hemorrhage, his mid-brain was compressed by a clot of blood on its surface. This occurred in a space where there is not a lot of extra room, for the mid-brain is confined to a rather narrow cavity. His mid-brain's anatomy was distorted and very likely remained so as a result of his injury. Activities such as lifting or straining, by virtue of their effect on the cardiac output and the return of blood to the heart, can increase intracranial (within the skull) pressure very significantly, and it takes no difficulty to accept that a change in pressure could further distort already disturbed anatomy and produce pain. Watching an emotional movie or TV show, however, does not in itself create increased intracranial pressure. Therefore, we are quite unable to explain his increasing pain in those circumstances on the basis of pressure dynamics within the skull. I had a feeling, a very strong feeling, that we were about to strike gold.

At our next visit, I asked Mark how he was doing.

"I think I am better. My mood seems more even. I don't feel as stressed. Let me tell you something. A few days ago I shot a turkey and carried it a mile back to the car. That is the kind of lifting that used to give me headaches. I expected a bad night, but I had no pain at all. I slept very well."

"That's great! How much of the medicine are you taking?"

"I am taking two of the big ones and three of the little ones."

"Mark, forgive me for saying this, but I don't do little, and I don't do big, and I don't do yellow, and I don't do white, and I don't do blue. Can you tell me the names of the medicines you are taking and how many?"

"No, I am sorry, but I can't."

It is remarkable to me that university professors, lawyers, ministers, financial planners, and others of that ilk identify their medicines by their size or by their color, almost never by their names. I don't know why I let it bother me so, but it does—chiefly because the identification of medicines by their size or by their color can offer misinformation, and I hate that I have to tell my patient to increase the number of the big pills and diminish the little pills or vice versa. Mistakes could happen, but fortunately they don't very often. I told Mark to gradually increase the number of both his little pills and his big pills.

The victim of smiling depression is actually depressed but either doesn't know it or refuses to accept it. He doesn't feel sad, but he does feel pain.

He returned at the appointed time, and when I entered the examining room, he stood up, wordlessly took my hand, and stared at me, wide eyed. His look was that of a deer in the headlights, and I see it not infrequently in those who recover from chronic pain. It reflects, I believe, their difficulty in comprehending that something so profound and so wonderful could happen to them in a span of but a few weeks, and in some cases just a few days. Speech finally came to him, and with an air of wonder he said, "The last three weeks have been the best in many years. My headaches are gone, and my stress level—and that had been bothering me a lot—has diminished. I seem very peaceful and contented. Thank you, Doctor."

"I am happy for you, Mark. I am truly happy for you. Let's just continue your current therapy, and I will see you again in a month. If I may, I would like to ask you another question."

"Of course."

"Do you think, as you look back on it, that you have been suffering depression all these past five years?"

"Yes, I see that now. I didn't want to admit it to myself, but I see it clearly now. Thank you for recognizing it. Thank you for giving me the right medicine."

Recall that during our first visit, Mark exhibited easy laughter and a proclivity to deny, his painfulness notwithstanding, that anything really bad was wrong with him. "I am really not very sick. I am 75 percent improved from where I was five years ago."

There was a diagnosis popular many years ago known as atypical depression or, in the vernacular, smiling depression. It was a good diagnostic term then, and it still is now. The victim of smiling depression is actually depressed but either doesn't know it or refuses to accept it. He doesn't feel sad, but he does feel pain.

Clark, at age sixty-one, was badly arthritic. Both a knee and a hip had been replaced, and an ankle surgically fused into immobility in an effort to diminish the pain generated by the bones grinding together every time he walked.

He had been quite successful financially and was able to retire at age fifty-five and exercise his passion for reading and traveling. His personal and social history was, to me, compelling. He was three times married and three times divorced. After the second divorce at age thirty-three, he entered a depression. He did not consult a psychiatrist. Rather, he treated himself, successfully, with cocaine. After some three years of this activity, he sought revival by a trip to northern Africa. While in Morocco, he smoked heavily of hashish and opium. He told me that the experience removed him from any craving for cocaine, and he found it quite easy to give up the other drugs. He returned to the States, made a bundle of money, and married again. His arthritic pains began about age fifty. He began taking Hydrocodone. His hip was replaced some three years before he came to me, and he acknowledged that he experienced a significant depression following this. It lasted some two months and then abated. He never sought medical care for it. Knee replacement was done two years later, and Clark again suffered depression with profound sleeplessness, often going five or six days without any sleep at all. Wiser now than before, he consulted his internist and was prescribed Prozac, which he found extraordinarily helpful. He terminated its use after a few months without any recurrence of depression.

By this time Clark's pain, in both his replaced hip and knee, had become a significant issue. He was taking Hydrocodone to a maximum of three pills daily. He confided to me that sometimes that wasn't enough, and on those occasions he found that smoking high-grade Belgian marijuana gave him immediate pain relief. About this time his third marriage was ending, and he faced an operation to fuse the bones of an unstable, arthritic ankle. His internist prescribed Prozac again in hopes of preventing yet another depression. The fusion was completed satisfactorily, and Clark was finally able to walk without pain in his ankle and foot, but his other joints were a terrible bother, and he was referred to me.

He was a quick-witted and pleasant gentleman, obviously possessed of *joie de vivre*, and his pain problem notwithstanding, he smiled quickly and eagerly. I liked him enormously. He acknowledged sleeplessness and restless legs but adamantly denied depression. He told me he was still taking his Prozac.

"Clark, I am giving you prescriptions for Clonazepam and Nortriptyline. The two drugs seem to work well together, and I think there is reasonable possibility that they will help you. I think the first good thing that will happen is that you will begin to sleep better."

"I will do as you say."

"Clark, there is something else I want you to do for me."

"Certainly."

"I have written a book about chronic pain, and in it I explore the relationship of pain to mental illness. You told me that you like to read. I think my book might have some meaning for you. I encourage you to take a look at it."

"I will certainly do that."

I wanted Clark to read my book so he could begin to connect the dots and look into the possibility that with his recurrent depression, his drug use, his manic ability to make money, and his multiple marriages and divorces, that he just might be bipolar.

He returned at the appointed time and reported that he was taking, as I had instructed, 50 mg. of Nortriptyline and 1.5 mg. of Clonazepam nightly. He told me his sleep was somewhat better, but he had seen no change in his pain. He was, however, tolerating the drugs with no side effects. He told me he was reading *Understanding Chronic Pain*. He was excited about the treatment options that might be available to us.

"Yes, Clark, there certainly are some options before us, but for now I want you to increase your Nortriptyline dose up to 80 mg., and you can take a little more Clonazepam, also."

On his return, he told me that he had elected to discontinue his Prozac. He felt his depression was in good order, and that he could get by without it. After a week or so, he knew he had made a mistake, so he resumed his Prozac. His depression ameliorated, but his pain remained largely unchanged.

I wanted Clark to . . . [see] that with his recurrent depression, his drug use, his manic ability to make money, and his multiple marriages and divorces, that he just might be bipolar.

I had, over the course of two months, achieved very little other than restoration of sleep. I suspected that Clark might be a core bipolar—although the evidence for that was presumptive at best. Where to go from here? I could add Cymbalta or Effexor. They are kindred drugs to Nortriptyline, and the addition of either would be reasonable. Another option would be the introduction of a mood stabilizer such as Lithium or one of the anticonvulsants. Psychostimulant therapy would be another choice, although probably a bit down the line. There was one more option, however, and that was the introduction of more opiate therapy. We would know quickly if it was the correct choice, but it was a bit of a dicey decision.

Clark and I were crossing the Rubicon. It is much easier to discontinue a failed therapeutic trial with a mood stabilizer or anticonvulsant than it is to discontinue a therapeutic trial with an opiate. If the additional opiate helped him even a bit, I would be hard-pressed to deny him its ongoing usage. Still, my instincts told me this was the way to go, and I have learned to trust my instincts.

I chose Methadone, the most unpredictable of the opiates. Its metabolism is erratic and varies greatly from one person to another. It can do some very bad things (as can any drug), but it can also do some wonderful things. I prescribed 10 mg. three times daily, and hoped to see positive results by our next appointment.

"Good morning, Clark. What do you have to report?"

"I feel better. My pain is much better, and I feel relaxed. I haven't felt that way in a long time. I am just not quite as driven as I used to be."

"That's wonderful, Clark. I am very happy for you. I think we got lucky on this one."

"Call it what you will, Doc, but I am very very happy."

There were some bumps left in the road. About two weeks later, I took a call from Clark's girlfriend. She said that Clark was very sedated and unsteady on the Methadone, and she suspected that, given his history of drug abuse, he was overusing it. I suggested that she accompany Clark to my office at the earliest possible time.

Clark appeared the next day, unaccompanied. He came on his on volition, he told me. He recounted that his girlfriend had been alarmed by his unsteadiness and slurred speech.

"Are you taking the medicine as I directed, Clark?"

"Absolutely."

"You are not overusing it?"

"No, I am taking it just as you told me, but I am afraid it is too much for me. I hate that because the drug really was helpful to me. It did more than ease my pain, it just seemed to make me feel more even. I stopped it three days ago, and the pain has come back badly. I am feeling very restless, and I am not sleeping well at all."

I told Clark I was going to keep working with him, and I accepted the fact that he was not overusing the medicine. I certainly wasn't going to deny him a drug that had been of such remarkable benefit. I suggested he try a half a 10 mg. pill every eight hours and demanded that he be alert to any problems with sedation. I told him to return in two weeks. I wrote a prescription for twenty-one Methadone pills, sufficient for two weeks at a dose of one-half pill every eight hours.

He did not keep his appointment, and I feared that I had lost him or perhaps worse, that he had lost himself. Methadone is available on the street, and for a drug of abuse, it is relatively inexpensive. As if that mattered; Clark had lots of money. Maybe I had made a horrible mistake by introducing a former cocaine addict to a new drug of abuse. It is easy to take the counsel of your fears when you are a pain doctor, but in spite of it all, I still had a good feeling about Clark. Six weeks later, I was thrilled when I saw his name on the appointment book.

> *Maybe I had made horrible mistake by introducing a former cocaine addict to a new drug of abuse.*

"I am so glad to see you, Clark. I have been worried about you. How are you doing?"

"Doc, I am doing great. I am sorry I couldn't keep my appointment, but I had an opportunity to go with a friend to work on his cabin in Nova Scotia. I helped him put a new roof on it. That was lots of fun."

"You were able to do that even with your pain?"

"Easy, Doc, I am having no pain at all."

"Okay, I will accept that, but tell me about the Methadone. Are you still taking it? You should have been out of it long ago."

"I just have a few left, Doc. Let me tell you what I have done. I have found out that taking just a half a pill of Methadone at bedtime is all I need. I sleep well, and I have no pain. What you have me on now is the perfect combination."

"Believe me, Clark, I have heard that kind of thing before." And I have. When I am administering opiate therapy, and my patient tells me we have hit on the perfect combination, Methadone always seems to be in the mix.

It is most curious to me that Methadone is the only painkilling opiate that my patients sometimes choose to take in quantities *less* than prescribed. Clark's dosage of 5 mg. daily is ridiculously small and by any standard quite insufficient to produce significant analgesia. That dosage is, however, I believe sufficient for the treatment of bipolar disease. Was Clark bipolar? Almost certainly so, and it is his response to low-dosage Methadone that tells us so.

John was sixty-seven years old and still worked in a sawmill. He had undergone bilateral knee replacement some four years before. He got a splendid result on the right, but the left continued to hurt and occasionally gave him the sensation that it was slipping out from under him. He was taking the opiate codeine with only moderate success.

He was wearing the habit of his trade, overalls and a heavy wool shirt, and he was whiskered, poorly groomed, and unclean. He sat quite still, his poverty of movement broken only by the occasional rubbing of his fingers across the top of his thighs.

"Tell me about your pain, John."

"It's my knee," he said. "It hurts a lot when I climb stairs and ladders."

"Do you have to do that a lot?"

"Yes, there are lots of ladders in sawmills."

"How are you sleeping?"

"Good enough."

"The pain doesn't keep you from sleeping?"

"No."

"How is your mood, John?"

"What do you mean?"

"Are you in a good mood or a bad mood?"

"Good, I suppose."

I continued my interrogations, and his responses, either in the affirmative or negative, were mere grunts. I soon realized that John was not a verbal or expressive man. My attempts at interview were moving at a glacial pace. In my younger years as a physician, I would have let this bother me. By the psychologic process known as transference, I would have put the blame on him. He was a "bad" patient, which is certainly more emotionally acceptable than considering that I am a bad doctor. I would have viewed him as perhaps an unintelligent and uncomplicated human being. I now know that there is no such thing as an uncomplicated human being.

I kept plugging, searching for some clues. I was unable, however, to get any kind of emotional reaction from him. Even when I moved into sensitive areas such as his sexual energy, his responses were, in the main, noncommittal.

> *I now know that there is no such thing as an uncomplicated human being.*

We will see in later chapters that my interview often gives offense. This is because, of necessity, I probe sensitive areas. I make every effort to pursue my questioning with civility and tact, but nonetheless I pursue it relentlessly. This is because if I am going to prescribe pharmacy, I must have some sense that I know what is going on. This I demand of myself. I stepped it up with John, getting a little more aggressive.

"John, can you read?"

He hesitated, and as his finger movements increased, he replied, "No."

"I'm sorry. I know you wish you could read."

He looked at me and said, "I appreciate you saying that."

"John, I see you have a son. How old is he?"

"Eleven."

"Oh, very young. I am sure you enjoy your son. Is he a good boy?"

Hesitation. "Yes, he a good boy," and then his voice tailed off as if he wanted to say more.

I placed my hand on his restless fingers and said, "John, you want to tell me something. Tell me what is in your mind."

He spoke slowly. "He is a good boy, but when I am around him, I feel nervous. My boy makes me nervous."

"Why is that?"

"Don't know, just don't know. He is always asking me questions, and that gets on my nerves."

"Does he ask you questions that you don't know how to answer?"

He looked up and said, "How did you know that?"

"Are there other things that make you nervous?"

He shook his big head back and forth and began crying. "Yes. Sometimes I am so nervous that I want to get up and run away. I want to be by myself."

"How long have you been this way?"

"Four years."

"That is when you had your knee operations, wasn't it?"

"Yes, sir."

"Anything else going on in your life back then? Any troubles?"

"Yes, sir, that was when my brother died. It was right before my knee operation. I still think about him a lot."

"Keep talking."

"I dream about my brother. I dream about him every night. Every night. I see him in the casket, and I talk to him. I say, 'Brother, are you cold down there? I don't want you to be cold.'"

"Does he ever answer you?"

"Yes, sir."

"What does he say?"

"He says, 'John, come on down with me.'"

"Any other kind of dreams?"

"Yes, sir, lots of them. They are all bad. I dream about dead people. My family and my friends. I dream of ghosts. That's what they are. They are ghosts."

"Do you ever see ghosts during the day?"

"Sometimes I think I see my brother out of the corner of my eye, but when I look over, he's not there."

"Do you ever hear your brother?"

"Sometimes I hear him talking to me. That happens a lot."

"What does he say?"

He put his head into his thick hands and said, "'John, come down here with me, come on down, John.'"

John's knee was painful, but he was also in a major, mind-bending depression with visual and auditory hallucinations. What to do? Which drug to choose? Clonazepam and a tricyclic? That is my favorite combination, and it worked very well in two of the men I have just described. Perhaps an antipsychotic to control his hallucinations? We certainly have lots of those, and they almost certainly would have restored his thought and arrested the hallucinations. But would they help his pain? More opiate therapy? Perhaps by diminishing his pain I could relieve his depression and all the rest.

I chose Zoloft, the SSRI antidepressant, and I am really not sure exactly why I did. Only rarely will I initiate therapy in the painful with an SSRI, for they have modest analgesic effect. They can, however, be marvelously effective in the treatment of depression, and I thought that that was John's core disease. There would be time later to treat the pain and hallucinations—if they needed to be.

I saw him three weeks later. He was smiling, he was clean, and he was talking.

"Everything is better. Everything."

"Even your pain?"

"Yes, sir, even my pain."

"How about your ghosts?"

"They are gone. Everything is better."

When the patient says, "Everything is better," the doctor has chosen the absolutely perfect drug.

Sory could not remain still. She was constantly seeking to ease her pain by rubbing against any object she could find. She would use the back of the chair for a while, and then she would lean forward and rub herself with the back of her right hand. I examined her and saw that her back was scarred from heating pad burns and excoriated and skin-thickened by incessant rubbing. Remarkably, the back of her right hand, which she used to rub against her back, was also reddened and excoriated. It hurt to watch her. She was one of the most pathetic creatures I have ever seen.

Her daughter provided the history. Sory was seventy-eight years old, ten years widowed, and living alone. Shortly after her husband's death, she began to experience pain on the right side of the low back. She was told she had osteoporosis, and treatment for that disorder was begun. Her disease evolved into a very strange pattern of behavior. Over the course of ten years, she would be stricken with pain—always in August. And yes, I was told, that was the anniversary of her husband's death. Her sieges of pain at first lasted for a few weeks, but over the course of time, they became of ever longer duration and of greater intensity. Emergency room visits for narcotics became necessary, and her current siege, which began in August, was by far the longest, for she was coming to see me in January. Over that five-month interval, she lost weight from 140 to 116 pounds.

In early December, she was admitted to the hospital for a two-week stay as her physicians tried valiantly to find some way to control her pain. Epidural steroid injections were done, but they were ineffective. A Duragesic patch was applied in the standard manner, one every three days, but it was of little benefit. Even intravenous Dilaudid, one of the strongest opiates, gave her incomplete relief. Then, after two weeks in the hospital, her pain suddenly and inexplicably went away. Sory walked out of the hospital pain-free. It was not to last. On Christmas Day with family, it struck again— even more bitter than before. Her frustrated family took her for consultation with yet another physician, an orthopedist. His evaluation showed osteoporosis but no fractures or any accountant for her extreme pain. He referred her to me.

Thought was bent into the delusion of pain, the obsession with pain, and the compulsion to rub ceaselessly against the pain.

I asked her daughter if she thought Sory was depressed, and she told me no, that when she was without pain she was quite happy. I was told that she was a very self-reliant person and insisted on remaining in her own home rather than move in with her children. When the flares struck her, however, she would call family members at all hours to come sit with her and rub her back. First-order clue-giving.

It didn't take me long to process all this. Osteoporosis does not flare up and cause pain lasting weeks or months every August. Only a disease of the mind can do that. Only a disease of the mind can make pain appear and disappear so rapidly and inexplicably, and only a disease of the mind can demand the attention of family members to attend at all hours.

I will, I am sure, startle the reader when I tell you that Sory was *imagining* her pain. It was actually being created by her mind and was, I believe, independent of the osteoporosis or any other injury to the body. I suspect that each August, on the anniversary of her husband's death, she would enter depression and delusional pain. Her pain was an abnormal belief, a disorder of thought. Thought was bent into the delusion of pain, the obsession with pain, and the compulsion to rub ceaselessly against the pain.

All this may seem highly conjectural, but I submit that it was correct because it led me to choose the perfect drug: Seroquel, the thought-correcting antipsychotic. I chose also to give the anticonvulsant Clonazepam. It was an empiric choice. That is, my experience suggested to me that it might be helpful.

When she came to see me a week later, there was but little evidence of the bitter angst I had seen but a few days before. She could sit relatively still in the chair, only occasionally rubbing her back. She was even able to lie on the examining table sufficiently still to allow an electrocardiogram to be done, an exercise not even attempted on her first visit. For the first time, she engaged me in conversation.

"Dr. Cochran, you are really helping me. My pain is much better."

"I am thrilled that I have been able to help you, Sory. Continue taking the medicines and come back and see me in two weeks."

She was having no pain at all, and I could see that the excoriations over her low back and her hand were clearing. She was still on the Duragesic, and she told me she was ready to taper it. Over the course of two months her dose was diminished, and then the drug was discontinued. She was doing quite well—cheerful, pleasant, and exhibiting none of the mannerisms that had so dominated our first encounter. I wrote a long-term prescription for her Seroquel and Clonazepam and told her that I did not need to see her for six months. If there was any recurrence of her pain, however, she was to call me immediately. It is near the end of August now, and I haven't heard a thing from her.

Let's review the five cases presented in this chapter. The first two, Richard and Mark, suffered pain and depression (although both were in an element of denial regarding the latter). Both were cured by the administration of Clonazepam and Imipramine. The next, Clark, suffered pain and also bipolar disease, and he was cured by the administration of the opiate Methadone. John suffered pain and hallucinatory depression. He was cured by the administration of the SSRI Zoloft. Lastly, Sory suffered pain, depression, and delusion. She was cured by the administration of Clonazepam and the antipsychotic Seroquel. Such is the incredible variety of pharmacy we have for the successful treatment of chronic pain!

What is the relationship of pain to depression, bipolar disease, hallucinations, and delusion? Clearly they can exist together (comorbid is the medical term).

I will introduce a metaphor from mythology, that of Hydra, the nine-headed monster that so challenged Hercules. Let's name some of the heads. One is pain, another depression, and then bipolar disease, delusions, and hallucinations, and as we shall see shortly, there are many others including narcolepsy, attention deficit disorder, and post-traumatic stress disorder. Each of these terrible heads are, as it were, appendages of the same body, and—this is quite important—they are highly interrelated and interdependent. It is because of this interdependence that we can, remarkably, often cure with a drug that simultaneously strikes several heads. When I treated Clark's bipolar disease with Methadone, his pain and depression went away. When I treated John's depression with Zoloft, his pain and his hallucinations went away. When I treated Sory's delusional obsession with Seroquel and Clonazepam, both her depression and her pain went away.

Hercules had it tough with Hydra. Every time he cut one head off, the monster grew two more. We have it much easier. We can cut off one head with pharmacy and in the process sometimes make several others wither away.

CHAPTER FIVE

Demons and Ghosts

C hris was thirty-two years old when he came to me. He had suffered a work injury some four years before, and in spite of surgery on a ruptured disc in his neck, he continued to be painful. He was directed to an examining room in the company of his worker's compensation caseworker, who whispered to me, "I am sorry to have to bring this to you; he has been a problem for everybody. You are his third pain doctor."

I rose to the bait. "Good, I like a challenge." I turned to Chris.

"Chris, I've got lots of records here from your previous doctors. Let's just talk our way through them."

"Okay, I'll do whatever you want."

"It seems your injury occurred in September 2002, and you had surgery some six months later."

"That's right."

"And you had a real problem with depression after the operation. Is that correct?"

"Yes, I was very depressed. There were a lot of things on my mind."

"Tell me about it."

"Well, even before I got hurt, I was having a lot of problems." His gray eyes became misty. "My wife left me, and I didn't like the way she was treating our son."

"Any other problems—financial, job?"

"Well, there are always financial problems, but my job was really very good. I was an assistant manager at a Dollar General store here in town. I was doing real well there, and they offered to send me to management training if I would be willing to move to Arkansas and open a store there."

"Did you?"

"No, that would take me away from my son, so I went back into construction work."

"And then the injury?"

"Yes, and I haven't worked since."

"When did you first go to the pain clinic?"

"About six months after my operation."

"What did they do there?"

"They did some injections in my neck and gave me physical therapy."

"What medicines were you taking back then?"

"Hydrocodone for pain, and they also gave me some Wellbutrin for my depression."

"What was the depression like?"

"It was terrible, and it still is. I cry a lot, I don't have any energy, I am tired all the time, and I don't have any appetite. I have lost a lot of weight."

"Did you ever think of suicide?"

"No, I could never do that, but there are lots of times when I think I would be better off dead."

"And your sleep?"

"I can't."

"Is it your pain that keeps you from sleeping? Does your pain get worse at night?"

"Yes, but there is something else. When I try to go to sleep, my mind starts racing. I can't turn it off. I feel nervous and my legs jerk."

"I see in the records that there is something about you flushing your supply of morphine down the toilet. Tell me about that."

"The Hydrocodone wasn't working, and the pain clinic started me on morphine. I took a pretty big dose."

"Did it help?"

"Yes, it helped a lot at first. But you may not believe this. I started feeling very angry. I was mad at everybody."

"Chris, I believe everything you tell me. I want you to know that." And I did. I have learned to accept everything the patient tells me without reservation. By doing so, I acquire their trust. That is the first step to getting well. Besides that, I have found that by believing what the patient tells me, I can learn a lot.

"Keep talking, Chris. Tell me about the morphine."

"Well, one day I had my son at home, and we were playing. All of a sudden, this rage came over me. For no reason, I grabbed him and started shaking him and shouting at him. I made him cry, and then I started crying. I let go of him, and then I went to the bathroom and got my morphine pills and flushed them down the toilet."

I acquire their trust. That is the first step to getting well.

"And then?"

"I had a real bad withdrawal, real bad."

"Nausea, vomiting, cramps, sweats?"

"No, it was something else. I felt like I was going out of my mind. It was like there was a demon in me, something controlling me."

"What do you mean? Were you seeing or hearing things that weren't there? Were you hallucinating?"

"No, nothing like that. I just felt like I was going out of my mind. I can't really tell you any more than that."

"How long did it go on?"

"Two or three days. Most of it I don't even remember."

"Did you talk to your doctors about it?"

"Yes, I did, but they wanted no more of me. They said I was irresponsible, and they fired me from the clinic."

I was studying Chris carefully. He was a rather small man, clean, but carelessly dressed and groomed. His eyes were reddened, and he sat still in his chair almost motionless. He didn't make eye contact with me. There was a flatness to his affect (emotional bearing), and his speech was robotic, void of inflection.

"And then a new pain clinic?"

"Yes. I told them that I was afraid of the morphine, so they gave me some Hydrocodone."

"Did they make any other changes in your medicine?"

"Yes, they started me on Prozac."

"Has that been helping you?"

He cast his eyes down and started crying.

"Not much. I feel so bad. I cry like this a lot."

"I am sorry, Chris, but we are going to keep talking. You left that pain clinic?"

"Yes, they did a urine drug test on me and couldn't find any Hydrocodone, so they fired me."

"Were you taking it as prescribed?"

"No, they would give me a month's supply, and I would hurt so much that I would take it up before the time of my return visit. That is why my urine test was negative."

"I want to change the subject a little bit, Chris. Tell me about your childhood. Were you happy as a kid?"

"Yes, I think I was happy. Some parts of my childhood I don't remember, but I do get good memories every now and then."

"Were you abused in any way?"

"No. I don't remember anything about that."

"How was school? Did you have a problem with nervousness or depression when you were young, when you were a teenager?"

"No, but I was a poor student. My parents had no education at all, and they weren't able to help me much. I left school after the ninth grade. I just couldn't do the work."

"And then?"

"I did odd jobs here and there, and then I got into construction work."

"But the Dollar General store?"

He brightened up and his speech lost some of its monotone. "Dr. Cochran, I want you to know something. I have always wanted to make something of myself. I went back to school and got a GED when I was twenty-four years old. After that, I found a job at the store. I did real well there."

"Any problem with drugs or alcohol?"

"No, none at all."

"Well, just a few more questions. Still having trouble sleeping?"

"Like I told you, when I go to bed, I feel nervous. I can't stop thinking. I keep worrying about my son."

"How is your mental focus, your ability to remember?"

"Really bad. I can't seem to keep my mind on one thing for any length of time."

I wrote him a prescription for Clonazepam and Nortriptyline to take in addition to his Wellbutrin, Prozac, and Hydrocodone. Lots of medicines, but sometimes that is what it takes.

I excused Chris from the room in order to go over his treatment plans with the caseworker. Before I could, he arched an eyebrow, offered a vague hint of a smile, and asked, "Well, what do you think about Chris?"

I responded that I really wasn't sure what I thought. The interview had gone well, and I commented on what I already saw as a paradox. His complaints of lack of mental focus notwithstanding, he seemed to be able to organize his thoughts rather well, and I suspected that he was an intelligent young man, but one badly depressed. I sensed the boy didn't have much left in him. We would just have to see what the medicines would do and then take it from there.

The caseworker nodded his acceptance and suggested that I review the records of the psychologic evaluation with some care. I promised to do so.

First, from the pain clinic:

> He stated the medicine turned him into a different person. He describes holding his child and realized that he was possibly hurting his child. He says this with tears in his eyes, and he decided to flush the morphine. He went through withdrawal, but he was unable to give much detail, just stating that he felt like he was 'going out of my mind, that there was a demon in me.'

From the psychologic evaluation, the conclusion:

> Chris was referred to determine whether or not he suffers from a substance abuse, emotional, or personality disorder. The examinee is a thirty-two-year-old male who alleges difficulty working due to chronic pain. His injuries were corroborated by prior medical records. He reported treatment for depressive illness following his

accident. He reported no mental illness among his relatives. He walked gingerly and moved his neck about frequently, as if in pain. He appeared to want to dominate the discussions, to be dramatic, and to minimize his role in his current difficulties. His scores on a symptom inventory were consistent with examination impression that he was overly dramatic about his difficulties. A projected technique suggests the presence of thoughts and feelings in common with those who suffer personality and/or characteriologic disorders.

Diagnostic Impression:

Axis I   Adjustment Disorder with Mixed Anxiety and Depressed Mood
Axis II   Personality Disorder not otherwise specified

An adjustment disorder is a psychiatric disease defined as an emotional and physical maladaptation to stress that usually disappears when the stress is removed. In other words, adjustment disorder is usually a transient and self-limited phenomenon. I am not sure that after four years of unremitting, sleepless, painful depression the diagnosis should still hold, but nonetheless, it fit pretty much with my conclusion that this was a young man who was simply overwhelmed by his circumstances.

Unlike the self-limited adjustment disorder, a personality disorder is ingrained and lifelong. There are many types—paranoid, histrionic, obsessive-compulsive, avoidant, borderline, and in Chris's case, the waste-basket—not otherwise specified. The various personality disorders have certain defining features, but in the main they are all characterized by lifelong maladaptations and difficulty with interpersonal relationships. They are, unfortunately, one of the most refractory of the psychiatric diseases, for they are rarely amenable to pharmacy.

I was interested in the psychologist's report that Chris's behaviors during the interview were overly dramatic with an apparent need to dominate the discussion. This was quite different from his behavior with me, polite, quiet, and deferential. I reflected on all this. Was his throwing away his morphine an act of nobility or simply an act of impulse? And the strange reaction to opiate withdrawal—"going out of my mind, a demon controlling me." Was that some kind of disassociation where he entered another personality, one which he could not even remember? Whatever it was, it is simply not something we expect to see with opiate withdrawal.

He was a slow learner. He only achieved his GED at age twenty-four. But within a short while, he was an assistant manager at a retail store with prospects of becoming a manager. And his complaints of thought-racing—what did that mean? I should have put it all together sooner, but I didn't, and when I finally did, it was almost dumb luck.

I saw Chris a couple of weeks later, and asked how he was doing.

"About the same—nothing has changed."

"Are you taking the medicines?"

"No, I haven't been able to get them."

"Why not?"

"Worker's comp won't buy them for me."

I addressed the caseworker: "What is going on?"

He rolled his eyes and said, "I'll look into it."

"I surely hope so. All we have done so far is waste two weeks."

Within a few days, I received e-mails from worker's compensation confirming that, contrary to Chris's statements, the prescribed medicines had been filled, and he had picked them up. They requested frequent urine drug screens and concluded with the comment, "He is notorious for getting Rx's filled on the weekend when worker's comp staff is unavailable to approve." Chris, it seemed, was a problem for everybody.

Personality disorders . . . are all characterized by lifelong maladaptations and difficulty with interpersonal relationships.

Why should he be lying to me? What gain was there in it for him? Maybe he wasn't lying. Maybe the insurers were making it hard for him. They certainly seemed to treat him with hostility. Maybe they were just frustrated by four years of expense and no response to anybody's treatments.

He returned at the appointed two weeks telling me he was taking his Imipramine and Clonazepam, and he was sleeping a little bit better, but his pain—and his depression—were unchanged. I prescribed transcutaneous electrical nerve stimulation (TENS), a device that administers an electrical current to the skin over the area of pain and creates a "buzz," if you will, in an effort to override the pain. Later, Cymbalta, newly arrived on the scene. Then, in turn, Neurontin and its derivative, Lyrica, and then Topamax, all anticonvulsants sometimes useful in the treatment of pain. None of them made any significant impact and time was passing by. A few months into his therapy, the caseworker told me that worker's compensation was tiring of my efforts and wanted consultation with a neurosurgeon to see if a dorsal column stimulator could be placed.

The dorsal column stimulator is like a TENS unit. The electrodes are placed not on the skin, but through a surgical incision onto the dorsal (back) surface of the spinal cord and then connected to a battery pack implanted under the skin of the flank. It is not a very graceful form of therapy, but I'll admit, it does sometimes work. There are problems, however. The electrodes sometimes displace, and although the batteries are getting of greater and greater capacity, they periodically have to be replaced through a surgical operation. Chris was very young. He had another fifty years of life in him, and the notion of electrodes on the spinal cord and a battery implanted under the skin for that length of time was not very appealing. Odds of some mischance, be this in the form of malfunction, displaced electrodes, or infection were quite high.

"Chris, go ahead and see the neurosurgeon and see what he says, but you have the right to refuse the procedure. You have the legal right to stick with me as long as you want."

The caseworker nodded his head in agreement.

"I want to stick with you."

"Chris, I am going to try a medicine on you that really may not work at all, but it is worth a try. I am writing you a prescription for Lithium. I want you to take one pill a night for a week, and then, if you are not having trouble with it, go up to two every night. If it disagrees with you, gives you nausea, tremors, or sedation, go ahead and stop it and call me. In the meantime, see what the neurosurgeon has to say."

"Thank you, sir. I will do what you say."

The caseworker rolled his eyes.

Lithium has proven usefulness in the treatment of bipolar disease and also in some forms of migraine. It is also occasionally useful as augmentation therapy combined with tricyclics and other antidepressants for the treatment of depression. It is not used much for that purpose anymore, but at least there was a precedent. I had legal and ethical grounds for administering the drug. Besides, I was beginning to suspect that Chris was bipolar.

I saw him a couple of weeks later and everything had changed. He was more engaging and animated. His demeanor was almost joyful. He directed his gaze to my eyes and said, "I like that Lithium, Dr. Cochran. It is the perfect drug. I feel much better."

"Tell me more."

"I am not as depressed, and my neck doesn't hurt as much. It is a lot better."

"Keep talking."

"My sleep is good, and I am not nervous anymore. You know, it is really strange, my mind doesn't race the way it used to. I can control my thoughts. I can stay on track now."

Chris and I had a nice talk, and I enjoyed glancing out of the corner of my eye at the caseworker whose jaw was slack and mouth was open.

"I want to get back to work. I don't think I can do the construction work anymore, but could you help me find a job? I have always wanted to be a surgical technician. Do you think I could do that?"

"Well, I don't know, Chris, but I can send you to Vocational Rehabilitation, and maybe they can help you."

"Would you really do that for me? I would appreciate that so much."

"I'll try to set something up. Now, Chris, let's talk just a little bit more. You told me that when you stopped the morphine, you felt like you were going out of your mind, like there was a demon in you."

"That's right."

"I want to ask you something very personal because I have been thinking about you a lot. Is it possible that you have always had a demon inside of you?"

He hesitated for a long while then stood up, directed his gaze out the window away from me, and said, "Yes, yes, yes! There has always been a demon in me. I've always known that something was wrong, that I was not right. But I think that demon is gone now."

"What was the demon doing to you?"

No hesitation now. "The demon kept me from relaxing. The demon directed my thoughts. The demon made me angry."

One of the delights of the pain business is the rapidity with which its practitioners can learn new things. Had I seen Chris in 2007 rather than 2005, it would not have taken me nearly so long to diagnose his bipolar disease. His unprovoked anger and rage at his child, and his impulsively flushing his morphine were typical bipolar behaviors. And his dissociation into another state of being of which he was able to remember but little was surely an episode of bipolar mania (a glutamine storm if there ever was one).

Bipolar disease is the great imitator.

Bipolar disease in its classic form, alternating emotional highs and lows, has been recognized for a long time. We now know that it is much more complex than that. It is a spectrum of diseases. It may present as hallucinations, mimicking schizophrenia. It may appear as mind-busy distractibility, as in attention deficit disorder or, surprisingly, as the daytime sleepiness and nightmares of narcolepsy. It may even mimic (recall Chris's psychologic evaluation) personality disorder. Bipolar disease is the great imitator.

I will suggest, and we will explore this together, that there is no aberrant emotion, thought, or act that cannot be dictated by bipolar disease. I will suggest also that there is no form of pain that cannot be dictated by bipolar disease.

Regina was tearful throughout our interview. Maybe she had right to be. She had been painful for most of her life. Some four years before, her primary care physician had referred her to a pain clinic. At age twenty-six, she was started on opiates, Hydrocodone and then Oxycontin, which disagreed with her, and then morphine in the form of MS Contin. She also was given Topamax for her migraines. Several months into her care there, she became pregnant for the first time, and all of her medications were withdrawn. As often happens, her pain, including her migraines, abated during her pregnancy. Shortly following the birth of her son, her many pains reappeared, and she resumed Topamax and morphine but within a short while was requiring escalating doses of the latter. Fearful of the morphine, she terminated the pain clinic's care and sought me out. She acknowledged that she was sleep disturbed and fatigued, but she denied adamantly she suffered depression. I prescribed Nortriptyline and Clonazepam. She was still tearful when she left.

Regina returned on the appointed day and handed me a letter. I will share it with you because it expresses, in the first person, the plight of the painful and the frustration, despair, suspicion, disappointment, and perhaps most of all, the self-doubt and confusion that comes to those who suffer chronic pain.

Dear Dr. Cochran:

I want to thank you for the opportunity to get a few things off my mind that I did not get the chance to do during my initial consultation with you.

First and foremost, most of my emotional reaction that day was due to the fact that I was once again (albeit by choice) in yet another doctor's office trying to determine why I am in constant pain. I've seen numerous orthopedic doctors, neurologists, chiropractors, physical therapists, and anesthesiologists (pain therapy/management), etc. I've tried countless exercises, procedures, injections, medications—all to no avail. Sure, I may get some relief for a brief period of time, which always seem to indicate to the doctor that, "This means something is wrong with you and we can do something to fix it." So, yes, I tend to get very emotional when I am speaking to a doctor about my past medical history and everything I've been though.

For example, with my knee surgeries, the first time around I was in pain for months before anyone could figure out what it was. My pediatrician had no clue, so he sent me to an orthopedic specialist.

He said it was called osteochondroma, and I needed surgery to remove the bone spur thing. I asked if I should ever worry about it happening to my other knee, and he said no. It was a one-in-a million thing—rarely ever happened. Six months later I am having surgery for the same thing on the other leg. Of course before either surgery, six adults had to hold me down on a bed so the doctor could remove the fluid under my kneecaps and inject cortisone.

With my jaws, Dr. Henderson said his surgery should do the trick, but I had to change my lifestyle to make it work too—quit my job, watch my stress level (in other words, marry someone rich and move to Tahiti—not something everyone has the opportunity to do)! So, three years later, after little to no relief from his surgery, I was under the knife again having the cartilage removed from my jaw joints because they were badly deteriorated and not worth leaving in. I grind my teeth in my sleep—what can I say? Now I wear a guard every night to prevent any further damage to my jaws and my already cracked teeth.

Believe it or not, I have a very high tolerance for pain. I must have after dealing with what I've been told are "several types of migraines that typically attack at the same time or in succession" and may last anywhere from three days to one month. There is no pain medicine I've found that knocks those—only sleep and Phenergan to keep me from vomiting until I burst blood vessels in my face and look as though I've been beaten. Unfortunately, because of everything that has been done to me, I also have a very high tolerance for pain medication. That is why the pain clinic put me on MS Contin three years ago after I finally got to the point where I could not walk, sleep, sit, or bend comfortably. Even on this medication, you cannot touch my lower back without me nearly dropping to the floor. At times, other areas of my body, such as around my ankles, wrists and hands, neck and shoulders, spine, etc., cannot be touched by anyone without me cringing in pain.

Now, you asked me about my childhood. At the time I was very frustrated with your line of questioning because it seems that every doctor I've been to complaining of pain wants to know if I'm depressed, stressed, etc., probably because I'm typically crying while I'm talking to them. As many patients as you see for chronic pain, I'm sure you realize as well as anyone that if you've been in pain for any length of time with no significant relief, it can be depressing in itself. I don't, however, see that as a reason to automatically, in just one thirty-minute visit, *diagnose me as someone chronically depressed and chronically painful. Can you explain that to me?*

But back on track—my childhood. I told you my mother was manic-depressive, and it took most of my childhood to get her medicine straightened out. I played "mom" to my younger brother and two younger sisters while going to school and, once I turned sixteen, worked part-time after school. I was responsible for most of the housework and a lot of the cooking because my dad worked so hard to support all six of us. My childhood was not unhappy— it just wasn't much of a childhood because I was always sick or very busy.

You also asked how my husband was taking all this. He has been great! He's said all along, "I married you in sickness and in health and I'm not going anywhere"—but I'm going to be very candid with you here, because this is a concern I've always had with anti-depressants. When I came home that day and told him the new meds you were starting me on, his statement was, "Great, there goes what little sex life we had left!" As I told you, it seems that ever since I had my son, I've not been very sexually motivated, although I didn't realize it was as bad as my husband says (apparently only six times the past year). Part of that was due to my back hurting, and part of it due to just being plain tired at the end of the day working full time and then coming home to cook dinner and chase around a very active two-year-old. But I don't doubt that all that medication I've been on played a role in my being tired as well. I'd rather not add another factor to the mix if I can help it.

My point in telling you all this is that I want you to find a way to help me deal with this very real, not imagined, not psychosomatic, pain, particularly in my back. I'm not a hypochondriac. I never asked for this and would give anything for it all to go away so I could roll around on the floor with my son without having to worry about him kneeing me in the back and putting me in the bed for days afterward on icepacks. I also want to have another child someday, so I don't want to be on a bunch of pills that could harm my child. I don't like this "narcoleptic" feeling I've had every day for past few months. I feel as if I'm becoming a danger to myself and others, as I cannot keep my eyes open sometimes, and I don't know when that feeling is going to hit me.

All I'm asking for is someone's help, not criticism, and if you know of a miracle cure besides drugs, please count me in! I'm only thirty years old; I've got a long life ahead of me, and I'd like it to be as pain free as possible.

Thank you for taking the time to hear me out, and please forgive me for being a basket case at our first meeting. Chalk it up to stage fright and past experience!

Sincerely,
Regina Green

I thanked her for the letter, and I read it in her presence. It was obviously important to her, so it was important to me. She had something on her chest, and she needed to get it off, and I was glad she did. I know well that frustration and hopelessness are companions to chronic pain. However, I reacted as I usually do to epistles such as this—dispassionately. In doing so,

I am trying to tell my patient that we are not looking back at what has been, but rather to the future and what will be. Then I asked her how she was doing on my medicine.

"Pretty good. I can tell a difference. I am sleeping better, and I think some days I don't have as much pain."

"That's good—that's great! Are you still taking the Topamax?"

"Yes, I like Topamax. That is one good thing the pain clinic did. My headaches are doing well."

"Okay, we will continue that. Now, how about the MS Contin. What dose are you taking now?"

"30 mg. a day—down from 90, and I want to reduce it some more. Can you help me do that?"

I wrote a prescription for 15 mg. MS Contin and told her to take one daily and to increase the dose of Nortriptyline and Clonazepam.

It went quite well for a few weeks. Pain and sleeplessness were both abating. She continued, however, to have a problem with a sense of daytime sleepfulness. I made note of that but made no change in her therapy. I was quite pleased at how well she was doing, as was she. Then I received a phone call from her.

I know well that frustration and hopelessness are companions to chronic pain.

She was pregnant! The obstetrician had advised her to come off all the medicines, and I instructed her how to do it. I was not to see her again for two years.

"Dr. Smith told me to come back to see you. She said you had helped me before, and she thought you could do it again."

"I am happy to see you again, Regina. You have a new child now?"

"Yes, a daughter."

"Healthy?"

"Yes."

"Did you have a difficult pregnancy?"

"No, just like the first one. It went just fine, and I had very little pain, even off the medicines."

"And then what?"

"Well, it all started coming back. Within a few weeks of Dawn's birth, the headaches, the fibromyalgia, the back pain and everything came back. I am back to square one, just like when I first saw you."

"Regina, why did it take you so long to come back to me? Your pain has been going on at least a year or so, hasn't it?"

"Yes, it has been there a good while, but you probably don't understand this. I want to be free of pain without medicines. I don't want to be taking pills for the rest of my life."

"The diabetic doesn't want to take insulin the rest of her life."

"I know, and you are right. Can you help me?"

At this juncture it was a no-brainer. Go back to what had worked before. I reinstituted the Nortriptyline, Clonazepam, and Topamax. She started getting better right away. She and I were both happy with her progress, but then she began a series of problems that are so common, unfortunately, in those who suffer chronic pain—side effects from the medicines. She began to develop sweet cravings and weight gain. I discontinued the Nortriptyline and tried Cymbalta. It worked for a while, but within a few months she developed some new symptoms, restlessness and sweatiness. These can occur with Cymbalta, and I told her to stop the drug. Fortunately, there were a few left we could try, and I prescribed Effexor. It worked rather well, and for several months she did nicely. Her sleep was restored, and her pain diminished. Her migraines were infrequent and not severe. I was happy with her progress, but she kept reminding me that her sleepiness during the day was becoming more and more of a problem. Probably another side effect of her medicine I thought. I suspected it was due to the Topamax. The drug is certainly capable of producing sedation, so much that in the vernacular it is called *Dopamax*. I told her to reduce the dose.

I had uncovered an unsuspected neuropsychiatric illness, narcolepsy, in a young woman who also suffered chronic pain in many dimensions.

"It is not working. I still fall asleep during the day, and my migraines are getting worse."

Maybe her sleepiness was not due to the drugs. Maybe in my concerns over her migraines, her fibromyalgia, her back pain, her temporomandibular joint disease, and her depression, I had over-looked something.

"Regina, do you just feel sleepy all the time, or does it come on you just periodically?"

"It just strikes me out of the blue during the day, I will suddenly nod off. I don't really feel sedated, just all of a sudden I go to sleep."

"How are you sleeping at night?"

"Pretty good with your medicines, but I want you to explain something to me."

"Go ahead."

"I have a ghost that comes to me at night."

"What do you mean?"

"I hear things and feel things that are not there. I have had it for a long time, and it frightens me."

"Does it happen when you are awake or when you are asleep at night?"

"I am awake, I think."

"Could it be a dream?"

"I've wondered, but it is so real. It can't be a dream. I am awake, and I hear things, like the sound of my husband walking through the room. That has happened to me even when he is out of town. Sometimes I can feel him sitting beside me on the bed even when he is not there."

"Do you ever see him?"

"No, I just hear something, and I feel the presence of something that shouldn't be there. It is my ghost."

"Regina, after your ghost comes to you, do you ever have the sensation that you are frozen, that you are paralyzed, that you can't move?"

"Oh, my God! How did you know that? It happens almost every time. It is scary!"

"How long does it last?"

"It seems like forever, but I suppose it is just a few moments."

Regina was suffering from, and the term is a beautifully alliterative one, hypnagogic hallucinations. Hypnagogic refers to that twilight interval between wakefulness and sleep. Hallucinations, of course, refer to the ghost and feeling of the presence of things that are not there. It is a sort of a dream, but so vivid that it seems to the victim to be real. In tandem with that she suffered sleep paralysis. It can be a horrifying experience. The mind is awake and imagining strange things, and the body is still asleep, immobilized, and unable to move. Fortunately it is a transient thing and, in the large scheme of things, harmless.

Hypnagogic hallucinations, sleep paralysis, and sleep attacks during the day are diagnostic of narcolepsy. With the history of that triad, it is just about the easiest diagnosis in the world to make. I prescribed Ritalin, long established in the treatment of narcolepsy. She was better in just a few days. Not just her sleepiness but her pain. Her pain actually went away on Ritalin therapy! It does happen.

I was happy for her and proud of myself. I had uncovered an unsuspected neuropsychiatric illness, narcolepsy, in a young woman who also suffered chronic pain in many dimensions. By treating the underlying disorder, I had relieved her discomfort. But, perhaps, it took me too long. In my focus on Regina's pain, her sleeplessness, and although she was in denial, her depression, and also her frustration, her perceived mistreatment, her suspicion, and her fear of being branded as somehow weak and depressed, she and I both forgot that in her letter to me, she had written, almost as an afterthought, about her "narcoleptic" feelings.

CHAPTER SIX

Remembered Pain

In this chapter, I want to explore the role of memory in the generation of illness, painful or otherwise. All of us have suffered unpleasant experiences, including pain, that we would like to forget. Most of the time, by the psychologic process known as repression, we are able to do this. Unpleasant memories are placed into subconsciousness where, most of the time, they unobtrusively remain. However, as we all know, they can, under provocation, reappear. This probably occurs most commonly during sleep when the conscious brain is at rest and the subconscious is uninhibited. Our dreams are often expressions of memories, both remote and recent. Another provocation, as many of us surely know, is depression. Unpleasant memories are often returned to consciousness during depressive interludes.

Sometimes, when the unpleasant experience was truly horrific, and I will offer examples such as a life-threatening accident, combat, or sexual trauma, the memory is so unpleasant that it cannot remain permanently in the subconscious. It periodically reappears in the form of the re-creation of the event, a phenomenon known as flashbacks. Flashbacks are hallmarks of post-traumatic stress disorder. They are often generated by exposure to some stimulus or trigger that incites the resurrection of memory. A war movie will incite flashbacks in those who have endured combat, and the sight of an automobile accident will re-create that experience. In those who have suffered sexual abuse, a certain sight, sound, or smell that reminds of the event restores it vividly to consciousness.

There is another disease in which memory plays an important role. Panic disorder, which is characterized by overwhelming, fearful anxiety and a sense of impending death, appears (at least early on) randomly, that is, without obvious provocation. It quickly becomes a remembered experience and a fearful one at that. The victim will do anything to prevent recurrence of the experience, and this leads to avoidant behavior. Let's offer an example. If a person experiences a panic attack on entering the nave of a church, that person will avoid entering a church's nave again, or perhaps even going near a church out of fear that the panic will recur. This leads to that symptom known as agoraphobia. Literally, it means fear of the marketplace. Figuratively it means fear of leaving the home. A remembered experience dictates our behavior and our symptoms.

Post-traumatic stress disorder and panic disorder derive from profound emotional memory. Now let's look at remembered sensory experiences such as touch and pain. I have worn a pager

Unpleasant memories are placed into subconsciousness, where . . . they unobtrusively remain.

for many years. It is attached to my belt and overlies my right hip. I prefer to keep it in silence rather than sound mode, and when my pager alerts me, it is by vibration. Thus, a small area of my anatomy has been sensory stimulated in the same vibratory manner, repetitively, for many years. Sometimes, and this is not rare, I feel the vibration and reach for the pager only to discover that I am not wearing it. We can certainly surmise that there is a small area on the surface of my brain that is dedicated to the perception of vibration over my hip, and that small area has been stimulated repeatedly through the years. It has, in a sense, been invigorated by repetition, a phenomenon known as kindling. It has acquired a life of its own, and it sometimes expresses itself even in the absence of any real reason to do so.

It is probably a kindred phenomenon that accounts for the well-known phantom limb syndrome. An amputee sometimes may appreciate the presence of his absent extremity by the appearance of a remembered sensory experience such as an itch, the perception of hot or cold, or pain.

Now let's go back to Bill, introduced in chapter three. Long after his lingual nerve injury had healed and the numbness in his tongue had gone away, he continued to feel a not-unpleasant sensation of tingling in his lips at night. A memory of pain was transmuted into a more pleasant sensation, a symbol perhaps of love lost and love gained, but nonetheless, certainly a remembered sensory experience. Now, back to Mark of the subarachnoid hemorrhage in chapter four. His was a painful and life-threatening experience and one not easily to be forgotten. For many years his remembered pain would strike him, often under the trigger of some emotional circumstance.

In *Understanding Chronic Pain*, I suggested that remote but remembered pains of different origins may be melded together to create a hybrid pain, particularly if the past pains were in the same area of the body. I gave an example of a lady who, through the course of her life, had suffered trigeminal neuralgia (neuritic pains in the face) and also migraine, which occurred on the same side of the head as her neuralgia. Her neuralgia was cured by surgery, and her migraine went away (as it often does) as she grew older. Then, under the provocation of late-life depression, her pain reappeared. It had some features of neuritic pain and some features of migraine, but it really wasn't quite either. It was a new disease, a hybrid of two old ones, and I believe that is exactly what happened in the case study that follows.

Jack was hurting again, only this time it was different. It was in his neck, arms, low back, and legs. He had certainly known the experience of pain before because, over the span of some twenty years, he had required operations for the repair of four separate spinal discs and also one for a blocked abdominal aorta.

"Jack, you have had a number of operations. Were they successful?"

"Yes, they certainly were. The disc operations were very successful. The one on my artery also, but it took me a longer time to recover. It was two months after that before I was able to go back to work."

"Tell me about your operations."

"My first was in 1985. I was having a lot of neck pain, and it would shoot into my left arm down into my hand. It was kind of like being shocked with electricity. The surgeon told me I had a ruptured disc pinching on a nerve, and he operated on me right away. As soon as the surgery was done, my pain went away."

"And the next time?"

"Almost exactly the same, except that the pain was in my back and my left leg. It was shooting again like electricity. After the operation the pain went away."

"And the next?"

"On the neck again. Just like before—the same kind of pain. If I remember correctly, it was going into the right arm that time."

"And the next?"

"The back. Same thing except the pain would shoot down into both legs and into my feet. Looking back on it, it seems like I would rupture a disc, either in my neck or back, every three or four years, but after the operations, the pains went away. I can't tell you how thankful I am for that."

"And then the problem with your artery—what was that like?"

"It was pain again but of a different sort. First I noticed it only when I had walked a long distance, maybe a half-mile or so. I would get a pain in my calves, and they would seize up and cramp. I would have to stop walking, and when I did that, the pain would go away."

"And then?"

"It got worse. As time went by, I got where I couldn't walk more than twenty yards without hurting. I talked to my doctor about it, and he checked me over. He said he couldn't feel any pulses in my feet. He told me that my pain wasn't coming from pinched nerves. It was coming from a blocked artery. He sent me to a vascular surgeon who cut me open and restored my blood flow. The pain in my legs went away, and I could walk just fine."

"How long ago was that?"

"Almost exactly three years."

"But you are hurting again—tell me about it."

"It began about a year ago, maybe more. I started hurting in my neck and both arms and my back and both legs. It is queer. Most of the time with my disc problems, my pain would be worse on one arm or one leg, but now it is the same on both sides, exactly the same."

"What is the pain like?"

"It is a constant pain. It is squeezing and boring. There is no electricity feeling to it, and there is no cramping to it. It is different from the pains I have had before."

"Does your pain change any when you walk, bend, or move your neck?"

"No, it is there all the time. It never changes."

"And what do your doctors say is causing it?"

"They don't know, that's why they sent me to you."

"Are you able to work?"

"No, I wish I could, but I can't. The pain is just too bad. My doctor gave me some Hydrocodone, and it helps a little bit. But I really want to get back to work. I enjoy being a policeman. Can you help me?"

Jack's pains, first in his neck and arms and then in his back and legs, had occurred repetitively. In the beginning they were from ruptured discs and then from a blocked artery. The experience of pain was reinforced by repetition (again, kindling) over the course of some twenty years. The remembered experience of pain was certainly susceptible to recruitment into consciousness, but our memory is often imperfect, and Jack's painful experiences were assembled to a new kind of pain, different, but derivative from separate prior pains.

> *A remembered experience dictates our behavior and our symptoms.*

"Jack, I have some more questions for you. Are you depressed?"

"No, I am not depressed. I don't sit around and cry. I don't think about suicide. Let's just say I am frustrated, and I am worried. I don't know whether I will be able to go back to work. Let's just say that if I didn't have this pain, I would be great. I would be better than good."

"Okay, I understand. I have heard lots of people say the same thing. But let me ask you this, have you ever in the past had a problem with depression?"

He hesitated and then said, "I think maybe I did a couple of years ago. I really was depressed for a while. It was after my father died."

"Tell me about your father."

"He was my best friend. We lived together on my farm west of town. He died suddenly of a heart attack."

"You grieved?"

"Yes, a lot. I had some crying spells, and I had to stay off work for two or three weeks. I have never had anything hit me like that did."

"Did you see a doctor about it?"

"No, I figured it was normal for me to grieve, but it did take a long time to get over it, several months. Work was my release. Without my father around, the farm kept me busy, and that was my outlet. I worked myself out of depression, but I still miss him, and I think about him a lot."

"Are you married?"

"No, I've never been married."

"Do you mind telling me why?"

"Well I guess I am kind of a loner, and I enjoy my independence."

"You've had some relationships?"

"Yes, I was in a very nice relationship for many years. We talked about getting married, but after my artery operation, it changed. She has two teenage children. They are great kids, but I was worried about my health. All those back operations and then the artery operation. It just kind of changed things. I guess I was worried about the responsibility of trying to raise those children. And then my father died, and I felt like I had to break it off."

"You are happy with your decision?"

"I think so. It saddened me, it really did. But now that I am having this pain, I think it was the right thing to do. I wouldn't have been a very good father."

"Jack, how are you sleeping?"

"I don't."

"You mean since you have been painful?"

"No, I mean I have never been able to sleep."

"Tell me about it."

"Three or four hours sleep is about all I've ever gotten. It doesn't seem to bother me. I have more energy than most people, I just don't need sleep. When I get in bed at night, my mind starts racing. I can't seem to slow it down. I will just lie there thinking about different things. Sometimes I get up and watch television. It is usually about 1:00 or 2:00 AM before I go to sleep, and I will wake up at 4:00 or 5:00."

"How do you feel when you wake up?"

"Pretty good. I am ready to go."

"Do your legs jerk at night? Are you a restless sleeper?"

"Yes, I've been told I am a very restless sleeper. Janet told me that many times she had to go sleep in another bed because I was jerking so much."

"Do you get fidgety when you go to sleep? Do you feel restless?"

"I sure do. When I go to bed, my legs start moving. I can't hold them still."

"How long have you been that way?"

"For all my life, as best I know."

"That is called restless legs. Have you heard of it?"

"Yes, I have seen ads on television about it. That is what I have. That is a perfect description. I have restless legs."

"Jack, your history of insomnia is very interesting to me because many people who have chronic pain tell me the same sort of story. I would like to pursue that a little bit with some more questions."

"Fire away."

"You tell me that you are energized, that you don't need sleep. Is it always that way? Are there ever occasions where you lose your energy and need more sleep?"

"Well, you know, I have never thought about it much, but every now and then I seem to lose my energy. When that happens, I'll sleep well. I'll sleep too well. Ten or twelve hours sometimes. I just figure my body needs to catch up from all the loss of sleep."

"Do you feel different when that happens?"

"Yes, I do feel different. I have a sense of fatigue, and I feel irritable and cross."

"Tell me about it."

"I don't want to be around anybody. I don't like the way I feel. When I get that way, I try to stay by myself. I won't even answer the phone."

"Do you feel depressed when that happens?"

"No, just cross and irritable. It kind of comes over me in waves."

"How often does it happen?"

"Oh, maybe three or four times a year."

"Do you see any pattern to it; can you explain why it happens?"

"No, no pattern, except it seems to happen more often in the winter."

Jack was mood labile, that is, his moods swung from high-energy sleeplessness to a sleepful want of energy with fractiousness and irritability. His moods were cycling, but he assured me his pain was not. Could Jack be bipolar? In its classic form, almost certainly not, but perhaps he had some fragment of that disease, a phenomenon known in medical parlance as a *forme fruste*. It was worth a try. I gave him Lithium and then Seroquel, both mood stabilizers, but neither worked. His illness was probably that which we recognize as cyclothymia—that is, cycling mood. It is a lesser form of, indeed the least form of bipolarity. Cyclothymia, in the true sense, is hardly a disease at all. Shifts in mood are a part of life, but their curious appearance in wintertime was certainly an expression of body time and its ability to influence our health.

> His moods swung from high-energy sleeplessness to a sleepful want of energy.

Jack did not suffer bipolarity, but he did suffer mood shifts and disordered sleep. He did have a psychiatric illness, and modest though it was, the psychiatric illness must be treated in the painful. I tried several different antidepressants, but they didn't work at all. They seemed to make him worse. He was intolerant of Clonazepam, one of my favorite drugs for restoring sleep and treating pain, but he did tolerate a kindred drug, Lorazepam. He lost his mind-racing, and he began to sleep. As he did, his remembered pains diminished significantly. At the time of this writing, some three years into his care, he requires an occasional Hydrocodone, but his pain is much relieved and, he tells me, he no longer experiences his winter-predominant episodes of irritability and sleepiness.

Lucy was an attractive but somewhat obese fifty-year-old. She suffered recurrent back pain through her thirties and early forties and had endured five back operations, each giving pain relief for a few years. Fortunately, the last one (eight years before) was quite successful. She was restored to a life of comfort until she was seized, a month before coming to me, with another attack of excruciating back pain. It was just like those she had known before, but this time her neurosurgeon could find no cause, and he referred her to me. She told me that she had been given Hydrocodone, and she found it helpful but was fearful of the drug and resistant to taking it on a regular basis. She also told me, tearfully, that she really wasn't depressed, only frustrated by her inexplicable painfulness. I inquired about her sleep, and she said that she used to sleep quite well, but with the appearance of pain, her sleep had become very disordered. I continued my inquiries, and she denied any problem in the past with drug or alcohol abuse, depression, or childhood trauma. She was divorced and lived alone, but her two adult children were attentive to her. She emphasized with the tears flowing that she had been very happy with her life and her church work until her pain struck.

Each time in the past when she had back pain, she told me, her neurosurgeon had found a ruptured disc and fixed it. This time he could find nothing. She didn't understand why, and she was afraid of a lifetime of pain. I asked about her family history, and she told me that her father and one of her sisters had bipolar disease.

I prescribed Imipramine and Clonazepam, and over the course of several tearful visits, I gradually increased the dosages. Her response was quite slow.

It was several weeks before Lucy could speak to me without crying and expressing her despair. I offered her Lithium therapy because I was very taken with her family history of bipolar disease (always important!). She was quite frightened of the drug but finally consented to take it. It was without benefit, and she discarded it. Then, some three months into my treatments, her pain gradually diminished. Her response to pharmacy was, in my experience, quite unusual. Many of the drugs, particularly the tricyclics useful in the treatment of pain, take a while to kick in, sometimes a matter of a few weeks. Her recovery months into treatment perplexed me. Nonetheless, it went well for a good while, but then she began to develop side effects, almost certainly due to her tricyclic therapy. She began to experience sweet cravings and memory impairment and also problems with word finding and periodic speech arrest. There were times when she simply couldn't talk for a few moments. I tried to reduce her Imipramine dosage, but every time I did, the pain reappeared. Then I added Neurontin, but that was without benefit.

Over the course of time, she evolved into a periodic flares of pain in the back. With these, she would inevitably become sleepless. Her behaviors during these intervals were quite predictable. She would become restless, anxious, agitated, and would catastrophize obsessively about her pain and the dismal prospects for the future. Strange, I thought, that her pain and her emotional behaviors should reappear in such a stereotyped and cyclical manner. I couldn't quite get bipolar disease out of my mind. I elected the anti-convulsant Topamax. It has analgesic effects and also the property of mood stabilization.

She would become sleepless and very frustrated with these attacks, and with each one would drift into almost a personality change.

It was a breakthrough drug. She reported great improvement in her pain and was delighted with the arrest of sweet cravings that came with it. Topamax can do this. It is one of the very few neuropsychiatric drugs that actually diminish appetite. Most of the others increase it. Lucy was thrilled with her progress. She felt well enough to proceed with gastric stapling, an operation she had been thinking about for several years.

The operation was successfully performed, and Lucy began to experience rapid weight loss—but desired weight loss became alarming weight loss. She had no appetite at all. She felt disgust for food. The gastric stapling had done its job, but I suspected that the Topamax was doing a number on her. I told her to discontinue the drug, and her appetite returned, albeit controlled, and she continued, happily, to slowly lose weight. She remained on Imipramine, Clonazepam, and an occasional Hydrocodone.

She did fairly well without the Topamax, at least for a while. Perhaps this was because she was so happy with the weight reduction she had achieved. She, to my eye, had always been a handsome woman. With her weight loss in the magnitude of a hundred pounds or so, she had become really quite stunning. I was not surprised when she told me that she has recently married after some ten years of living alone.

It is never perfect, though. She continued to have weeks-long attacks of pain in the back, and her neurosurgeon could still find no cause. She would become sleepless and very frustrated with these attacks, and with each one would drift into almost a personality change, ruminating and obsessing about her pain and her future. I continued my prior therapies, and periodically gave her a cortisone injection and a big dose of reassurance. She would seem to improve, but over the long haul we were losing ground. She requested that we resume the Topamax, the wonder drug. I did it cautiously, beginning at low dosage, and she achieved a high level of stability. Notably, and most curiously, she did not have any appetite reduction with reinstitution of the drug, and this is the way it goes. Hard to believe, but drugs behave differently at different times in people's lives depending, we suppose, upon the way their neurotransmitters are behaving during that particular interval. She had her last flare of pain about two years ago, and of her own accord, without asking me, increased her Topamax dosage from 100 mg. twice daily to three times daily. After a few days, the pain went away.

We talked about her attacks of pain, and she told me, "You know, it is really strange, these things seem to come on me in October almost every year."

I scanned my records and noted that she was correct. I wrote a note in the chart about her observation. She laughed at me when she saw me do it and said, "Don't do that, if anybody ever sees that, they will think I am crazy."

Lucy's pain was, I believe, the recrudescence of the remembered experience of recurring back injury kindled over two decades. But why did it occur only periodically? What brain force was exciting it into expression every October? I don't know, but I will offer a speculation. Lucy had a strong family history of bipolar disease. Moreover, her pain was cycling in the manner that depression and mania cycle in the bipolar. Is it possible that she did have bipolar disease, clinically silent for most of her life, but finally expressing itself as periodic attacks of remembered pain, sleeplessness, and a behavior pattern characterized by obsessive worry, anxiety, and the expression of hopelessness? Maybe it wasn't really bipolar disease, but it was certainly something like it—a *forme fruste* perhaps. After my initial therapies with their incomplete control of her symptoms, I chose, in turn, Lithium, Neurontin, and finally Topamax. All three are mood stabilizers, useful in the treatment of manic-depressive illness. Two of them did no good, but with the third we struck gold.

Frank suffered pain in his mid-back. He also suffered the Wolff-Parkinson-White Syndrome (WPW), a disorder of the heart's electrical system that is characterized by recurring tachycardia (rapid heart action). Just a few days after I saw him, I received a long letter. It relates a forty-one-year-old man's voyage of discovery, and I will share it with you. I am sure you will agree that this is marvelous stuff.

Dear Dr. Cochran:

I enjoyed our visit on Monday past. You have offered me a new avenue of hope, and God only knows I need at least hope. I went home and devoured your book and finished it the following evening and felt compelled to provide you with some additional insight about myself. I must admit I was a little bit skeptical and uncomfortable with the lines of questions concerning any past depression. Nevertheless, I hope the following provides you with some insight into who I am and how I got to this point.

There was so much of me in these pages—the sleeplessness, irritability, fatigue, and depression. The latter three, I guess in my mind, have developed as a direct result of the pain. Irritability and fatigue have been something that has been occurring over the past two to four years as I have been increasingly unable to manage the pain. Sleeplessness has been something that has been going on for years. Depression, this is a hard pill for me to swallow, and you and

I need to explore this further. I have always considered myself a strong, self-reliant person. And as I look back on the past, I do not see that depression has been an integral part of my life. Yes, I have had those low-light seasons, typically around February, when I get a little indifferent and lack motivation—mostly around job-related activities. These episodes do not happen every year, and the German in me does not want to call them depression. The past month, when my ability to cope with the pain lessened, I will admit that I had been exhibiting signs of depression.

After reading your book and attempting to understand some of the root causes that may have shaped my painfulness, I hope to provide you with some historic insight.

There are three areas (early learning disability, alcohol use, and WPW) that I feel may have shaped my mind in a negative way. The first, an early learning disability, was something that had a big impact on me during my school years. The root of the problem was that I could not seem to develop the capacity to read. As a result, I was labeled a less-than-intelligent person. By third grade, I was reading at early first-grade level, and at this point I was required to go to summer school. I recall one time when my mom visited my fifth-grade teacher, she was told in front of several people, "Your son is just a dumb cluck." I remember how it hurt my mother so. By the time seventh grade rolled around, my reading had gotten to the point where I was finally able to learn, and my whole school experience changed from that point forward. I became an A and B student in eighth grade and for the most part got A's in high school. I went to college and graduated with a BS degree in civil engineering and an MS in geology. Pretty good for a dumb cluck, but needless to say, the experience had an impact on shaping me as a person.

Though I had overcome the issues related to learning, I was still a relatively shy person and out of a need to belong with the in-crowd,

I began my experience with alcohol. I began drinking heavily at age sixteen and continued through high school. Once I went on to college, the drinking continued, but heavier. During the summer following my sophomore year in college, I received a DUI and lost my license for a year. This was a turning point for me. Now I rarely drink at all.

Layered on top of all this was my experience with WPW. I remember as a kid lying in bed and being able to hear my heart beat in my ears at night, and it always seemed that my heart beat louder than normal. It was not until age ten or eleven that the WPW started to manifest itself as tachycardia. My heartbeat would race, and sometimes I would get what I called grayouts. Usually before the onset of the tachycardia event, I would experience heart palpitations and pain in my left upper chest and the left side of my neck. I also experienced a very sharp pain in the middle of my shoulder blades in the same area where my pain radiates from now. Is there a connection? Once I reached the age of twenty-eight, my body started having difficulty handling the tachycardia, and my wife caught me passing out in church. She forced the issue, and I was diagnosed with WPW. I was medicated with beta-blockers to control the tachycardia. However, they caused me to live in a state of fatigue for the four years I was on them.

Then one night I was watching PBS and saw a program reporting the use of heart catheters and radio frequency to ablate the unwanted nerve tracts in my heart. I found a specialist who was doing this on an experimental basis. I weighed the risk and decided to undergo the procedure just to get off the beta-blockers. I really felt that I was less than whole, fatigued while I was on the medications (not too dissimilar from what I am experiencing today with my painfulness). The operation was a success. The tachycardia was gone, and I was free of the beta-blockers, but I was not quite whole. I was still experiencing some of the periodic palpitations and upper chest pains; however, the sharp pain in the middle of my shoulder blades was gone. I had attempted to track this heart stuff down for ten years now but to no avail. The heart pain I get is like a hollow ache in my left upper chest. Typically, when I have these episodes, I go home and go to bed, and it passes by the morning. They happen periodically throughout the year; however, I have not had one in several months. The funny thing in looking back on it is that I have had my worst episodes around the month of February. Any connection?

Let's delve into my painfulness. As I indicated when I spoke with you, this all started back in November 1994. I was visiting Nashville on a house-hunting trip. After spending the night in a hotel, I awoke with a stiff neck and pain in the center of my shoulder blades. This was the first real back pain that I had experienced. At the time it was just an annoyance, but it persisted for a few months. I finally went to see a doctor about it and was referred to an orthopedist. He indicated that I had some degenerative disc issues in the area of concern. He prescribed a round of pain meds and physical therapy. The meds helped, but the therapy did nothing; all this happened in 1995.

Frustrated with the results and not wanting to take the pain meds on a long-term basis led me into thinking that this was just going to be a part of me, and I was just going to have to deal with it. I did pretty well for a while. The pain was not as intense as it is today. I would deal with it until I would get tired of it and then go see my internist. She would prescribe Hydrocodone. I would take it for a while and then get off of it, sometimes for a few months maybe a couple of times a year. I cycled like this until 2002, when I was having a harder time managing the pain on my own. Since then I have consistently taken Hydrocodone to help manage it. In the beginning, one or two pills a day would work, but I seem to have built up a tolerance, and now I am taking about three to four per day.

Not really liking this scenario, I tried to get aggressive with my problem in 2003. After speaking with my internist, she sent me for an MRI, and the results came back that I have osteoarthritis (diffuse bone spurs throughout my upper spine and lower neck). So I asked her what this means. She tearfully looked me in the eye and said there was nothing that could be done. This was not an acceptable answer. So she sent me on my way with a six-month prescription of Hydrocodone and said to call her if I needed more. I know she was sincere, but this was not an acceptable answer.

Just some general facts: I have been a light sleeper as long as I can remember. I usually go to bed about 10:00 PM and wake up by 5:30 AM. It usually takes me thirty to forty-five minutes to fall asleep. Generally I will be up two or three times a night to urinate. This does not count the times I will wake up and fall back to sleep. Often I will wake because I cannot get comfortable due to the pain. On occasion, I will experience what I call night terrors. I will find myself in a semi-awake state and be aware that I am paralyzed. During these times, I perceive the presence of something or someone evil in the room. Whatever it is, it is a terrifying experience. This only happens a few times a year.

I am three days into your initial drug therapy and seem to be sleeping better; however, I have been feeling somewhat hung over during the day. No real opinion on the pain yet. I look forward to seeing you on my next appointment March 1.

Sincerely,
Frank Roth

I receive my share, maybe more than my share, of notes of appreciation and even praise from my patients and readers. I accept these for what they are, expressions of gratitude. Their impact on me, however, pales next to Frank's and those of others who invite me into their very souls. I am humbled and honored when I receive such correspondence.

My heart tells me to stop at this point and let you savor what Frank has written without any intrusion, but he tells us so much that I must, for lack of a better word, dissect what he has written and explore its meaning.

He expresses skepticism and discomfort with my lines of questions and particularly the suggestion that he might suffer depression. Later in the letter, he expresses the frustration and even the anger that befalls so many who suffer chronic pain. "She tearfully looked me in the eye and said there was nothing that could be done. I know she was sincere, but it was not an acceptable answer." Tellingly, he struggles with denial, saying, "The German in me does not want to call it depression." Nonetheless, he offers, either consciously or subconsciously, marvelous clues that he thinks might be helpful to me.

Frank was subject to frequent life-threatening attacks associated with near faints, the apprehension of death, and pain in the chest, neck, and mid-back.

He says that many times in February he will become indifferent and lack motivation. He opens up later and acknowledges that he really was struggling with depression at the time of our consultation. He described his strange heart palpitations and a sense of heaviness in his chest even ten years removed from the successful ablation procedure, and with incredible insight tells us, "The funny thing in looking back is that I have had my worst episodes around the month of February—any connection?"

He describes for us the cardinal features of chronic pain, the sleeplessness, irritability, fatigue, and depression. He tells us that throughout his life he had had difficulty with sleep—a very important historical feature in those who develop chronic pain. He tells us also that he abused alcohol when he was younger—another cardinal feature. He describes his restless legs and his need to get up two or three times at night to urinate. A rare symptom indeed in a forty-one-year-old man, but it does occur with some frequency in those who suffer chronic pain. He tells us about his learning difficulty as a child, and I really don't know if that relates to his painfulness. It would seem unlikely, but I am going to start asking other patients if they had a similar problem. There just might be a connection. Lastly, he tells us about the presence of something or someone evil in the room at night. An incredible clue!

Now I want to move into the timeline of Frank's illness, and I will suggest to you that that which ended up at age forty-one with back pain, depression, fatigue, and irritability actually began at age ten or eleven when his WPW was first manifested as rapid heart action. His descriptions are beautiful. With the tachycardia event, the cardiac output falls, the brain is deprived of oxygen, and grayouts or faints may occur. The blood supply to the heart muscle itself is compromised by the diminished cardiac output, and the experience of chest pain, and for that matter the neck and back pain he described, are symptoms similar to the well-known angina pectoris of coronary artery disease. Referral of such pains away from the heart into the neck or the back is quite common.

Just think about it. From age ten to age twenty-eight, Frank was subject to frequent life-threatening attacks associated with near faints, the apprehension of death, and pain in the chest, neck, and mid-back— remember that, mid-back. At age twenty-eight, the issue was confronted, and he began therapy with one of a group of drugs known as beta-blockers. They are heart sedative, and they can be very effective in slowing the heart rate. The drug, it seemed, helped Frank, but he suffered the common side effect of fatigue. It was so bad that on his own initiative, he sought out a new and at that time still rather experimental ablation procedure for the control of tachycardia. It was successful, and Frank was able to remove himself from fatigue-producing beta-blocker drug therapy. To keep the timeline going, this was at age thirty-two (1993). He tells us the operation was a success and the tachycardia was gone, but he tells us also that "I was not quite whole." He continued to experience palpitations and chest pains, and even ten years later when he came to see me, he was having spells of heart awareness that forced him to leave work and go home and rest. This in spite of the fact that his cardiologist could find nothing wrong with his heart.

The course of Frank's illness is really, I believe, quite understandable. For reasons that he alone must address, he chose to ignore very important and very distressing symptoms over the course of nearly twenty years (such is the human capacity for denial). The issue was finally addressed and his illness successfully treated, but after that, he suffered four years of incessant drug-induced fatigue. These experiences were, I can assure you, ensconced in his memory, and they were powerful forces within him, and they continued to assert themselves.

I will suggest that Frank suffered something like post-traumatic stress disorder. It is an imperfect diagnosis in this case, but it is pretty close to what really was happening. Very fearful experiences in his past, kindled by repetition, would not remain in the subconscious, and on provocation (strangely with the predilection for February) he would relive them and continue doing it for ten years. I hope this thesis is not hard for you to accept. It seems eminently reasonable to me. I doubt that any of us could have come through Frank's heart experience, over the course of more than thirty years, without occasionally reliving it.

I respect Frank in many regards. I am very taken with his intelligence and insight. He connected many of the dots and made many of the associations as he reviewed his history, but there was one connection he tried to make but didn't quite pull it off. He told us that his palpitations and chest pain continued to occur after his ablation procedure, but he tells us also that his back pain went away. It did—but for only one year, and that is a short interlude indeed in a thirty-year illness. His ablation was done in 1993, and he relocated to my city in 1994. While visiting on a house-hunting trip, he awoke with pain between his shoulder blades *in exactly the same place he had experienced his heart pain*. A memory, a powerful memory of pain had not abandoned him. When he got to me ten years later, he was suffering incessant mid-back pain, periodic heart awareness, and enervating fatigue. I will suggest to you that all of these were an exercise of memory of disturbing events long before.

Frank and I have been at it now about three years. I began by introducing Clonazepam and Imipramine. He was very pleased with his improvement. He slept better, and his depression and fatigue diminished. He continued to have his heart symptoms and went through another evaluation by the cardiologist. He was reassured that all was well, but he admitted he still had trouble accepting it. As time went by, he began losing ground, and I had to make drug adjustments. The pain came back, not nearly so bad as before, but enough to require resumption of the Hydrocodone. I added Cymbalta and that helped—for a while. He began to complain of "mind fog" and a sense of distraction and daytime sleepiness. I made more adjustments by adding Zoloft, and when that failed, Celexa. It helped a bit, but we really weren't getting where we wanted to be. Frank did tell me that were it not for my medicines, he would be on disability, so I felt that to be a positive. Just a few months ago I had to add Oxycontin, a stronger opiate. I had him on a lot of stuff: Oxycontin, Hydrocodone, Imipramine, Clonazepam, and Celexa. It was more medicine than I would like him taking, but he was sleeping well, his pain was in moderate control, and he was at least not on disability.

At that juncture, I decided to write this book. I thought that Frank's story and his remembered pain would make an interesting chapter. I reviewed his chart and made a special point to re-read his letter. Going through it, I marveled at his capacity for expressing things that are often difficult to express. Near the end of his descriptions of his disordered sleep, I was astonished when he concluded the paragraph by telling me, "On occasions I will experience what I call night terrors. I will find myself in a semi-awake state and be aware that I am paralyzed. During these times, I perceive the presence of something or someone evil in the room. Whatever it is, it is a terrifying experience."

I had not paid it the attention I should have, perhaps with good reason. Frank was painful, sleepless, fatigued, and depressed. In my urgency to address those issues, I had ignored a clue. Frank was describing hypnogogic hallucinations and sleep paralysis! I called him the next day to have him come in to see me. I told him we had important things to talk about, and that I just might be able to help him.

Before continuing, I have to pause and share with you some truly remarkable coincidences. I'll ask you to remember Regina from the previous chapter. She expressed the same frustration as Frank. Their words are almost identical. Regina wrote that she was "frustrated by your line of questioning." Frank wrote that he was "skeptical and uncomfortable with the lines of questions." At the conclusion of her letter, Regina wrote about her "narcoleptic" feelings. I had overlooked her description just as I had overlooked Frank's night terrors and paralysis. There were, after all, in both of them more important things to think about at the time. Only later, as their diseases evolved, and we achieved some measure of control, was I able to explore nuance. Regina called her hypnogogic hallucinations and sleep paralysis her "ghost." Frank called them "the presence of something or someone evil." Is that not absolutely uncanny?

Both Regina and Frank were trying to share with me something that in their hearts they knew was important. I was not alert enough to pick up on the fact that in addition to their painfulness and all the rest, they both also suffered narcolepsy.

I prescribed Adderall for Frank, and his response was quite as good as Regina's had been with Ritalin. Within days his pain had greatly diminished to the extent that some days he used no Hydrocodone at all. He was more wakeful and energized, and his mental focus, he told me with pride, had returned.

What if I had not chosen to write this book—and to include Frank in it? How long would it have taken me to discover and treat his narcolepsy and with it, his pain? Call it what you will, providence or just good luck. Whatever it is, it is a wonderful thing, and I am privileged to be a part of it.

Jack, Lucy, and Frank teach us, I believe, that pain is often a remembered experience. The fact that Jack's pain improved when I treated his cyclothymic mood swings with Lorazepam, and that Lucy's pain improved when I treated her (perhaps) bipolar disease with Topamax, and that Frank's pain improved when I treated his depression and narcolepsy with Imipramine, Clonazepam, and Adderall is simply icing on the cake.

The pain doctor must be ever reminded to search diligently for the psychiatric comorbidities that travel so often with pain. They must be sought out and even if they exist in mere fragments, they demand treatment, for thereby the pain is often relieved.

I want to share with you one last thought. When I entered this pain business some twenty years ago, I realized in short order that disordered sleep was a fundamental part of the disease. I occasionally wondered why I was seeing so few pain sufferers with narcolepsy. It just seemed that I ought to be seeing more. I have now learned, and this dates over only the past year, that narcolepsy is not uncommon in the painful. Indeed, it is quite common. The reason I wasn't finding it was because *I didn't know to look for it*. I have learned a lot. I now routinely ask in interview if my patient experiences attacks of daytime sleepfulness or if they suffer ghosts or the presence of evil at night.

CHAPTER SEVEN

The Damaged Brain

S ophronia was frail and stooped, and she was obviously suffering badly. She chose to remain standing for the interview, braced on her walker. It was painful, she told me, to either sit or lie down. Her daughter supplied most of the history. Sophronia was eighty-two years old and a widow. She had not want for comfort or affection, however. She lived in an apartment in her daughter's home and received the frequent attentions of her three children and her several grandchildren and great-grandchildren. She had, until recently, kept her apartment by herself and even attended her vegetable garden, sharing its produce with her family. She read a lot and occasionally watched television even though she interrupted to say, "There is nothing on there really worth watching."

I was told her memory was good and told also that she saw the important things with great clarity. She brooked no nonsense, and she suffered fools poorly. She also suffered doctors poorly. She had, until the appearance of her severe back pain, not seen one since her last child was born fifty years before. She had never had a mammogram nor for many years a Pap smear. Her only medication had been Tylenol for her occasional backache.

Her back had bothered her for many years, but it was only an occasional inconvenience. A day or two in bed usually took care of it. In recent months, however, it had worsened, with pain extending to the buttocks and sometimes into the legs. She was unable to be on her feet for any length of time and had to forego her work in the garden. Her family prevailed on her to see an orthopedic surgeon. X-rays showed that her vertebrae were thinned by osteoporosis and many of them collapsed from compression fractures. Their alignment was disordered, one of them slipping forward over the one below. There was no reasonable hope for surgical repair. The orthopedist prescribed

Hydrocodone and suggested that Sophronia see a pain specialist, one skilled in the use of opiates for relief of pain. An appointment to see me was scheduled, but then there occurred an event that turned out to be disastrous.

Sophronia awoke at night with severe abdominal pain and vomiting. Testing in the emergency room showed that she had gallstones, and with them an infection of the gallbladder. Surgery was undertaken the following day. Puncture wounds were made in the abdomen for the insertion of tubes that allow fiberoptic visualization and cautery. The gallbladder was removed without difficulty, but Sophronia developed a bloodstream infection with high fever and heart and kidney failure, and a prolonged interval of confusion with delirium and convulsive seizures. She survived the ordeal and after nearly a month in the hospital, she was discharged to her home and the care of her family. Her back pain had become excruciating. She came to my office as soon as her strength allowed.

Curiously, the illogical answer is often the correct answer in those who suffer chronic pain.

"I'm sorry you are so uncomfortable, Sophronia. I'll try to make this as quick as I can, but I must ask you a few questions."

"Okay," she said, "but you must know I am really hurting badly."

"Are you able to sleep at night?"

"No, I can't sleep at all. The pain keeps me awake. I can't get comfortable in bed. I have to sleep in a recliner."

"How is your appetite?"

"I have to force myself to eat. I don't have any appetite at all."

"Sophronia, I can barely imagine what you went through those weeks in the hospital. That experience would strain anyone's emotions. Let me ask you, do you feel depressed?"

"No, I am not depressed. I have never been depressed, and I don't intend to get depressed, but I do need some help with this pain. It is almost more than I can bear."

Chronic pain is, as I have written many times, a disease of the mind. As my experience grows, I have become more convinced of the correctness of this belief, and it is people like Sophronia who have taught me so.

There are times, however, when the belief is so contrary to common sense that, it seems, it simply cannot withstand challenge.

There is an important medical adage that says, *when you hear hoof-beats, think of horses, not of zebras.* That is to say—look for the logical explanation, not the illogical one. Curiously, the illogical answer is often the correct answer in those who suffer chronic pain. But this was not the time for intellectualism and sophistry. Sophronia had a very bad back, she was suffering terribly, and there was urgency. I had to do something and do it quickly to give her some measure of relief.

I chose the time-honored, appropriate, and logical drug morphine. If she was able to tolerate it (always a fear), I anticipated significant measure of relief, and then I might be able to conduct a more extended interview and pursue some other treatment options. Although I was hopeful the morphine would help her, experience has taught me that it is not always the perfect answer.

She returned at the appointed time, and she looked worse, not better. She continued to rely on her walker, shifting her weight from one leg to another and said, "That stuff you are giving me for pain doesn't help at all. I could get as much relief by drinking a glass of water."

Well, it does happen. One has to live with the unexpected.

"I'm sorry, Sophronia, I am very sorry. I had hoped the morphine would work, but it didn't. We will just try a different kind of pain killer."

The daughter stood up next to her mother and helped support her weight as she embraced her with tears in her eyes.

"Mom is just not the same since she was in the hospital. She is suffering so much that it breaks my heart. She used to be so strong and independent and now she wants somebody around her all the time. She is afraid to be alone. She calls me up in the middle of the night to come sit with her."

"Is that right, Sophronia?"

She turned her eyes away and said, sadly, "Yes, that's right."

"Sophronia, I know you are uncomfortable, and I know this isn't pleasant, but I have to ask you a few more questions because I think I may be able to help you."

"Please do. Please do."

"Are you having bad thoughts? Are there things in your mind that you haven't told anyone? Are you having thoughts that scare you?"

She hesitated and then she began to cry. She took her daughter's hand and held it tightly and said, "Yes, I do have bad thoughts. Things are happening to me that I don't understand. Sometimes when I look at the television I see my husband. He talks to me."

"What does he say?"

"I am not sure. I recognize his face and his voice, but I don't remember what he says."

"Are you seeing or hearing other things? Are there things that are frightening to you?"

"Yes, sometimes at night I see strangers in the room, and they say bad things."

"What do they say?"

"They say they are going to rob me and hurt me. Sometimes I hear voices like that when I pick up the telephone to make a call. What is wrong with me? Please tell me what is wrong."

The door was wide open. My God, how I love this work!

Sophronia had a bad back—of that there is no question. And as she grew older, her back progressively deteriorated, and she experienced more and more pain. So far so good. No one would contest the logic of this simple observation. But I want to introduce another idea. As Sophronia's back was getting older, so was her mind. Some degree of senescence, however modest, is present in most eighty-two-year-olds. Moreover, her mind was burdened by an unhappy prospect, debilitating illness and a loss of independence. Few would debate that this kind of ideation can worsen pain.

Then, an intercurrent illness, and a very bad one at that. An operation on the gallbladder, then a bloodstream infection, and a failure of her organ systems. Her kidneys quit working, and her heart failed. Her mind also. The combination of age, bloodstream infection, heart failure, and uremic poisoning, the biologic equivalent of an earthquake, overwhelmed her resources. She became encephalopathic with delirium and convulsions. After three weeks in an intensive care unit (itself a mind-altering experience), she recovered—or so it would seem. Her cardiac function returned to normal, and her kidneys began making urine again. Her seizures arrested, and she awoke and became lucid and coherent. Her mind appeared to have been restored as well as her kidneys and her heart. We can easily measure the workings of those organs by laboratory testing. The workings of the mind, however, are much more difficult of assay.

She used to be so strong and independent and now she wants somebody around her all the time.

After a month in the hospital, at total bed rest, Sophronia's pain had become excruciating. Did her spinal anatomy get that much worse during her confinement? It seems unlikely. Sophronia's back did not deteriorate over the course of a month, but her mind certainly did.

I did not recognize this at first, and my choice of morphine was not a good one. Then came the dénouement, *mother is afraid of being alone.* Sophronia's encephalopathy had left a legacy. How could weeks of delirium and repeated seizures not leave a legacy in an eighty-two-year-old? She was experiencing a common clinical phenomenon known ungracefully as sundowning. When the light becomes dim, vision—that sensory experience which above all others keeps us in contact with our environment and reality—becomes less efficient and invites the development of strange imaginings.

Sophronia had a badly deteriorated back and, by virtue of brain damage, was subject to hallucinations. She also had that disease we know as chronic pain—derivative of and coexistent with the others but probably a thing unto itself, an independent agency of suffering, if you will. This conceptualization is important because it helps direct treatment strategies.

I told Sophronia to discard the morphine, and I was faced with an important treatment choice. The physician reader will certainly recognize that hallucinations are most appropriately treated by an antipsychotic drug. There are several of them, and any would, with great predictability, have terminated her hallucinations, but I am not sure at all they would have helped her pain. (They might have, but I will never know). I chose

Nortriptyline and Clonazepam, low choice for hallucinations—very low—but first choice for chronic pain. It was perhaps a risky choice, but my instincts told me to do it.

On her return a couple of weeks later, her entire demeanor had changed. She was smiling and moving about with a gracefulness unimaginable two weeks before. She told me her appetite had returned, and she had abandoned her recliner. She was able to sleep through the night painlessly in her bed. She was using Tylenol for pain, and she had nearly abandoned her walker. She told me, with considerable excitement, that come spring she planned to get back to her gardening. I didn't even bring up the subject of the hallucinations. There was no need to.

Sophronia suffered pain and a disorder of thought in the form of hallucinations. Recall John and Sory from chapter four. They, too, suffered pain and disordered thought: John, hallucinations and Sory, delusions. The reader will, I trust, recognize the similarities among these three people, and if knowledgeable in matters medical, will also recognize the dissimilarities in their treatment. The SSRI Zoloft for John, Clonazepam and the antipsychotic Seroquel for Sory, and Clonazepam and a tricyclic for Sophronia. I will admit that my treatment decisions were inconsistent, but they were, with the exception of misfiring with morphine for Sophronia, highly successful and quickly so. Chalk it up, perhaps, to good luck, or perhaps experience, or perhaps even to the hand of God—for I do believe that God is with me when I attend the painful. I wish I could give you a better explanation as to why I chose those particular drugs, but I cannot.

Fred was obese, and his round face was swollen with fatty cheeks. With the angles of his mouth pulled up into those huge cheeks, his features were those of a happy face cartoon. I soon saw, however, that his smile was frozen, as if dictated that way by nature rather than emotion. He exhibited no mirth or jocularity. His responses to my queries were measured and clipped, and his features changed but little when he spoke. His affect was constricted and flat. His physical features were those of happiness but his behavioral ones those of apathy and perhaps sadness. The presence of this strange combination was to lead me, for quite a while, down the wrong path.

His life had not been arduous, forty years in the civil service at a military base. His marriage had been quite satisfactory. His physical health, obesity notwithstanding, had been good. His pain had begun some two years before within a few months of his retirement from the federal government. With time on his hands and no particular hobbies or interests, he found employment as a red-vested greeter at a Wal-Mart Superstore. With the prolonged standing, an activity to which his body was unaccustomed, he began to experience a dull pain in his low back. He took over-the-counter analgesics, and they helped for a while, but after several months Fred elected to seek an orthopedic opinion. X-rays of the back demonstrated some signs of wear and tear, but considering his age of sixty-five years, they were really rather modest. The orthopedist opined that there was no major disease of the spine, and that the pain was coming from the muscles of

Weight loss in the obese is important . . . but I am not at all sure that it will cure backache. Maybe it has in a few people, but none that I have ever seen.

the back, overtaxed by supporting his massive weight. He advised weight loss and suggested that if Fred could lose seventy or eighty pounds, his back pain would surely diminish.

The advice was commonsensical and logical. It has been given, I am sure, by every orthopedist who has confronted an obese patient with a backache. So far so good, but what does the orthopedist say to the skinny patient with a backache?

The physician, encountering the person with an obscure symptom, and particularly obscure pain, often falls victim to the quest for the easy answer. That, unfortunately, entails putting the responsibility for the disorder on the patient. We do that when we tell our patient that the back is hurting because he is obese. It is an easy trap to fall into and we physicians, subconsciously perhaps, do it a lot. It absolves us of any responsibility for the failure of our treatments. I have had considerable experience in the treatment of backache, and I have never seen a backache go away with weight loss.

Don't get me wrong. Weight loss in the obese is important. It will help control or prevent the development of diseases such as hypertension, diabetes, and coronary artery disease, but I am not at all sure that it will cure backache. Maybe it has in a few people, but none that I have ever seen.

The painful disorder fibromyalgia is known to most readers. In its typical form, it is characterized by aching discomfort in the neck, the upper back, and the shoulders. It is more common in women, and women have breasts. Some of them have very large breasts. On the presumption that upper back pain could derive from the muscular stress imposed by carrying large breasts, some physicians advise reduction mammoplasty (surgically diminishing the size of the breasts) for the treatment of fibromyalgia in the large-breasted. A few of my patients

Depression need not present as despondency.

have actually had the procedure performed (certainly not on my advice). None of them really got any better. Chronic pain, at least the sleepless, depressed, fatigued, appetite-disordered chronic pain that I write about in this book is not the product of too-heavy postural mechanics. It is a disease of the mind.

Fred retired from Wal-Mart and at least tried to lose weight, but he couldn't do it. He had never been able to before, and he couldn't do it now. His pain continued—indeed it got worse and spread to his buttocks and mid- and upper back. After a few more months of painful frustration, he sought a second opinion, that of a neurosurgeon. An MRI showed no significant abnormalities, and Fred was referred to me for management of his chronic pain.

I searched for clues as to its origin but could find little. He did tell me his sleep was disturbed by frequent painful awakenings and also a couple of awakenings at night to empty his bladder. I continued my interrogations.

"Fred, are you sad or depressed?"

"No," he responded tersely.

"Have you ever been treated for depression in the past?"

"No, I have never been depressed."

"Have you ever had a problem with drugs or alcohol?"

"No."

"Can you tell me just how you feel?"

"I hurt in my back."

"Are you fatigued? Do you feel tired?"

"Yes, I feel tired."

"All the time?"

"Yes, all the time. I really don't feel very good," he said with that strange, mask-like smile. "What do you think is wrong with my back?"

"Well, I am not sure, but I know you are hurting, and I am going to try to do something about it. I am going to give you some medicine that I think will help your sleep and probably your pain."

He then asked me the question that I have heard from virtually every person I have treated for chronic pain. "What are the medicines for?"

"They are for you, Fred."

It was an unsatisfactory answer, perhaps, to a very reasonable question, but it is the one I routinely give because it allows me to explain to my patient just what a complex disease chronic pain and why its treatment is so uncertain and so subject to trial and error. The endocrinologist can tell his patient that he is giving them thyroid medicine to raise the thyroid levels in the blood or that he is giving them insulin to lower the blood sugar. The cardiologist can tell his patient that the medicine he is giving is to lower the blood pressure. The rheumatologist can tell his that the drug is to reduce inflammation in the joints. The pain doctor doesn't have the luxury of easy answers. He cannot tell his patient he is giving them one drug for pain, another for sleep, and another for energy. The pain doctor gives his medicines because, in the last analysis, he has seen them work in others with similar symptoms. Most (not all) of my patients are accepting of this explanation.

"Will I become addicted to the drugs?"

"I don't think addiction is our problem. Pain is our problem. The medicines I am giving you are reasonably safe, and if you take them as I instruct, we should have no problems."

"Will they make me feel sleepy and drugged?"

"If they do, you are to reduce the dosage and call me." I prescribed Imipramine and Clonazepam and watched him very slowly step off the examining table and shuffle his way down the hall.

I have written before about smiling or atypical depression, diagnoses much in vogue a few decades ago. Both refer to the person who, stated succinctly, is depressed but doesn't know it. Depression need not present as despondency. It may present as fatigue, insomnia, or anxiety. The most common presentation of smiling or atypical depression, however, is chronic pain. Fred, with his fatigue and sleepless painfulness and his strange smiling countenance fulfilled, quite literally as well as figuratively, the criteria for smiling depression.

When I saw him next, I detected no change in his demeanor at all. He was smiling as before but with little emotional display otherwise.

"How are you feeling? Have the medicines helped any?"

"Not much. My pain is just about the same. It really hasn't changed."

"Are you sleeping any better?"

"A little bit maybe. My bladder doesn't bother me quite as much, but I still have to get up most nights."

"Do you feel different in any way?"

"No, I don't feel any different at all."

Most of the drugs used in the treatment of pain are slow in their onset of action. I certainly didn't expect Fred to be well three weeks into treatment, but I expected some change, however subtle. He was sleeping a bit better, and I viewed that to be a positive, but I was concerned about his lack of progress otherwise. Nonetheless, I stuck with the going diagnosis, chronic pain and smiling depression. It did not seem illogical. Chronic pain (and depression) often appear after life events, and the termination of forty years employment at one place certainly qualifies as a life event. I encouraged Fred to increase the dose of the Imipramine and see me again in three weeks.

"How are you feeling now, Fred?"

"No different."

I then directed the question to his wife who had accompanied him on each visit. "Do you see any change at all, a change in his disposition or temperament?"

"No, I don't see any change at all. I don't see that the drugs have done anything."

Six weeks into treatment and nothing had happened. The drugs are a long way from perfect, but they almost always do something, if not for the good then for the bad. Fred's response had been neither. I was faced with two major possibilities. One, I had picked the wrong drugs or two, I had picked the wrong diagnosis.

I studied his frozen, placid face and his large and immobile body and saw something I had not noticed before—a tremor in the thumb of his right hand. The muscles of the thumb were contracting, repetitively, moving the digit quite slightly about two times per second. I moved over to him and took his arm in my hands and moved it through its range of motion. There was no stiffness or rigidity, and although I looked for quite a while, I saw no other tremors. It was confined to one digit of one hand. An idea, perhaps a very good idea, was percolating through, but at this juncture I kept my thoughts to myself and told my patient and his wife that we were going to try another drug called Prozac.

The drugs are a long way from perfect, but they almost always do something.

"That is dangerous, isn't it?" Fred said. "I am not sure I want to take that."

"It is no more dangerous than the drugs I have given you before nor is it more dangerous than the drugs I may give you in the future. I really want you to try it."

"Prozac is for depression, isn't it? Do you think Fred is depressed?" his wife asked.

"I am not sure, but it is a very real possibility, and it is important that he take it. If he has trouble with it, discard it and call me, but it is important that we try the medicine. It may help or it may not, but I need to know."

"I will take it like you tell me to," Fred said, his placid, happy face moving but little as he spoke the words.

I watched him more closely this time as he stepped very slowly from the examining table and walked slowly away. Just as his face showed no animus, neither did his body. His steppage was slow, and the movements of his arms as he walked was constricted and graceless.

Parkinson's disease is a rather common neurologic disorder. Certain cells deep within the brain that manufacture and employ the neurotransmitter dopamine, for reasons uncertain, die off, and Parkinsonism, a disease of movement, is characterized by tremor, rigidity, bradykinesia (slowness of motion), and masked facies (facial immobility and want of emotional expression).

There are many subtypes of dopamine differing only slightly from one another. They are distributed throughout the brain, and we might expect, probably naively, that each subtype has a specific function, but it doesn't work that way. The mind is a vastly complex place, and the notion that a single chemical or a subtype of chemical has a single specific function at a specific place within the brain can be dismissed out of hand. The workings of the dopamine system are highly interactive. They are mutually dependent, and the disturbance of one will almost invariably effect the others. Thus, Parkinson's disease, which begins as a disorder of movement, expresses itself as it progresses into disorder of memory, thought, mood, and also—you are certainly expecting this—the perception of pain. These effects tend to appear late in the game when the disease is advanced, but there is no law of nature which dictates that it must be so. Could pain not be an early symptom of Parkinson's disease?

On his return visit, he reported no change on the Prozac, and he certainly evidenced none. Two months into therapy with Clonazepam, Imipramine, and Prozac, and nothing had happened. His doctor had been treating the wrong disease.

Smiling depression it could and perhaps should have been. Remember, hoofbeats should make the physician think of horses, not zebras. Depression appearing as pain is quite common. Parkinson's appearing as pain is probably much less so. The physician should accept the most probable diagnosis, and he should also, if there is no urgency, accept the most favorable diagnosis. Depression is a more favorable diagnosis than Parkinson's disease, for it can be treated rather well with pharmacy. Parkinson's also, but it is nonetheless a progressive disorder, and with time the drugs work less well. It was my lot to address with Fred and his wife the very real possibility that he had a neurologic disease, something much more complex than a backache.

"Fred, let me ask you a few questions. I have seen you now over several visits, and it seems that you move rather slowly. Have you noticed that?"

"Yes, a little bit, but it is due to my back. It hurts when I move."

His wife offered her opinion. "He is slowing down. It takes him longer to get dressed in the morning. He seems to have trouble buttoning his shirt."

"Have you noticed that tremor in the thumb?"

"Yes," he said with hesitation, "I have. What does that mean?"

"Well, it may mean something important. It is possible, Fred, that you have an early form of Parkinson's disease. But I can't say that with certainty yet."

And I couldn't. There is no blood test or imaging study that tells us whether a patient has Parkinson's disease. The diagnosis is made by observation and most often by the employ of a therapeutic trial. I told Fred to progressively taper the dose of his medicines and then to discard them, and I instructed him to begin the drug Sinemet three times daily. Sinemet is, in a physiological sense, one of the simpler drugs. It consists principally of dopamine, the very chemical that Fred's brain was lacking. Its administration provides cells that are starved for the neurotransmitter their agency. The effect can sometimes be miraculous.

Fred was a different man when I saw him next. There was fluidity and grace to his movements. He was more voluble in his speech, more spontaneous. His smile remained, the angles of his mouth seemingly pulled upward by his fatty cheeks, but his expressions were less frozen. His features bore an emotional content that they had not before, and his tremor had gone away.

"Fred, you look like you are moving around a lot better."

"Yes, I am getting around a lot better. I can button my shirts better."

"How about the backache? Has that changed any?"

"It is gone."

"Gone?"

"Yes, totally gone. My back doesn't hurt at all. Can you believe that?" he said as he broke into a big, warm, expressive smile.

I have written already of the cure of pain by the administration of pharmacy for psychiatric disorder, be this depression, bipolar disease, narcolepsy, hallucinations, or delusion. Those are all diseases of brain function. Parkinson's disease is not only a disorder of brain function but also of brain substance. Unlike bipolar disease, narcolepsy, and all the rest, a portion of the brain actually dies in Parkinson's disease, and replacing that which has been lost by the administration of the missing neurotransmitter can actually relieve the attendant pain.

James was a successful businessman, now in his seventies, and recently retired. He had surgery for his chronic back pain a couple of years before, but it had not gone well. His pain continued, and he became sleepless. His wife told me that she thought he was depressed. He didn't think so, but he told me he was concerned about his memory. He was just not as sharp as he used to be.

I prescribed Nortriptyline and Clonazepam. Sleep was restored, but otherwise there was little change. Along the way I detected signs that bothered me more and more. James continued to complain of forgetfulness, and he performed poorly on the mental status examination (a brief office evaluation of memory and cognition). I obtained an MRI of the brain. It showed slight cortical atrophy, a shrinkage of the surface of the brain. Perhaps indicative of Alzheimer's disease, but not certainly so. Many healthy seventy-year-olds will show on MRI testing some cortical atrophy. I felt I needed some help on this one, and I referred James to a psychiatrist who had a particular interest in Alzheimer's disease.

My colleague sent me a letter stating that he thought James suffered mild cognitive impairment, a euphemism for senile forgetfulness. Mild cognitive impairment is not Alzheimer's, but it is getting close. The psychiatrist continued to treat James with antidepressants, even including Ritalin. Despite his efforts, however, James was becoming ever more painful, and his forgetfulness, he told me, was really becoming a problem. I saw him one day, and he told me that the psychiatrist had sent him to a clinical psychologist who performed a battery of tests.

"You know, Dr. Cochran, I really had trouble on those tests. I was surprised at how badly I did, and how much trouble I had with remembering."

A few days later, another letter from the psychiatrist. James had Alzheimer's disease and was prescribed the drug Namenda. Alzheimer's is in many ways similar to Parkinson's disease. For reasons unknown, those cells that manufacture acetylcholine, the brain's memory enhancing neurotransmitter, die off. And Alzheimer's, like Parkinson's, is not only a disease of brain function, it is a disease of brain substance. We have had, for a few years at least, a cluster of drugs for the treatment of Alzheimer's. They are no means perfect, but they do seem to slow the progression of the disease. The early ones increased the action of acetylcholine. Namenda is different. It antagonizes glutamine, the brain's excitatory neurotransmitter. Glutamine certainly plays a role in the function of memory, presumably destructively so, and for that reason, a drug such as Namenda, which antagonizes glutamine, can be helpful in the treatment of Alzheimer's. Glutamine is also a neurotransmitter of pain, and a drug that antagonizes it could, at least theoretically, relieve pain. It is for this reason that Namenda is being explored as an analgesic drug.

"How are you doing, James? Dr. Jones told me he had given you a new medicine."

"Really pretty well. I don't hurt as much as I used to. I can tell a real difference."

"He is not as depressed and not as tired as he used to be," his wife said. "Is that right, James?"

"Yes, that's right. I really feel a whole lot better, and I can remember better."

Over the course of several months, James has continued to improve. He has become quicker and wittier, and I welcome his visits, for he is delightful company. How long his improvement will be sustained, I do not know.

An important question: Did Namenda relieve James's pain because it arrested, and perhaps even reversed, his Alzheimer's disease? Or did it relieve it by a separate agency, its antagonism to pain-inducing glutamine? We don't know the answer to that yet. Regardless, I hope I have given you the message. Chronic pain is a disease of the mind, and it travels in company with other diseases of the mind.

Before I conclude this chapter, I want to share with you the story of another person whose damaged brain led him to suffer pain. It happened many years ago, and it changed the course of my career and led me to become a pain doctor. I did not appreciate it at the time, but now, in retrospect, I see it very clearly.

Bob was a chemical engineer. He had an outstanding academic record, and he climbed the ladder quickly. Anticipating sooner or later a job in management, he obtained a law degree through night school. He worked hard and went nearly to the very top. Then, after a disagreement, he left the manufacturing firm and entered, successfully, the practice of law. About age seventy, Bob began to lose ground. He became forgetful and his handwriting became less legible. He began to experience visual hallucinations. "I just saw a mouse run across the corner of the room." His deterioration from Alzheimer's was rapid. In that era, there were no drugs available to arrest the progression of the disease. As he became more demented, he began to experience incessant pruritis (itching).

Pruritis, as medical students of my generation were taught, is subliminal pain, and anyone who has endured the experience certainly knows that. There was little I could do for Bob's discomfort. I left that in the hands of his dermatologist. He was treated with ultraviolet radiation and cortisone injections and creams, but in spite of the best efforts of his doctor, his itching did not get better—it got worse. Bob failed rapidly, but in his occasional moments of lucidity, he would tell me, "This itching is more than I can bear." It broke my heart because Bob was very dear to me.

I thought about Bob a lot. Indeed, I could think of little else. I kept asking, why did this dreadful thing happen? Why did he experience such discomfort as his mind was deteriorating? Was there a connection?

Bob died after several months in a near-vegetative state. His death was a blessing, for his distress had been extreme. I am thankful for what I learned from him. He set me on a path that has led me to explore the role of the mind in the genesis of pain. He made me think, tentatively at first, perhaps, that his more-than-I-can-bear itching was one with his mind disease. I have learned much since that time, but nothing I have learned has dissuaded me from that belief. In suffering and dying, he taught me much, and I am grateful that what I learned so many years ago from him might be helpful to others.

Bob was the most wonderful man I have ever known. He was my father.

CHAPTER EIGHT

Pain Behavior

B arry grew up in a brutal environment. He was the youngest of thirteen children. He was beaten badly by his father and also his older brothers and sisters. Whether his epilepsy derived from head injury incurred in some of those beatings or whether it was a result of some genetic mischance is uncertain. He achieved a tenth-grade education, but his learning skills were limited and he is functionally illiterate. In spite of his handicaps, however, he found steady employment as a carpenter. He had a stable marriage of eighteen years and was the father of two sons.

His first back surgery for a ruptured disc was done at age thirty-eight. He recovered sufficiently to go back to work. The following year he became ill with an intestinal blockage that required several operations. During the course of this prolonged illness, he lost weight—from 245 pounds to 117. He became depressed and sleepless and remained so in spite of treatment with Effexor. His misfortune continued. He ruptured another disc and required surgery, but he failed to recover and entered a life of incessant painfulness. He began treatment with Hydrocodone and the muscle relaxant Soma. His pain spread all over his body into his shoulders, torso, hips, and legs. His doctors told him, he said, that his joints were "worn out from hard labor."

He moved about with hesitation, limping badly, and holding on to any available piece of furniture to help support his weight. His movements were restricted by pain, and it took him forever to gather himself onto the examining table and lie down on his back. He grimaced and winced frequently and sometimes screamed when a movement was particularly difficult for him. Finally, with Barry supine on the table, I attempted to perform the time-honored straight leg raising test. In this maneuver, the physician slowly lifts the patient's leg toward the ceiling, asking if and when he has pain. If pain occurs before the movement can be completed, it is a sign that the large sciatic nerve is damaged, most commonly by a ruptured disc (the term sciatica refers to pain radiating down the leg). I was able to get Barry's leg but a couple of inches off the table before he screamed in agony. I repeated the maneuver on the other leg, and the same thing happened. Almost any back-injured person, even with the worst sciatica, will tolerate their leg being lifted two inches without pain. Why couldn't Barry?

It is time now to talk about pain behaviors, that is, the exhibition of physical suffering. We have all done it. I certainly have many times with back spasms, leg cramps, or an acutely swollen gouty knee. With these illnesses I grunt, I wince, I grimace, and I resist any movement that will worsen the pain. The migraineur does the same when she goes into a room and turns off the light and closes the door to lie quietly alone. These are all understandable actions, and they are in many regards self-protective. We avoid that which makes the pain worse. Pain behavior is a part of our lives, and it is a common, even predictable reaction to injury. It is rather uncommon, however, in those who suffer

> *We avoid that which makes the pain worse. Pain behavior is a part of our lives.*

chronic pain. Only a few of the people I have described thus far exhibited any real pain behaviors during the course of my interview. The reason for this is, I believe, that pain behaviors are energy inefficient and energy wasteful. Sustaining them for weeks, months, or even years is exhausting and self-destructive. Nonetheless, it does happen occasionally, and I want to address this subject in some detail because my thinking of the matter has turned 180 degrees within the past few years.

When pain behavior persists beyond the time limits that the physician could reasonably expect from the injury, it invites suspicion. It suggests that the patient's exhibition of suffering offers him some gain—be this sympathy, attention, more pain medicines, or financial reward from litigation. These benefits are identified in the lexicon as secondary gain. In other words, the victim, by virtue of his behavior, gets something more out of his illness than he deserves. This, I emphasize, represents a high order of presumption. We don't really know that the victim is seeking something extra. We only presume it. It is an easy trap to fall into, and we physicians do it a lot. We ascribe what appears to be an overreaction to pain in pejorative terms, using descriptors such as attention-seeking, non-physiologic (and Barry's two inches off the table back pain was certainly non-physiologic), or symptom magnification. We compound what I believe is an erroneous judgment by frequently attributing it to some want of intellect or emotional strength. And Barry, we certainly know, had plenty of that. He was, after all, childhood abused, uneducated, illiterate, and epileptic.

I want to pause now and develop an idea that I think is quite important, perhaps one of the most important that I present in this book. There is a well-recognized psychiatric disorder known as conversion reaction. It is characterized by the loss of some neurologic function such as sensation, muscle strength, or vision that appears in reaction to stress and occurs in the absence of any identifiable abnormality of the brain. Conversion, certainly, is non-physiologic. For example, the victim of conversion reaction blindness says he cannot see, and yet his pupils constrict on exposure to light. Or he cannot move—he is paralyzed—but his reflexes are perfectly normal. We believe that conversion reaction is an act of the subconscious. It is not the product of will. That is to say, the victim does not knowingly create the symptoms. (If the symptom is created by an act of will, that is known as malingering).

Conversion reaction is one of several psychologic defense mechanisms, ways of coping, however maladaptively, to stress. I have already written at some length about denial as a defense mechanism and also, briefly, repression and transference. The defense mechanism of conversion, we have traditionally believed, usually befalls the less endowed, those who by dent of limited intellect and education lack the emotional resources to confront stress. They are not sophisticated enough to enter denial. They are forced to express their damaged emotions in a more vivid exhibition.

Now, back to Barry's extravagant pain behaviors. Could they not be a form of conversion reaction? Psychiatrists would be very reluctant to say so. Traditionally they are disinclined to view pain and its companions, including pain behaviors, as a form of conversion, but I really don't see why. If we could but accept the possibility that they are, it would be an enormous conceptual advance.

If pain behavior is indeed a form of conversion, it is (so far as we know) the product of the subconscious and, therefore, quite independent of will. How then can we use terms such as attention-seeking and symptom magnification when the victim has no control at all over his symptoms? How could he possibly magnify that which is beyond his control? How do we know that the patient is seeking gain? Really, we don't know that the patient is employing his symptoms for advantage. We only presume it, and that, I will suggest, may be as much a product of physician frustration as anything else because pain behavior is indeed difficult to put up with. It is distracting and time consuming, and most physicians have a lot of trouble with it.

> *How then can*
> *we use terms*
> *such as attention-*
> *seeking and symptom*
> *magnification when*
> *the victim has*
> *no control at all over*
> *his symptoms?*

Conceptualizing that pain behaviors can be a symptom of conversion has, I believe, made me a better physician and probably a better man because it has removed me from preconception and prejudice. I now view pain behavior/conversion as merely another symptom of chronic pain along with disordered sleep, mood, and all the rest. I have learned, and this is quite surprising to me still, that pain behavior is actually a very good prognostic sign. I suspect that very few physicians would agree with that, but I believe it to be true.

I completed, at glacial pace, my interview and examination. I prescribed Clonazepam and Imipramine, telling Barry to continue his Hydrocodone and Soma. He returned at the appointed time to report that his sleep was somewhat better, but his pain was absolutely unchanged. His wife commented to me, however, that she thought he was feeling better, and that his mood was certainly better. I enjoyed observing that he seemed to move about with a little less hesitation and a little less grunting. I scheduled him to return in three weeks, but it was three months before I saw him again. He was no longer encumbered. He moved about with ease, and I made a point to check his straight leg raising test. Both legs could be pointed directly above him to the ceiling, a full 90 degrees, with no pain at all.

"Barry, I was supposed to see you a couple of months ago. Why didn't you come in?"

"Well, Doc, I really didn't need to. I had enough medicine to last until now, and I was doing just fine. I feel a whole lot better, but I need some more of the medicine."

"How are you sleeping, Barry?"

"Sleeping real good, Doc, real good."

"And the pain, how is the pain?"

"Not so bad. The pain medicine keeps it in pretty good shape."

I saw him next six months later. He told me that he was doing just fine, and he had even gone camping and fishing with his boys—an activity undreamed of a year before.

I want you to think about something. If Barry's vivid exhibition of painfulness and suffering was the product of will from which he derived some reward (secondary gain), why did he stop doing it? Why did he abandon painful behavior if it was doing him any good? I suggest that he did not willfully abandon his pain behaviors any more than he willfully abandoned his sleeplessness, his depression, and his pain. They, under the aegis of pharmacy, *abandoned him* just as did his painful behaviors. Does that not make sense?

One last observation about Barry. His improvement at first was slow. It then gradually accelerated. In spite of no change in his drug therapy at all, he kept getting better and better. And I see this so often. Patients I have followed for years keep getting better, and I think this happens because with pharmacy, the infrastructure is restored (this happens over a matter of weeks), and then a brain, now integrated and resolute, exercises its own resources for recovery. What would happen if I elected to stop Barry's medicines? He just might maintain his improvement because his infrastructure had been repaired. I do not plan, however, to perform that experiment.

I saw Jim in company with his wife. He was a pathetic-looking man, disheveled and despondent. He was seated in a motorized wheelchair. He kept his gaze to the floor. I began my inquiries, and he said his trouble all began when he was born clubfooted. He had several surgeries on his feet, but they remained a source of pain. I asked him some details about the surgery—how many there were, at what age they were done, and the outcome of each of them.

He responded by asking me, "Do you want my mother to come in? She is outside, and she can tell you these things better than I can."

I was surprised by his comment, and I judged that Jim had, among his other problems, one of unusual dependency for a fifty-year-old man.

"If your mother wants to come in here, and if you want her in here, that is fine with me, but I am not sure that we really need her to provide the history. I believe you and your wife can do that very satisfactorily."

"Okay, we will let her stay outside."

I slowly extracted the history, and his clubfeet, it seemed, were repaired rather effectively when he was quite young. I discovered that he actually entered military service and performed satisfactorily in both active duty and reserve. I asked him how his feet stood up to that trauma, and he said only that he had to wear special shoes.

He described the appearance of back pain some twenty years before. Fifteen years into his painfulness, he finally came to unsuccessful spinal surgery. He then entered the care of a pain clinic where he was given epidural steroid injections and started on Oxycontin. Nonetheless, his pain gradually spread over his body, and the diagnosis of fibromyalgia was made. He was being treated with Amitriptyline and Oxycontin to a dosage of 160 mg. twice daily—quite a lot. He told me that he separated from the pain clinic at the prodding of his mother. He said she believed him to be a drug addict. He had reduced his Oxycontin to 40 mg. a day, and his pain had become excruciating. Formerly employing a cane to get about, for the past month he had been in a wheelchair.

"Tell me some more about yourself, Jim. What was your childhood like? Were you happy as a kid?"

"No, I was not happy at all."

"Were you abused in any way?"

He hesitated, his eyes down, and then said, "My father was alcoholic. He beat me."

"Tell me more."

"You see, Mother and Daddy had three daughters before I was born. Daddy always wanted a son, and he finally got that when he got me, but I was deformed, and he was ashamed of me. That is why he beat me. He beat me for several years, and then he left—he abandoned us."

"Were you sexually abused?"

"No, nothing like that."

"And your mother, tell me about your mother."

"Well, she has always been good to me, but I have a lot of stresses in my family. My mother says I am a drug addict. That is why I want to come off the Oxycontin. She is not going to let me have any peace until I do."

"And you are having more pain now as you have reduced the dose?"

"Yes, a lot more."

"How are you sleeping?"

"I don't."

"Are you depressed?"

"Yes, I am very depressed. I have been that way ever since the operation and probably before that." His wife nodded in agreement.

"Have you ever been suicidal?"

"Yes, I think about it a lot—but I am a coward. I couldn't do it."

"Have you ever seen a psychiatrist?"

"No, Mother said I really didn't need that. She said I ought to be able to get over this by myself."

I took a deep breath and reflected that I had seen few people who suffered despair like Jim.

"You told me you had been in the wheelchair for the past month since you started coming off the Oxycontin. Are you able to walk at all?"

"Yes, if you give me time, I will try to stand up and walk."

He performed the act with excruciating slowness, grunting and grimacing as he pushed himself up from the armrest and asked his wife to hand him his cane. He took a few hesitant steps, enough to tell me that there was no paralysis in the lower extremities. I asked his wife to assist him onto the examining table, and I excused myself—telling him that my nurse would come in and perform an electrocardiogram.

I purposefully delayed my return to the examining room. I often do this to allow my patient and their spouse or other family member time to think about my questions and share their thoughts with each other. It can be a pretty effective device. It was with Jim. He looked me in the eye for the first time and said, "I want to tell you that I was sexually molested by my father. I have never told anyone, not even my wife. She never knew about it until today."

Oh boy, sometimes I hear more than I want to and maybe even need to, but still it is probably better to get it out in the open.

"I am sorry, Jim, I am truly sorry. If it is any comfort to you, I have lots of people with chronic pain tell me the same thing. I assure you, you are not alone."

I performed my examination with particular reference to his very painful feet, which, it seemed to me, were the focus of his attention even though he had great pain throughout the rest of his body. His surgeons of many years ago had done a good job. His feet were not clubbed. They were quite normal in appearance. When I reached down to touch them, he writhed in pain.

"I am sorry I hurt you, Jim. I certainly didn't intend to do that."

"That's okay, I know you have a job to do."

"I will be as quick as I can, but I would like to check your ankle reflex. May I do that?"

"Yes, you may," he said as he gripped the sides of the examining table on which he was sitting, as if preparing for the torture. He screamed with pain when I struck the Achilles tendon on the right side. I elected not to do it on the left. There was one more test, I told him, and with that the evaluation would be complete. I put modest pressure with my fingers on the toenails of both great toes and asked him to push them upwards against my resistance. There was no movement at all. A total paralysis of dorsiflexion (up-going) of the toes. An interesting finding to be sure but incompatible with his ability that he had demonstrated so hesitantly early in the examination to take several steps across the room without slapping his feet in the manner expected of one with a foot drop. A conversion reaction if there ever was one. A form of conversion reaction also, I submit, was the extreme pain behavior invoked by merely touching the feet or tapping the Achilles tendon.

I told Jim that I was going to add Imipramine and Clonazepam to his therapy, and I also told him that the rate of his withdrawal from Oxycontin was unrealistic. I prescribed 40 mg. four times daily, about half of what he was taking before but certainly a step up from his current dosage. Jim was a train wreck, but still I had a good feeling. As I have written before, the presence of pain behaviors and conversion is usually a very good prognostic sign.

I was pleased but not really surprised when I saw him next. He walked into the examining room with the aid of a cane in each hand. He had abandoned his motorized wheelchair. He told me he was sleeping well and with Oxycontin achieving some measure of relief from his pain. He was more voluble and animated. I touched his feet—carefully and very lightly—and he evinced no pain.

Sometimes I hear more than I want to and maybe even need to, but still it is probably better get it out in the open.

On his next visit he came in using a single cane. His ankle reflexes were equal and appropriate, and my performance of the test gave him no pain at all. I asked him, as I had done before, to lift his feet against my resistance on his great toe, and he exhibited full strength and range of motion.

It was a month later when I saw him, for the first time in the company of his mother. He walked in without his cane and proudly introduced me saying, "My mother has her son back." We had a nice chat, and I elected to explore some issues—although there were a lot of issues I chose not to explore.

"How do you feel about your son taking these medicines?"

"I am happy he is taking them. I used to think he was a drug addict, but he is not, is he?"

"No, certainly not. I want him to continue taking them. They have a done a marvelous job for him. Do you have any problems with that?"

"No, I am happy to have my son back."

There was so much of Jim that I would like to know more about. His childhood traumas, his complaints of severe ankle and foot pain throughout his life even though he had been able to perform arduous military service for many years, comforted only by "special shoes." His remarkable dependency on his mother I chose not to explore, although I am sure there was much to learn. Jim continues to get better and better under my care, and I am satisfied with that. No need to look any further.

Carla's pain began some three years before she visited me. She had progressive discomfort in the back, but the orthopedist could find little to account for it. He advised physical therapy to strengthen the muscles of the back. Carla achieved a measure of relief, and she did rather well taking only an occasional Ibuprofen for flares of her back pain. Then, one day while vacuuming, her pain reappeared full force and radiated down her left leg. An MRI was done, but it was normal, and an electromyogram (EMG), which measures the performance of the nerves and muscles, was also normal. Carla's pain, which had become severe, sufficient to require the use of Hydrocodone for relief, was totally unaccountable. Such pain, be it in the back and leg or the stomach or the head, is the *bête noire* of most physicians. It is bread and butter, however, for the pain doctor because most chronic pains are, in the end game, quite unaccountable.

> *Most chronic pains are, in the end game, quite unaccountable.*

Carla was suffering badly. Her sleep was disturbed by her pain, for she was unable to find a position of comfort in bed. She lost her appetite and with it, twenty-five pounds of weight. She was unable to function as a beautician, and she took a leave of absence from work.

She was a comely brunette, but her face betrayed desperation, and the redundant skin of her neck was clear evidence of a recent and sudden weight loss.

"Carla, I know you are hurting badly. Let's see what we can do about it. I want to explore your illness and ask a few questions. They may seem a little beside the point to you, but they may be important."

"Go ahead. I will do anything to get well."

"You have suffered a great deal. Are you depressed?"

"No," she said emphatically and almost defensively. "I am not depressed. I am frustrated, and I am worried, but I am certainly not depressed."

Depression is, in the minds of many, a humiliating illness, a sign of weakness (we have already seen many examples of this). The notion that they are depressed, and therefore weak, is an affront to their sense of self-worth. This behavior is much less common now than it was a few decades ago. Lay persons now are much more sophisticated in matters medical than they have been in the past. The diagnosis of depression, and with it the prospect of recovery, is much less threatening now than in times past. Still, Carla's abrupt reaction to my simple and civil interrogation suggested that I had struck a nerve.

"Have you ever suffered depression in the past?"

"Yes, I know what depression is like, and I will never go through that HELL again!"

"Tell me about it."

"It came on all of a sudden. It was overwhelming. I could think of nothing but death. I was sure my husband and children were about to die, and I wanted to die. I was very anxious. The psychiatrist said I had panic disorder."

"When was this?"

"In my early thirties."

"Your treatment?"

"Prozac and Diazepam."

"Did they help?"

"My anxiety improved, but the depression didn't. It stayed with me. I tried several different drugs, but nothing really worked very well."

"But you did ultimately recover, didn't you? It seems you were well at the time your back began hurting."

"Yes, I eventually got better, but it wasn't due to the drugs. I made some adjustments in my own life and worked my way through the depression."

"Do you mind telling me exactly what you did?"

"Do we have to go there?"

"Yes, I very much want to go there."

"I don't like talking about this."

"I am sure, but please do. You will find me a sensitive listener."

"I had an unpleasant childhood. My father was very stern and demanding. I could never please him. He loved my brothers, but he didn't love me."

"You were abused?"

"Yes, I was emotionally abused, never physically."

"What was your relationship with your father like after you grew up and left the home?"

"Pretty bad. We could never get along. I went out of my way to avoid being with him."

"Keep talking."

"My psychiatrist suggested that I confront my father and tell him the way I felt about him. He thought that some kind of reconciliation would help me through my depression. He said that my depression and anxiety were a type of post-traumatic stress disorder."

"It seems, in my judgment, that the psychiatrist was probably correct. Did you and your father work things out?"

"Yes, quite well. He was understanding, and he apologized. It was a big thing to do, and I am sure it was hard for him, but we became good friends. That is when the depression went away."

"Do you still see your father?"

"No, I wish I could, but I can't. He died a few years ago."

"How did you handle that?"

"Pretty well, I think. I grieved a lot, but I was comfortable with my feelings about him and his about me. You see, my mother is very frail. She wasn't able to care for Dad when he was ill. I did most of the work. I was his caregiver for several months before he died, and he made me the executrix of his estate. Me, not my brothers."

"How did they react to that?"

"Not very well. There was some conflict, but I think that is mostly behind us now."

"A bittersweet experience, wasn't it?"

"Yes, bittersweet."

Chronic pain is a cruel illness. One of its cruelest ironies is that victims, traumatized in their youth by a parent, often, very often indeed, become caregivers when that parent grows old, infirm, and needful of help. I won't explore the psychologic mechanism that drives the abused to become caregivers to those who traumatize them, but it happens quite a lot. I am sure many readers have shared, and perhaps even benefited, by that experience.

"When did your father die, Carla?"

"Three years ago."

"That's about the time your back pain began, wasn't it?"

"Yes, come to think of it, it was. It was just a few months after he died." She paused for a few moments and then said, "You are not suggesting that my backache has something to do with my father's death, are you? Are you telling me my back pain is some kind of psychologic problem?"

"No, I assure you that I do not believe that your pain is a psychologic disease, but I think it may relate in some manner to some of the events that we have been talking about. Let me put it this way, your history is very typical. Chronic pain often appears after emotionally charged events. But you must understand this does not mean that pain is an emotional illness. Look at it this way, some people, and I sure you have heard of examples, suffer heart attacks or strokes during periods of profound emotional stress. That doesn't mean that their heart attack or stroke was a psychologic illness. It merely means that our emotions and our moods alter, sometimes in profound ways, the way our bodies behave. If a powerful emotion can actually induce blood to clot within the arteries of the heart or the brain, could it not also alter the way we perceive pain?"

"What you say makes sense, but I am not sure I can accept it."

"I am really not asking you to buy into it. Realize that I am just exploring your past history, and that is very important in helping me understand your illness. Not only understand it, but to treat it, probably successfully. The appearance of your pain shortly after your father's death may have been nothing more than coincidence."

I was lying.

Carla had a noticeable limp, favoring the left leg. I spent quite some time examining her. She had good strength all the way down from the hips to the toes. The reflexes were normal as was sensation. While I was examining her, she offered the observation that whenever she stepped with the left leg, she was unable to feel the presence of the floor on the bottom of her foot. She had that experience only when she put weight on the foot and at no other time. Strange indeed. One with a painful leg can certainly limp in order to protect that leg, but the appearance of numbness only when the foot strikes the floor was truly bizarre. I suspected that Carla just might be manifesting conversion disorder on top of her painfulness.

I prescribed Imipramine and Clonazepam. My intuitions told me that she probably was going to do well. I found myself liking her a lot. She had an engaging personality, and she had survived some of life's trials rather well, I thought. When I saw her again, she was not limping nearly so badly as before. I was expecting some kind of emotional embrace from her, but she surprised me. I was about to learn that Carla was not shy about expressing herself.

"I want you to know how angry I was at you when I left this office. I was angry at your suggesting I was depressed. I was angry that you thought I had some kind of psychologic illness. I told myself I wasn't going to come back to you, and I really wasn't. I had made up my mind, but about a week into my treatment, I woke up one morning and realized I felt better. I felt more energetic. My pain had lessened—a lot. I was astonished."

"I am happy for you, Carla. Let me thank you for sticking with me. I notice you are not limping as much. Are you aware of that?"

"Yes, I am certainly aware of that."

"And how about that numbness in your foot when it strikes the floor? Has that changed any?"

"It is not as bad, it's really not. Let me tell you something. I hate to say this, I really do hate to say it, but I think some of your ideas are right. I started getting better and was really pleased, and then something came up at home, and I had an argument with my husband. The pain came back just like before. It lasted about two days and then went away. I am afraid you may be right."

It went stunningly well for several weeks. I enjoyed my visits with Carla, and it was fun to watch her become ever more insightful and acquire some understanding of her illness. A few months in, we had a backset. Her son was arrested on domestic violence charges. When that happened, the pain all came back, as did the pain behavior limping and the numb foot. I elected to add a second tricyclic (heresy in the minds of some) in the form of Nortriptyline. She got better rather quickly. Whether it was the addition of my drug or simply the passage of time, I am not sure. She did, however, bring up an issue that concerned her.

"My husband says I moan and jerk at night and sometimes I talk in my sleep. He says that he often wakes me up to be sure I am all right. Is that an effect of the drugs?"

"Yes, it well could be. Are you aware that you are doing these things?"

"No, not at all. So far as I know, I am sleeping very well."

"This kind of thing can happen with the medicine, but if it is not bothering you, I think we can leave things as they are considering how well you are doing otherwise."

"I am quite happy with that, I just needed reassurance."

Sometime later, nearly two years into her treatment, she came at the appointed time in the company of her daughter. It was first time I had met any of her family. The daughter did the talking.

"The family wanted me to come in with mom today. We have concerns. Personally, I have not liked Mom very much the past couple of years. She has developed a mean disposition, and that is not like her. We think it is due to the antidepressants, and we want her to come off of them."

"Carla, is that correct? Are you having a disposition change?"

"Well, I suppose so. Everybody in the family tells me I have been grouchy and cross since being on these medicines."

"But didn't you feel better, a lot better, when we first started them?"

"Yes, I will admit I did, but I want to get off the antidepressants."

That visit was almost one year ago, and I remember it extremely well because it just seemed that something wasn't quite right. Carla had been doing, at least to my eye, extraordinarily well, and she exhibited great enthusiasm for her recovery. Why did it take two years to decide that the drugs were changing her disposition? And why the daughter's presence? It just didn't fit, and I had a feeling Carla wasn't telling me the whole story.

It didn't take long. Within a month, Carla limped into my office complaining of the reappearance of pain in the back and the leg and the reappearance, also, of depression and numbness in the foot. I prescribed Cymbalta, and a short while later she was back in fine form. It lasted three months. She developed, as people on Cymbalta sometimes do, sweet cravings, weight gain, sweatiness, and sedation.

"We are going to have to stop the Cymbalta, Carla. That is almost certainly the drug that is giving you the trouble."

"Okay, I am more than ready, but let's just stay off antidepressants. My family is really opposed to them."

"Why is that?"

"I think they are ashamed that I have to take them."

"But they helped you! They did help you, didn't they?"

"Yes," she sighed, "they really did help, but I want to go without them."

I was several months before I saw her again. She came in then to request that she go back on the Imipramine and Clonazepam again. We had a good chat. She told me that the medicines really didn't change her disposition. She thought them very effective, but her family wanted her off them. She was, she told me, merely submitting to their wishes. I recalled to her the visit of a year before when her daughter attended.

"She was just there to be sure I said the right things."

She went on to talk about her husband's verbal and emotional abuse, his insensitivity to her illness, and his need for control. She told me she intended to confront him, as she had many years before, her father. I wrote the prescriptions that she requested.

"It went well," she told me. "I am afraid my family just didn't understand how bad I hurt and how much the medicine was really helping me. I think they are going to be more sensitive to my needs now."

"A happy ending, Carla?"

"Yes, I really believe a happy ending. My husband and I have a very good relationship now, and looking back on it, it hasn't been very good for a long time. Now I have a question for you."

"Shoot."

"Are you going to write another book?"

"Yes."

She took my hand and squeezed it, her eyes widened, and her voice became angry.

"Then write about me! Tell people what it is like to suffer pain and to be made ashamed of it. Tell them what is like to feel guilty because you are sick. Tell them what it is like to be manipulated by your family when you are ill. Tell people they don't need to be ashamed because they are taking medicine. That is so important. It is important to me, and I know— I absolutely know—that it is important to lots of others out there. I want you to do this for me, I want you to write about me."

"I will, Carla. I promise you I will."

CHAPTER NINE

Drugs of Abuse

T om was fifty-five years old, and he had suffered with back pain for many years. He was referred to me by a psychiatrist I knew quite well.

"How long have you been seeing Dr. Hildebrand?"

"About four years."

"That's quite a long time. Could I ask why you are seeing him?"

"Because I work with him. I am a psychologist. I help him with many of his patients."

"Oh, I am sorry. I just presumed . . ."

"No apology necessary," he smiled, enjoying my embarrassment.

"I understand you have a problem with your back. Have you seen other doctors about it?"

"Only once. I went to an orthopedic surgeon a few years ago. He told me I didn't have any pinched nerves or ruptured discs. He said the pain was due to arthritis of the facet joints."

The facet joints are the articulating or moving joints of the spine, and like any other joint they can degenerate with arthritis and cause pain.

"Did he suggest treatment?"

"He told me that the joints could be injected, but I told him I didn't want anybody putting a needle in my spine. So he told me to take some Ibuprofen and live with the pain."

"How have you done with it?"

"I get by. I still work regularly, but I have an awful lot of pain. Sometimes I have to use a cane to get about. The pain seems to get worse at night. It really interferes with my sleep."

"Have you taken any kind of opiate or sleeping pill?"

"Most certainly not! I work at a drug treatment center, and I see many people who are addicted to drugs because of back pain. Besides, I am in recovery myself."

"From opiates?"

"No, alcohol."

A painful psychologist with a history of alcoholism. The plot was getting thicker. I asked Tom to tell me about his life, his career, and his alcoholism. We could get to the backache later.

"I am an only child, and I had a very good family. My father was a surgeon and my mother a chemist. She did some of the early work on Prozac."

"That is interesting."

"Yes, I am very proud of what my parents achieved with their careers. My aptitudes were a bit different. After I received my PhD, I began work for a drug company, mostly doing animal testing."

A painful psychologist with a history of alcoholism. The plot was getting thicker.

"Did you enjoy that?"

"Yes, at first I did. I was young, recently married, and making a very good salary. After a while, though, I became bored with it. It really was unfulfilling, and I started drinking. It took me a long time to realize I was an alcoholic. You would think a psychologist, of all people, would recognize the disease. I see it easily in others, but it took me a while to see it in myself. One morning I woke up and went into the kitchen, and instead of fixing a cup of coffee, I had a drink—whiskey—and that is when I knew I was in trouble."

"You entered a treatment center?"

"Yes, I have been in recovery ever since, almost twenty-five years now."

"What did you do then?"

"I made a big change. I moved to Sedona, Arizona, to work at a wellness clinic."

"I know Sedona rather well. That is sort of an epicenter for spiritualism and holistic medicine, isn't it?"

"Yes, and that is why I wanted to go there. I have always been attracted to the power of the mind to control the body and its discomforts. I do believe that there are energy forces that allow us to channel our emotional resources into wellness. I am a firm believer in yoga, and I practice it daily. I believe it helps my back quite a lot. Meditation is a powerful tool. Do you agree?"

"I certainly believe that yoga can be very helpful."

"And acupuncture, do you believe in acupuncture?"

"Let's just say I accept acupuncture. I am not quite sure I believe in it. I have had a few patients who have found it helpful, but most have not. Have you tried it?"

"Yes, and I'll have to admit it didn't help much. It has helped many of my patients, quite a few in fact, but it really didn't help me."

"I can understand that. Nothing works on everybody."

"I quite agree."

"You came here from Sedona?"

"Yes, my wife died six years ago. It was a very bad time. We had been together for thirty years. I rebounded and got married again, but too quickly. I soon realized that I had never come to grips with my wife's death, and I was agonizing over my decision to get married again."

"And that is when you decided to move?"

"Yes, there was a nice opportunity here. Half time at Dr. Hildebrand's office and half time at a very good treatment center."

"Are you comfortable with your professional life here?"

"Yes, quite. And I have been pretty successful in working through some issues about my marriage. We are doing well now."

"Let's talk about your backache now. When did it begin?"

"It is really hard for me to say, but it probably started shortly after I moved to Sedona."

"That was when you entered recovery, wasn't it?"

"Yes, come to think about it, that's correct. Do you think there is some sort of connection there?"

"Perhaps," I said. "It is strange, but I often see people whose pain began after they entered recovery from drug or alcohol abuse. I don't think it is coincidence. I just see it too many times."

"That is curious, indeed."

"Let me ask a few more questions. Have you ever suffered depression?"

"Yes, I am subject to depression. I have to work on that issue a lot."

"Have you ever taken drugs for it?"

"Yes, I have experimented a bit. I have tried Prozac, and it seems to help, but once I get in control, I stop it. I really think most of us can get by without drugs for the treatment of depression."

"I agree, many of us can, but some cannot. There is irony here, isn't there?"

"Yes, irony indeed. I am taking the drug my mother helped create, but I will admit I am ambivalent about using it."

"Tom, I have a big question for you. You have had pain for many years, and you have struggled with it, but you appear to have accommodated to it rather well. You are working and, I gather, enjoying your work. You seem to be inconvenienced by your pain, but you are getting by. You have seen, I gather, very few doctors. Why have you elected to come to me at this point in time?"

> *I often see people whose pain began after they entered recovery from drug or alcohol abuse.*

"Good question. I came because Dr. Hildebrand told me that you could probably help me. He told me you had good luck using antidepressants and anticonvulsants for pain."

"Well, I do have some success, but I don't think it is due to luck."

He smiled and said, "My apology."

"No apology necessary. I do think I can probably help you, but you must understand that some of the drugs I use carry the potential for addiction. Do you have concerns about that?"

"Obviously I do, and I am not going to take opiates. Nor am I going to have a back operation. Otherwise, I am certainly willing to consider your suggestions."

"I respect your concerns, and I assure you I will be very careful also about the administration of the drugs. But before we get into that, I would like to explore your past history a little bit more. Are there any other medical issues, particularly painful illnesses that I need to be aware of?"

"I have really been right healthy. I have had a problem, however, with interstitial cystitis."

"That is certainly a strange illness."

"It surely is, and painful. It hurts when I empty my bladder, and I have to do it very frequently. I wake up three or four times at night to void, and it always hurts. Do you know anything about interstitial cystitis?"

"Not a lot. I don't think anybody really understands the disease. It is certainly a painful condition, and it doesn't totally surprise me that you have a problem like that. Many people suffer multiple painful diseases simultaneously. I am not sure that is a coincidence."

"That is an interesting observation. I had never thought about it, but I see a lot of people that seem to have many different kinds of pain at the same time."

"When did your cystitis begin?"

"When I was in Sedona."

"It began about the same time your back pain began?"

"Yes, come to think of it, about the same time."

"Any other problems I should know about?"

"Irritable bowels, and that didn't begin when I moved to Sedona. I have had that all my life."

"How much of a bother?"

"It crops up under stress. When I have to meet a deadline or when I am pressured, I will have a lot of diarrhea and cramping." He smiled and added, "I had diarrhea all the way through grad school."

Painful arthritis of the facet joints, painful cystitis, painful bowels, alcoholism, and depression—all, as is so often the case—comorbid with one another.

"Tom, I want to start treatment with Imipramine, a drug with which I know you are familiar."

"Yes, I have no problem taking that at all."

"And also Clonazepam. You know that drug well, I am sure. It is potentially addictive, but in my practice I find that problem quite rare. I think the Clonazepam in combination with the Imipramine may help you a lot, not just your back pain but perhaps even your bladder and bowel discomfort. You may also find it helpful for your depression. I really think the risk of abuse is quite low. How do you feel about it?"

"I am sure I can manage the Clonazepam. I will be very careful with it."

Tom was taking a big step, accepting the use of drugs that for so many years he had told others to avoid. I told him that I respected his courage and that there was a fair chance he would be greatly rewarded.

Within weeks his sleep had restored, and his back pain diminished. His painful nocturnal voidings were reduced from three or four times nightly to one, and occasionally none. Even his bowels were calm. Two years into his treatment, he continues to do well. I see him only every six months for prescription refills.

Anne was a sprightly matron with two years of pain in her mid-back and left flank. Her internist and consulting neurosurgeon performed their obligations and found evidence of arthritic change in her spine appropriate to her age of eighty years. Epidural steroid injections were administered in a series of three. They were without effect, and the internist prescribed Hydrocodone 10 mg. four times daily. It did nothing, and Anne requested a stronger analgesic. Oxycontin was given, 20 mg. three times daily. Faced with the unhappy prospect of providing increasing quantities of opiates to an elderly lady, her internist referred her to me.

She was an utterly charming woman, graceful, alert, and intelligent. Her husband of many years had a successful career in the insurance business, and she was both socially and economically quite comfortable. I began my inquiries by asking if she was depressed.

"No, I am terribly frustrated, but I really don't feel depressed, and for that matter, I have never had that particular problem. Lots of my friends do, and I have always considered myself lucky to never suffer depression. It must be a horrible illness."

When I inquire about depression, and I invariably do, I am, of course, interested in the affirmative or negative answer but also in the manner in which my patient responds. Many victims of chronic pain are in depression but are either unaware of it or in denial. In the latter case, they often become, as we have already seen, defensive and over-reactive. Anne's response, given so circumstantially, suggested that depression was not a central issue. Yes, you can suffer chronic pain and not be depressed. It doesn't happen a lot, but it does happen.

"How are you sleeping? Does the pain keep you awake at night?"

"I sleep quite well at night. I take Oxazepam at bedtime, and it works quite well."

"How long have you used it?"

"Oh, I suppose thirty years or so. I've had a problem with insomnia for a long time, but the drug works just perfectly."

Oxazepam is one of the benzodiazepine drugs, akin to Clonazepam. It can be a very effective sleeping aid, and her physician made a very wise choice many years ago. It is remarkable when you think about it—that the drug could continue to work so well for thirty years.

I asked her about her energy, appetite, and mental focus. She denied any problem. Except for her history of disordered sleep, and that well controlled with pharmacy, she had absolutely none of the major symptoms that attend a state of chronic pain.

"Anne, you are taking both Hydrocodone and Oxycontin now. Are they helping you?"

"Very little, and that surprises me. I have never taken painkillers before, and I would have expected a lot more relief than I am getting. Can you explain to me why they are not working any better?"

"Not yet. Another question, please. Does your pain get worse when you are active, and does it get better when you rest or when you lie down?"

"Well, of course, if I am very active, it seems to bother me more. But most of the time it stays about the same."

"Is there anything at all that you can do that makes the pain better?"

"Yes, there is one thing that works every time—vodka."

"That really relieves your pain?"

"Absolutely. It removes the pain totally."

"How much vodka does it take?"

"Two vodka on the rocks will do it, but usually a third one helps even more. I drink them in the evening with my husband. They relieve my pain, and for a few hours I am quite comfortable. Then I take my Oxazepam at bedtime, and I sleep quite well. The pain is bad, though, when I wake up."

"So you have been drinking three vodkas every night since you have been painful?"

"Well, yes, but you need to understand that I have been drinking three vodkas a night for my entire adult life."

"That is a lot of vodka, Anne. Do you feel like it has ever been a problem for you? Have you ever felt like you were drinking too much?"

"Well, to be honest with you, I do occasionally feel guilty about it. But I never drink during the day, and I never get any sense of inebriation. It is just the way I relax."

"Let's go back in time, Anne. You've had this pain now for two years. Was there anything going on in your life when it started—difficulties with your children or your husband? Was there any kind of change in the way you lived?"

"Well, I suppose you could say so. My husband and I enjoy traveling. We go to Europe at least once a year. We were in Germany on the occasion of the 9/11 attack. We were stranded there and had to extend our stay for several days. I suppose I had time to ponder about certain things, and I don't really know why I did this, but I decided to stop drinking."

"You stopped drinking on 9/11?"

"Yes, I did. I didn't tell my husband about it. I just drank water while he was drinking his vodkas. A month later I told him about it. At the time I was quite proud of myself."

"Did you have any kind of withdrawal symptoms? You've consumed a lot of alcohol in your life. Did you develop insomnia or nervousness or tremors when you stopped drinking?"

"No, none at all. I really didn't feel any different. I didn't feel better, I didn't feel worse, but I was happy that I had stopped."

"Can you tell me with any precision when your pain began?"

"You know, I remember being uncomfortable on the flight home. It wasn't very bad, and I didn't think much about it, but over the course of a few months it got worse and worse."

"So your pain began shortly after you stopped drinking?"

"That is correct."

"And now you have obviously resumed your vodka habit. When did that happen?"

"It was maybe three months after I started hurting. The pain was so bad, and the pain medicine wasn't doing anything, so I took a couple of drinks. The effect was just miraculous. I wish I could drink during the day because I know it will relieve the pain, but I am not an alcoholic, and I don't want to become one."

Anne's termination of alcohol after many years of its use should have produced some kind of withdrawal. In the worst case this would have been hallucinations and convulsions (delirium tremens), but more likely it would be less serious—perhaps an interval of anxiety, tremors, or at least insomnia. She had none of these. Just why her good fortune is uncertain, but I suspect it was because she continued to take her sleeping pill each evening. Alcohol and Oxazepam are quite different drugs, but they both stimulate the neurotransmitter GABA, the brain's calming chemical. I am rather sure that if she had stopped both her vodka and Oxazepam at the same time, she would certainly have experienced a withdrawal, perhaps even a convulsive seizure. Fortunately, she continued her Oxazepam, and she had no problem at all except that she developed chronic pain. And that, I suggest, was a symptom of alcohol withdrawal, just as it was

Anne's termination of alcohol after many years of its use should have produced some kind of withdrawal.

in psychologist Tom. I have seen this scenario play out hundreds, if not thousands, of times. Usually the pain appears within a short while following the cessation of the drug, but I believe also it can occur years later.

Anne offered me some interesting treatment decisions. Although she achieved temporary relief with the reinstitution of alcohol, it was incomplete. I was faced with the prospect of treating an eighty-year-old woman who was doing poorly on the combination of Hydrocodone, Oxycontin, Oxazepam, and vodka. I wanted to find a happy answer as, fortunately, I had found in Tom. It was not to be. She did get better ultimately, but in way I had hoped to avoid.

I told Anne to continue her Oxazepam, and I added Imipramine, the same drug that had been so successful with Tom. It didn't work at all. In turn, I tried Cymbalta and Effexor. These are splendid drugs for the treatment of depression and pain. In the absence of depression (and Anne really was not depressed), they work less well. I then undertook an exercise that was intellectually attractive to me but turned out to be futile. I believed that Anne's use of Oxazepam had protected her, albeit incompletely, from alcohol withdrawal. Perhaps a bigger dose of Oxazepam, administered throughout the day, would relieve her pain. It didn't. I then prescribed in its place Clonazepam, a kindred drug but one with anticonvulsant properties and often helpful in the treatment of pain. It did no good either, and I had nowhere else to turn but to use more opiates. I offered Methadone.

Anne recoiled at the suggestion. "No, not Methadone, that is for heroin addicts. I am not going to take Methadone."

Many patients fear Methadone just as they often fear Lithium. Why these two drugs are so odious in the minds of the lay person is, I suppose, the connotations they invoke. Methadone for heroin addicts and Lithium for crazy people. I increased her dose of Oxycontin from 40 mg. to 60 mg. Just a week or so later, I received a note from her.

Dear Dr. Cochran:

I have been having second thoughts about increasing the dose of Oxycontin. The first dose I take in the morning makes me so drowsy, I doze off while trying to read the paper, and I fear that taking more would be a bad idea. If you agree, I would like to change to Methadone as we discussed on a previous visit.

Thank you for your help and patience,
Anne

At our next meeting I prescribed Methadone in a tiny dose, 5 mg. three times daily in addition to the Oxycontin and Hydrocodone. It worked—and beautifully.

"The perfect combination," said Anne. "There is no sedation, and I am comfortable now. I have almost no pain at all."

Years later, Anne remains well on Methadone, Oxycontin, Hydrocodone, Oxazepam, and three vodkas daily. It reads badly, but it is really not. She is happy, functioning well, and free of pain. The outcome wasn't perfect, but it was pretty close. In the pain business, you take whatever you can get.

I want to pause now and return to some of the material on neurotransmitters presented in chapter two. Let's look again at those systems that provide us with the sensations of comfort, pleasure, reward, and elation. These wonderful experiences occasionally occur in the course of our lives, when we fall in love or have some sort of spiritual revival. Recovery from serious illness (including recovery from addiction) often generates this kind of feeling, known as the flight to health. It can also be generated, and most commonly is, by the administration of pharmacy, both legitimate and recreational. The major neurotransmitter systems that are involved are GABA, which calms; opioid, which relieves pain; and dopamine, which is actually the reward or pleasure neurotransmitter. These three systems can, under provocation, collaborate and make us feel very good. They work with each other and work through each other. They are interdependent.

Now let's look at two recreational drugs, marijuana and alcohol, both of which can relieve pain (this effect is widely recognized). Marijuana stimulates the cannaboid receptors, and alcohol the GABA. In turn, both cannaboid and GABA stimulate the opioid neurotransmitter system, and it is the release of opioids that actually relieve the pain. We know this because Naltrexone, the opioid antagonist, will block the analgesic effects of marijuana and alcohol.

Marijuana and alcohol cannot only relieve pain, they can make us feel very good. This is because of the opioid release that they engender stimulates, in turn, dopamine, the pleasure and reward and sometimes craving inducing neurotransmitter. It is for this reason that Naltrexone, which antagonizes opioids, is actually being used for the treatment of alcohol addiction. Because of the blocking of opioid systems, dopamine cannot be stimulated, therefore, the pleasure derived from alcohol and marijuana—and the cravings—are diminished.

Now let's turn it around. If alcohol and marijuana can stimulate the opioid system and relieve pain, could not withdrawal from alcohol or marijuana create pain? Yes, almost certainly. Look at it this way. The frequent user of alcohol or marijuana is constantly stimulating the brain's pain-relieving opioid transmitters. As a result of this constant stimulation, the opioid system becomes, in a sense, fat and lazy. It is incapable, physiologically, of reacting as it was designed to do—that is, respond to the experience of pain. And this is exactly what happens on withdrawal from alcohol and marijuana abuse. The opioid system has become insensitive and nonreactive. It can no longer respond with the accustomed and nature-ordained purpose, and therefore the drug abuser in recovery may face, following painful injury or illness, a life of chronic pain.

The drug abuser in recovery may face, following painful injury or illness, a life of chronic pain.

I know I may have tested you with some of this, but I assure you the conclusions are physiologically quite sound. There are many examples of vital body functions that grow lazy and unresponsive when they are no longer required to exercise their proper functions by the administration of pharmacy that gives them no need to do so.

Candy escaped from her abusive, alcoholic father at age sixteen. She moved in with an older man, who she was soon to discover was a pedophile. That is when she started drinking, a habit that was to continue for some twenty-five years. She worked as a bartender and waitress and entered a lifestyle characterized by promiscuity and risk-seeking diversion. She was an aggressive mountain biker and rock climber. She told me she handled her liquor well—no DUIs, no loss of jobs. She was married for a few years, but it was unsuccessful and was terminated about age thirty. That was when her depression first appeared. She remained under psychiatric care off and on until I saw her some fifteen years later. She had been on several different antidepressants—Prozac, Wellbutrin, and Effexor—first one and then another. She was also on Alprazolam to control her progressive, alcohol-fueled anxiety. About age forty, following a drunken impulse to suicide, she made a phone call to Alcoholics Anonymous. Under the sponsorship of that organization, she entered sobriety and remained there for several years. She experienced, as many in recovery from drug or alcohol abuse do, the flight to health. She felt empowered by her achievement (as well she should have). But her demons were not to be assuaged, and she continued to recklessly seek excitement and danger. The end to her happiness came suddenly. She fell while rock climbing and suffered a ruptured lumbar disc. Surgery was performed. The disc was removed and pressure on the nerves relieved, but Candy continued to hurt in her back. Her depression reappeared, and therapy with Effexor and Alprazolam was reinstituted. After a couple of years of painfulness and depression, she resumed her alcoholic habit. Alcoholics Anonymous came to her rescue again, and she once again entered recovery, albeit painfully. Her internist started her on Oxycontin and then sent her to me.

This scenario is very typical. The victim of childhood abuse is, by virtue of that experience, scarred—emotionally and physiologically (if we must make the distinction between the two, and we shouldn't, for they are a single integer). Addiction in the young and depression in the young both often stem from childhood trauma and so does death-defying, risk-seeking, prove-you're-something behavior.

I pondered my options for Candy's treatment with care. She was on Effexor, Alprazolam, and Oxycontin when she came to me. She was depressed, unemployed, and painful in the back, and she had a history of recurrent alcoholism.

There is general agreement among those who practice pain medicine that a history of addiction to any substance of abuse does not preclude introducing drugs of potential abuse, but it does demand great caution. Candy was still attending AA meetings and encouraging others in the avoidance of alcohol, but at the same time she was taking Oxycontin and Alprazolam, both carrying the potential for addiction.

I elected to start her on Nortriptyline and Clonazepam. There was some redundancy in my choice of the latter because she was already on Alprazolam, and the simultaneous use of two benzodiazepines is viewed with some disfavor by those in the know—psychiatrists. She began to sleep better, but her sleep was disturbed by nightmares. I adjusted her drugs a bit and discovered that her nightmares were due to the Nortriptyline. I discarded that, and she achieved restorative, dreamless sleep—quite an achievement. Her pain, however, was unimproved.

"My psychiatrist said I cannot take the Clonazepam and the Alprazolam together. He refused to renew my Alprazolam."

"That's okay. You are sleeping better, and I am grateful for that. I will write a prescription for both drugs. Hang on for the ride. I am doing the best I can as quickly as I can."

We spent several weeks trying this and that drug. Along the way she requested Soma, a muscle relaxant and a potentially addictive agent (derivative of the long-ago Equanil). Reluctantly, I prescribed it. Give the patient the benefit of the doubt but remain ever vigilant. Several weeks into her therapy, Candy, the recovered alcoholic, was not only on Alprazolam, and Oxycontin but also Clonazepam and Soma. Nonetheless, she was sleeping through the night, and her depression had lessened at least a bit.

A few months into treatment, I elected to try Cymbalta. It is approved for the treatment of neuritic (nerve) pain, but I, and everybody else in the pain business, will use it for almost any painful state. It worked, and in spades! Her pain diminished, and her mood and energy improved. She was able to go back to work as a server in an upscale restaurant, her first employment in nearly five years. It took a lot of medicines, but I was happy with our achievement.

She did, however, offer me a little surprise just a few months ago. She told me that she was having problems with attention and mental focus and asked that I write her a prescription for Strattera, a drug she had been given in the past for attention deficit disorder (ADD).

"Candy, why didn't you tell me about this before?"

"Oh, I don't know. At the time it just seemed unimportant. I had bigger problems, but now that I am working, I am aware that my mental focus is not what it should be. Can you please give me the Strattera?"

"Happily, Candy, happily."

In a later chapter we will explore the relationship of chronic pain to childhood abuse, attention deficit disorder and its parent, bipolar disease, which is what I believe Candy had.

Will had experienced progressive back pain over the course of several years. A month preceding his visit to me he had undergone a lumbar fusion operation. The spinal fusion, whether in the low back (lumbar), the mid-back (thoracic), or in the neck (cervical) is performed to arrest the slippage of one vertebra away from another and to prevent damage to the spinal cord or nerve roots. Chips of bone are placed between the vertebral bodies to fuse them together and then the vertebrae are trussed with metallic rods and screws. It can be a huge, many-hour operation, particularly in the low back when the stabilization of multiple vertebral levels is necessary. A lot of bad things, including chronic pain, can appear after a spinal fusion.

Will did quite well for a while. He was given Oxycodone for post-operative pain, but after a few days had little need of it. His rehabilitation was uncomplicated, and within a couple of weeks he was walking two miles a day without difficulty. Then he suddenly developed intense pain in his back and numbness and weakness in his left leg. He called his orthopedist and was admitted to the hospital on an emergency basis. He required intravenous morphine to control his pain. A reevaluation of his spine was performed, and no cause for

As every physician knows, sometimes we have to confront God-knows-what.

his pain could be identified. His orthopedist called me, recounted the recent events, and asked if I could see Will that very day as soon as he was discharged from the hospital.

He was a handsome fifty-three-year-old. With morphine still floating in his veins, he was in a state of relative comfort, and the interview went well. He was many years married and had two children. He made a good living in the plumbing supply business. I asked a few leading questions, and he responded with great candor. He acknowledged that he was a many-year abuser of methamphetamine, cocaine, marijuana, and alcohol. He terminated their use some four years before his back surgery. He acknowledged that he had been subject to depression along the way, and since his pain had reappeared he was quite sleepless. He also told me that his pain was unbearable, and that I must provide him some kind of opiate therapy.

There was clear evidence of damage to several of the nerve roots of the lumbar spine. He had numbness over the left side of his calf and the top of his foot. He also had a foot drop—that is, he was unable to lift his toes off the floor. It is quite hard to understand exactly what caused Will's pain and the numbness and weakness in his leg to appear so suddenly a month after seemingly successful spine surgery. I have seen this kind of thing happen a few times. It is a God-knows-what. And, as every physician knows, sometimes we have to confront the God-knows-what. I prescribed Imipramine, Clonazepam, and Lyrica, a drug of proven value in the treatment of nerve pain. I also prescribed morphine.

I do believe that Will's pain related in some manner to his long history of drug abuse, even though it did not appear until a few years removed from his cessation of the drugs. I believe this effect is comparable to post-traumatic stress disorder. The flashbacks, anxiety, and depression of that disease usually begin shortly after the triggering event, but occasionally they appear years removed from the stressor.

Will returned at my instruction just a few days later. I saw him in the company of his wife. He reported that he was sleeping better on the medicine, and the morphine was doing a fair job of controlling his pain. However, there had been no change in his strength and sensation in the leg. I increased the dosage of his medicines and elected to give him cortisone for a few days on the suspicion that his nerve injury might have been some kind of allergic phenomenon, a reaction perhaps to the metal hardware implanted to stabilize his spine.

At the conclusion of the visit, his wife offered the judgment that even before the operation he was getting depressed, and that this remained after the operation. He was, in her words, "in a state of extreme fright and anxiety when the pain struck him." I thanked her for the information and invited the two of them to take a look at *Understanding Chronic Pain,* in which I devoted a great deal of attention to the appearance of inexplicable pains after recovery from drugs of abuse. They promised to do so.

I saw Will three weeks later. I entered the exam room to find him flushed and tearful, obviously upset. He hesitated to speak, and he handed me some notes scribbled, I suspected, while he was in my waiting room. Clue-giving if there ever was!

- *Lost confidence in myself*
- *Depressed*
- *Full of guilt and shame over drug abuse*
- *Emotions wild*

- *Cry a lot*
- *Thoughts of suicide*
- *Sold our business in order to use drugs, forcing my wife to find employment, and now she works all the time and I can't*
- *Empty nest. Both children moved out of the house*
- *Major surgery, afraid of outcome!*
- *Everything that I do, I do in excess. Working full speed, cannot take a break*
- *When doing drugs, I always try to do more than anyone else*
- *At least once a week a quick thought of suicide or killing somebody*
- *Short attention span at times*
- *I am just not the leader I once was*
- *Since surgery, my emotions are a wreck. I cry very easily. FULL OF GUILT AND SHAME!!!*

"Will, thank you for giving me this. I think it is going to help us a lot. It looks like you have had a problem with your emotions for a long, long time."

He hesitated and then whispered, "Yes, all my life."

"Do you think your drug use was an effort to control your emotions?"

"Yes, I am sure that is what I was doing."

"What happened to your emotions when you stopped the drugs a few years ago?"

"Really bad. More and more thoughts of suicide, more strange thoughts, less and less sleep. Thinking back on it, that is when my back pain began. I had lots of depression, and I hate to admit this—fear. I was frightened to death of that operation. I just knew something bad would happen."

"You have given me a lot to work with, Will."

"I read in your book about using Lithium. Can you give me some? I am sure I have bipolar disease."

"Demon there a long time, Will?"

"Yes, all my life."

"I will prescribe Lithium for you. I think it is a very appropriate choice. Be advised that if it is going to work, it will work pretty quickly— you will be able to tell a difference within a week or so. Continue the other medicines as before."

Will's notes told me a lot about his life and his drug use. They also told me a lot about his bipolar disease. "Depressed—emotions wild—short attention span—everything I do in excess—at least once a week thoughts of suicide or killing somebody."

Will was much improved when I next saw him.

"Everything is better. I really like the Lithium. My thoughts don't race through my mind anymore. I am not as restless. It is strange, but I don't feel as driven as I used to, and I am not nervous anymore."

"How about the pain?"

"It is definitely better."

"Still using the morphine?"

"Not so much, and I really don't like it. It is kind of sedating to me. Could we use another drug?"

"Sure—we will try some Hydrocodone."

"Okay, I have taken that before, and it doesn't disagree with me."

We are over a year into Will's treatment. He still has some weakness in his left foot and some numbness over his calf, but his pain is much diminished. He is using two or three Hydrocodone a day, and he has gone back to work.

When I wrote *Understanding Chronic Pain* and began giving talks on the subject, I anticipated resistance to some of the subject matter. I felt that my suggestions that pain may be the product of childhood abuse, which is certainly one of the most traumatic and sensitive experiences a being can endure, or that pain may be a symptom of manic-depressive illness (certainly an unnerving prospect for those who suffer chronic pain) would create offense. This has not happened. Most readers, the great majority, welcome the insights. My suggestion, however, that pain may be the product of drug abuse, and that it may appear as one enters recovery has indeed often given offense. I suppose the issue is so sensitive and the struggle to achieve sobriety so difficult that the notion that nature can extend a payback for past indiscretions is so disheartening that it is unacceptable.

CHAPTER TEN

Why I Fail

L ucas was a realtor. His back was progressively painful from spinal stenosis. The degeneration of multiple lumbar discs and the overgrowth of bony spurs had narrowed the spinal canal, compressing the nerve roots. Lucas was told that an operation was feasible, but there would be a possibility of nerve injury and perhaps even paralysis. The surgeon prescribed Hydrocodone and advised deferring the operation. Lucas found the drug quite helpful, and he was able to continue his active career. Repeat imaging studies done a year later showed no progression of his disease. The surgeon once again suggested delaying the operation. Lucas requested a second opinion, and his doctor endorsed the idea.

The consultant reviewed the original studies and did some of his own and reached the same conclusion. Lucas would be best served by waiting it out, taking the opiates, and submitting to surgery when his pain became so bad that he was unable to work effectively. He suggested referral to me, telling Lucas that perhaps a pain doctor could help keep his discomfort under control for a while, perhaps even a few years, until the operation became absolutely mandatory.

Lucas was in his fifties, well groomed, and handsome. He evidenced no distress as he moved about on and off the examining table. There was good range of back motion, and the reflexes were preserved. I commented that he seemed to be enjoying his vocational life, and aside from the inconvenience of pain, was not in any real way restricted from earning a living. He acknowledged this to be true.

I explored for the typical concomitants of chronic pain and found almost none. He slept well at night. His appetite was satisfactory. His energy was quite good, and he denied depression or any history of depression. His personal life, it seemed, had been exemplary. "I really have no vices," he said, jokingly. My instincts told me that he did not have the disease chronic pain. Prospects for success with neuropsychiatric drugs was low indeed.

Lucas interrupted my thoughts by saying, "I think if you just provide me with Hydrocodone, I will be fine. The neurosurgeon said you would do that, that you were a specialist in the treatment of pain, and I certainly have that. Do you think I should have an operation now?"

"Lucas, I can't make that judgment. That has to be left in the hands of the neurosurgeon. You are to remain under his care, and I will treat your pain as best I can."

"With the Hydrocodone?"

"Yes, with the Hydrocodone. Tell me how much you need."

"However much you want to give me."

"Lucas, that is unacceptable. You know how much pain you have. You have been taking Hydrocodone for many months, and you know how much you take. You must tell me how much you want, and if that is acceptable to me, I will prescribe it."

"Gee, I am not really sure."

This type of response may seem a bit strange to the reader, but it is a very common one, as if the simple declaration of the need for opiates in a specific quantity is an embarrassment. Understandable, perhaps, but also a clue about which there will be more in just a little bit.

"Well I guess four or five a day would be okay."

"That's okay with me. I will write it for every six hours, that is four a day."

"Well, let's make it five."

"Okay, I am writing you a prescription for Hydrocodone up to five times daily. That is one hundred fifty a month. I am providing them for you without question, and I will continue to do so as long as you are compliant with my instructions. I will see you again in a month."

"Thanks, this seems very reasonable to me."

It went nicely for quite a while. Along the way, at his request, I increased his Hydrocodone to six pills daily. He reported improvement on this program. He was able to continue his career, interrupted only by occasional visits to me for observation and refills. Respecting the demands on his time and comfortable with his compliance with my therapy, I moved his office visits up to every three months instead of one.

A digression here. I had the option of changing Lucas's opiate therapy from the short-acting opiate Hydrocodone to a sustained release preparation such as Oxycontin or MS Contin or even the naturally long-acting opiate, Methadone. Any of these, at least in theory, would have given him a more even level of analgesia and spared his liver the possible damaging effects of the Tylenol that is included in most Hydrocodone preparations. I elected to not do so because Lucas, to all appearances, was doing well. He was getting satisfactory analgesia, and he was tolerating the Hydrocodone without significant side effects. A cardinal rule in dealing with the human machine and its pharmacy is to leave things alone if they are working well.

Several months into his treatment, I received his latest MRI report and also a covering letter.

Dear Dr. Cochran:

I want to express to you my respect for your professionalism. It has been a privilege to meet you, and I am quite comfortable with your care. I want to advise you also that your staff is invariably courteous and pleasant, and I request that you offer them my appreciation for their many kindnesses.

Sincerely,
Lucas Gregory

A very nice note from an appreciative man, it would seem. But things are often not what they seem. The letter was a little too ingratiating, and ingratiation from a person dependent on me for the long-term prescription of opiates always gets my attention.

I receive many gifts from patients—home-cooked foods, flowers from the garden, hand-crafted items, or notes of appreciation. I accept these expressions of gratitude and affection with delight and humility. The physician is like everybody else. He enjoys being recognized for a job well done. However, when the notes are too fulsome in their praise—"you are the best doctor I have ever had"—or when the gift is of some, however small, financial significance, it is a warning. I occasionally receive gifts such as a pen or a pocketknife. Sad but true, most of the time these come from patients for whom I provide opiates. Nonetheless, I try to accept them as sincere gifts (although I always discourage such giving in the future). It is perhaps too easy to be cynical, and I try to avoid it. Nonetheless, boundaries are sometimes exceeded. The too-large Christmas basket with a bottle fine wine given to the "best doctor in the world" should and does invite my suspicions. Sometimes the gifts can be ludicrously generous. I have been offered the use of an apartment in New York City, a ranch in Colorado, and a villa in Acapulco, all by people receiving opiate therapy from me. There is absolutely no doubt about the intentions of these offerings.

> *A cardinal rule in dealing with the human machine . . . is to leave things alone if they are working well.*

Insurers that provide pharmacy benefits are able to track each of their clients' drug usage. When appropriate, they share this information with the prescribing physicians. The simultaneous use of drugs that have the capacity for dangerous interaction is called to the attention of the prescriber (or prescribers). Called to attention also is the simultaneous prescription of controlled substances, drugs with the capacity for addiction, by several doctors. Thus, if a person is receiving opiates from several different physicians, and particularly if that person is getting prescriptions filled at a number of different pharmacies (an almost certain sign of deceitful behavior), the information is shared with the physicians under high anonymity. The physician is not given the names of the other prescribers, only the dates and quantities of drugs prescribed. I had received a printout of Lucas's drug usage the same day I received his letter. I did not study it in detail, but I placed it in the chart to reference it when I saw him on his next visit.

Just a few days later, I took a call from Lucas's neurosurgeon.

"I need to talk to you about Lucas. I am afraid we have a problem here."

"Tell me what you've got."

"I got a pharmacy printout from his insurer. He is taking drugs from several different sources. I am supposing you are one of them since I referred him to you."

"Yes, I am prescribing. Go slow until I get his chart in my hands."

"I gave him a prescription for one hundred twenty Hydrocodone in January and another one in February. He also got a prescription for one hundred eighty Hydrocodone from another doctor in February. Was that you?"

"No, it wasn't me. I didn't start seeing him until mid-March."

It didn't take long to discover clear evidence that Lucas was receiving Hydrocodone from several different doctors. It looked like he was getting close to four hundred pills a month. He was also getting them from several different drugstores.

"Thanks very much for calling me. Where do we stand with things now? Have you seen Lucas? Have you confronted him with this information?"

"Yes, I just have. He and his wife were in here to go over the last MRI. I discussed the problem with them."

"How did they react?"

"The usual—outrage, anger, and denial."

"What do you plan to do now?"

"Well, I am sure not going to operate on him until we get this business straightened out. Do you have any ideas?"

"Well, we are in a no-win situation. The operation sure wouldn't help him. He would be taking more opiates after it than he did before."

"I agree."

"I guess the best thing to do is to see if we can prevail on him to see an addictionologist, and if we can't get him off opiates, at least we can control their usage. Maybe then you can think about doing an operation."

"Maybe, only maybe."

"Is he still in your office?"

"Yes, I wanted to keep him here until I talked to you."

"Let's strike while the iron is hot. Send him and his wife over here to me. I will work them in and see what I can do."

"Thanks, that is what I wanted. I will give you a little advice. Lucas is in absolute denial. He wife seems to have a little more insight. Maybe you can work on her."

"Thanks for the advice. While you are on the phone, let me ask you a question."

"Sure."

"How bad is that spinal stenosis? Is an operation absolutely imperative?"

"Not really. He has got some spinal stenosis but not a lot. Frankly, he shouldn't be hurting nearly as much as he says he is. He ought to be able to go several more years before he really needs an operation."

I prepared myself for one of the most unpleasant tasks a physician has to do: confronting the drug abuser. None of the attributes that the physician holds most dear—intelligence, the ability to measure evidence, and to treat his patient with sensitivity and compassion—is worth a hoot on the first confrontation with the drug-addicted patient. I knew I would meet hostility and resentment. Very probably I would be accused of being the problem. I was hopeful that Lucas's wife might be able to help me, but I discovered in short order that she had changed sides.

"It is just terrible to have to come to a doctor and be treated this way," she said. "It is horrible being told the things we have been told."

"I am very sorry, but sometimes people come to doctors and get very bad news. Sometimes people come to doctors, and they are told they have cancer."

"I know that. I have had cancer."

"I am sorry, I hope you are doing okay with it."

"I am," she said coldly. "Thank you."

I was already on the defensive.

"We have some data here that I need to go over with you. The pharmacy service has provided me with a record of Lucas's prescriptions. It looks like he is taking about four hundred Hydrocodone pills a month. That amounts to more than twelve a day. I was prescribing them at the rate of six a day. He is getting the rest from other doctors."

The wife was doing all the talking. "There has to be a mistake. Those records are wrong."

"They may be. I will accept the possibility of error. Here, I want you to look at the record and when you leave, give it to my receptionist so she can make a copy for you, and you can address that with the pharmacies or, if you wish, the insurer. If there is a mistake, I will certainly offer you my apology, but these records are usually pretty good. The pharmacies are very careful about that."

"This is humiliating."

"I know it must seem that way, but my intent is neither to humiliate or embarrass. Lucas has a problem, and it is my intent to help him through it."

"You don't understand. Lucas doesn't have a *drug* problem. He has a *pain* problem. You have no idea how much he hurts. I often see him crying in pain. He has to spend a lot of time in the car, and that is very uncomfortable. If he is with a client and having extreme pain, is he supposed to excuse himself and call you to see if he can take another pill? The idea is absurd!"

> *I prepared myself for one of the most unpleasant tasks a physician has to do: confronting the drug abuser.*

"No, he doesn't have to call me every time he needs an extra pill, but an extra six pills every day is unacceptable. If my prescription says six pills a day, it means six pills a day. It doesn't mean twelve. And both you and Lucas should surely recognize that. You should also certainly recognize that receiving opiates from several physicians simultaneously without their knowledge that you are doing so is not only deceitful, it is dangerous."

"So you are going to quit giving Lucas the drugs?"

"No, I never said that. Please listen to me. Lucas has a problem. It is an enormous problem, but it is solvable. There is way out of this, and I would like to help you find it."

"What do you propose?"

"I want Lucas to see an addictionologist. I want his input on where we go from here. I do need his advice before prescribing any more medicine."

With that statement, Lucas shouted at me, "Oh, my God! I am not a drug addict! I have spinal stenosis."

"I didn't call you a drug addict. I said you had a drug problem, and you do."

"You are abandoning me. That is what you are doing. You are abandoning me. You are supposed to be a pain doctor. You are supposed to help people with pain. You are not doing that at all."

"I am not abandoning you. If I were abandoning you, I wouldn't have asked that you come in to discuss all this. Please, Lucas, listen to me. There is a way to get well. I wish you would work with me."

"I will never work with you. You are a poor excuse for a doctor. You have no compassion at all."

His wife echoed the accusation. "You are the most insensitive person I have ever met. Your bedside manner is pathetic. I have never had to endure anything like this, and I am leaving. I want no more of you."

She left, the pharmacy letter in her hand. Lucas followed her, and on the way out turned to me and said, "You will hear from me about this. I assure you of that."

Lucas is at a crossroads in his life. He has ample resources for recovery. He has a successful career and a wife who obviously cares very much for him. He could achieve, with the aid of the drug Subutex, a comfortable withdrawal from Hydrocodone. Aftercare would be critically important, and this includes the ongoing support of physicians, his family, and most especially those who are themselves in recovery. This is easily possible of achievement but cannot be done until he abandons denial and accepts the horrible reality of his condition. If, however, Lucas does not come to grips with his disease and continues to suffer a pain problem rather than a drug problem, he will go from doctor to doctor. Sooner or later he will come to spinal surgery and his brain, constantly bathed by opiates, will lack the resources to recover from that painful operation, and his opiate need will ever increase.

It is perhaps hard to believe, but there is a very real possibility that following withdrawal from opiates his pain might actually diminish and also a possibility that he might never even need an operation. We have come, in recent years, to recognize the phenomenon of opioid hyperalgesia. That is to say, the administration of opiates can actually increase pain! This strange effect seems to occur in some people who have been on the drugs for extended periods of time. There is some thought that it might be prevented by rotating opiate therapy from one type to another. We don't know how often opioid hyperalgesia occurs, whether it is common or rare (it is probably somewhere in between), but the phenomenon does exist, and that is reason that termination of opiate therapy can diminish or even relieve pain.

Rebecca was an attractive sixty-nine-year-old with neuritis. Her feet and the lower portion of her legs were constantly and bitterly painful. I reviewed her past history. Her first husband had died some seven years before. She had become depressed and was given Paxil, it seemed with some benefit. She acknowledged that depression had been an issue with her several times in her life, but she didn't seem very eager to talk about it. She had remarried, happily she told me, and she and her husband wintered each year in Florida.

Her leg and foot pain had begun some three years before, and as is often the case, the exact cause of her peripheral neuritis was uncertain. Her therapy, initiated in Florida, had been rather aggressive. A dorsal column stimulator had been placed, and she described benefit from it. She was started on opiates early on and was currently taking Oxycontin at the moderate dose of 40 mg. every twelve hours. I asked her who had been providing her medicine before she came to me. She told me the doctors in Florida during the winter and her primary care doctor the rest of the time. He was, she said, reluctant to continue prescribing opiates and on that account referred her to me. I asked if she had any medical records with her. She said no.

A very frustrating answer. I did not really suspect that my patient was drug seeking. Her relatively advanced age and her evident affluence spoke against that possibility, but, as we have already seen, one never knows for sure. I admonished her to obtain some documentation regarding her drug use and her compliance with therapy. If she was not able to do so, I would be unable to continue providing her care. That said, there was no need for her going into withdrawal from Oxycontin on my watch, so I wrote a prescription for a month's supply and also a prescription for Nortriptyline and Clonazepam because she was sleepless and, I felt, still depressed.

She came back a month later to request some more Oxycontin. As she did so, she returned the other prescriptions I had given her telling me that she didn't feel that she needed any kind of antidepressant therapy. She had not obtained any of her medical records. She told me she was going to Florida in another month and would consult with her pain doctor there. I gave her another month's supply of Oxycontin and told her that I felt it best that I not continue her care.

Will Rebecca be a better person and a healthier person off opiates? Will I be a better doctor if she is off opiates? The answer to that is that we really don't know.

It was spring, and Rebecca was back. She appeared about as before, well groomed, quite pretty, and dressed colorfully and expensively. I guess she had a good memory, though, because she handed me a copy of her medical records from the doctor in Florida. The dorsal column stimulator had become progressively ineffective and had been removed, and she was now taking 300 mg. of morphine daily. An enormous dose! And certainly an escalation from the 80 mg. of Oxycontin she had been taking only a few months before. Nevertheless, her records indicated that she had been very compliant with this therapy.

"I know we didn't get along that well when I first came to you, but I really do need you. You must understand that I am having very little pain now, and I am asking that you provide me with the morphine."

"Well, okay. Rebecca, I am writing you a prescription, but that is an awfully big dose. I am not sure you really need that much."

"I know, but it is working well. My pain is not nearly as bad as it used to be."

We would probably be at 300 mg. of morphine a day yet but for an intercurrent event that turned out to be quite fortuitous. Rebecca developed pneumonia and was admitted to the hospital. Her internist, concerned about the high dosage of morphine and its depressant effect on respiration, certainly an issue of significance in a person with pneumonia, reduced her dosage while she was in the hospital and instructed her to follow up with me for further reductions.

This happens not infrequently. General physicians, unused to the quantity of opiates that pain doctors prescribe, are often alarmed. They will initiate a reduction in drug dosage and advise their patient to follow up with me for further detoxification. As if it was all so easy! It rarely works, but in Rebecca it did. She was taking 240 mg. of morphine when she came back to me and told me she felt better. She was eager for further reduction. We went down to 180 mg., and she told me her pain was actually diminishing. She was sleeping better and, she said, her mood was better.

We are down to 60 mg. a day now. Rebecca tells me that she has little pain. She was actually able to drive down to Florida with her son without making frequent stops to get up and walk about.

"Rebecca, you are going great! Let's keep going. Let's see if we can get by on 45 mg. a day."

"I would really rather not. I think I am at the right dosage. I don't want to change a thing. Can you understand that?"

"Yes, Rebecca, I do understand. We will stay at 60 mg. if that is what you wish."

I know, reader, that you want me to get Rebecca off opiates altogether. But why? Will Rebecca be a better person and a healthier person off opiates? Will I be a better doctor if she is off opiates? The answer to that is that we really don't know. As we go along, I may try to reduce the morphine some more, but Rebecca is happy with her treatment. Her pain is controlled, and she is doing more. I don't want the quest to remove her from opiates to become an ego trip for her doctor. I am happy to leave her where she is, at least for now.

The take-home lesson is that Rebecca suffered opioid hyperalgesia, and her pain diminished when her opiate therapy was reduced. How often could this kind of thing happen? The answer is—we really don't know.

Troy was a high school basketball coach until his automobile accident. His low back was badly damaged, and he required a spinal fusion. He was left with chronic painfulness. His orthopedist prescribed Oxycodone at the rate of one every four hours. Troy was unable to work, and several months into his slow convalescence, he took to drink. After an alcohol and Oxycodone debauch with furniture throwing and an attack on his wife, he was referred to me. Back braced and slow of gait, he nonetheless was an imposing, square-jawed, physical presence.

"Troy, I understand that you have been taking too much Oxycodone and mixing it with alcohol. Tell me about it."

Powerful and imposing though he was, Troy was not skillful with the use of words. "Aw shucks, Doc, that was nothing. They are making way too much of it. I just had a bad day. I was hurting real bad. I won't do it anymore."

"Troy, it may not have been much to you, but your orthopedist was very concerned about it. He wants me to manage your Oxycodone."

"Doc," he said, "that's not necessary. I don't have a drug problem. My problem is back pain."

"Troy, how much Oxycodone do you take?"

"Aw, Doc, I don't really know. I don't keep count."

"Troy, that is not an acceptable answer. How much of the stuff do you take?"

"I take a much as I need—sometimes maybe eight a day."

"Have you had a problem with alcohol along the way?"

"Doc, why do you have to bring that up?"

"It may be important."

"Yeah, I went into detox five years ago. I had been clean since that time, but, gosh, my pain was so bad the other day, I just had to do some drinking. It was the only way to stop it."

"And you took a lot of Oxycodone too?"

"Yes, I took a lot of Oxycodone."

"It looks like there really is a problem. Your orthopedist wants me to prescribe the Oxycodone. He doesn't want to do it."

"Well, if you want to do it, that's okay with me. I don't care where it comes from, I just know I need it. I really have a pain problem."

"Well, Troy, I'll do it, but we have to begin with a consultation with an addictionologist. I want his advice."

"An addictionologist! I am not a drug addict. Hell, you talk like I am some kind of horrible person."

"You are not a horrible person, but you have had problems before with drugs. Alcohol is a drug, and you had a problem with that. That is why you went into detox."

"Aw, that was nothing. This Oxycodone is nothing too. I just need a little bit to keep me going. I am sure not going to see an addictionologist. That is an insult!"

"Okay Troy, I won't be able to treat you. I am sorry it didn't work out. I wish you every success. I hope you get well, but unless you cooperate with me, I can't treat you."

"Shucks Doc, don't do me that way. Don't make me go see an addictionologist."

"Troy, the choice is yours. Either the addictionologist or back to the orthopedist. Maybe he can find somebody else to treat you. I am not going to do it."

It was hard not to love Troy. He carried frustration, but he didn't personalize his anger. Unlike Lucas, he never really got mad at me. He shook my hand and said, "Thanks for your time, Doc. I will go back and see my surgeon."

Troy's surgeon, who had been one of the most commanding figures of his life and the man who had seen him through the greatest travail, told Troy he would have to come back and see me if he wanted any more Oxycodone.

Nothing like a united front.

"All right Doc, I will go see the addictionologist. I don't want to, but I guess I have to."

"Troy, you are going to like the man. Just listen to him. I am not saying that we are going to deny you the use of opiates. You need pain relief, but we have to do it with some measure of control, and I need advice on how to do that."

"Okay, I will do it for you."

"No, damn it, Troy, you are not doing it for me. You are doing it for yourself—and your family—and you need to get that into your thick head."

"Okay, Doc, you are right. I understand."

I gave him a measured quantity of Oxycodone sufficient to last until his appointment with the addictionologist, and waited to see the results.

"I really like that guy. He didn't put me down. He told me he understood. He told me that he had been drug addicted. He knew what it was like. He made me realize I really do have a problem, that I could get in trouble real easy."

"What specific advice did he give you? Share it with me."

Troy gave me his signed drug contract. Under its terms he was to see me at frequent intervals and be given medication sufficient only until the next visit. He was to receive the drugs from a single pharmacy. If extra drugs were needed, I was to be informed, and absolute compliance with my instructions was mandatory.

"I can live with that. I hope you can."

"I can live with that just fine, Doc."

Troy and I had connected. I was charmed by his boyishness. I sensed that with a lot of time on his hands, he enjoyed his visits to me as much as I did.

"Troy, you are a young man. You have got a lot going for you. What are you going to do with the rest of your life?"

"I don't know, Doc. I want to do something, but I sure can't coach."

"Do you have any particular skills to help you find a job?"

"No, nothing outside of sports. Playing ball and coaching are the only things I really know."

"What do you enjoy doing? Are there pleasures in your life, are there things that really make you happy?"

"Being with my family makes me happy. I enjoy watching my kids play ball."

"How are you and your wife doing? She has been through a lot, almost as much as you."

"Yes, she has been through a lot. I love her dearly. She has stuck with me."

"How is your sexual energy? Are you performing okay there?"

"Aw Doc, not worth a shit. This is embarrassing. I hate to talk about it, but since you have asked, I am not worth two cents in bed."

"Is that a problem for her? Does it cause some discord?"

"Yes, I know it bothers her, but she never talks about it."

"Troy, have you ever read about Viagra?"

"Sure, everybody has heard about Viagra. I don't want to fool around with that stuff, Doc. That is embarrassing—having to take a pill for sex."

"Are you embarrassed about having a back injury?"

"Of course not."

"Are you embarrassed about taking Oxycodone?"

"No. I don't like it, but it is sure not embarrassing to me. I have got plenty of reasons to take it."

"There is no need for you to be embarrassed about taking Viagra. Sexual dysfunction is common after spinal injury like you had, and the Oxycodone you are taking can lower your testosterone level."

"Gosh, really?"

"Yes, really. I am going to give you some samples of Viagra. You can take them if you want. If you don't, that's fine with me, but I suggest you do. It is really worth a try."

"I tell you what, Doc, I am going to take one, and I am not going to tell my wife about it."

"Do as you wish."

I gave him two packs of Viagra samples and a prescription for another month of Oxycodone.

When he returned, he had a smile on his face and said, "That's good stuff, Doc."

"Did you tell her you were taking Viagra?"

"I didn't have to. She knew I was taking *something*!"

"It has been good?"

"Real good, Doc. Really good. It did her as much good as it did me."

"Did it hurt your back when you had sex?"

"Not near as much as I thought it would. You know, it is kind of funny. My back hasn't been hurting as much the past month. I am taking a little less Oxycodone."

People with chronic pain . . . don't need distrust. They need trust.

Troy and I had come so far. I wish the story had a happy ending, and maybe it does, but I suspect not. The months went by, and there were more and more calls for extra Oxycodone. Then, another alcohol-induced, life-threatening event. What should I have done? Should I have given him more opiate? Would that have relieved his pain and diminished his need to seek relief in alcohol? Or would it have merely increased his risk of killing himself—or perhaps somebody else? Or should I have sent him back to the addictionologist for a detox? Would taking less opiate have diminished his pain as it did in Rebecca? Or would it only have made his pain worse?

Troy solved the problem for me. He left me to find another doctor. Whether he has improved as a result of that exercise, I do not know, but I am not terribly proud of my performance.

A word now about the drug contract. Its use is standard operating procedure in virtually every pain clinic in this nation, and I don't like it. It demands, in my judgment, that the signer supplicate himself to the prescriber. Moreover, it doesn't just imply distrust; it articulates it. And people with chronic pain, even those on opiates, don't need distrust. They need trust. If they are taking advantage of me, I will discover it sooner or later, but I don't like telling my patients that I distrust them. I have never had a patient who has signed a drug contract for me get better. And I have had a lot of them who didn't sign a drug contract get a whole lot better.

Antonio was a medical corpsman. After a tour of duty in Afghanistan, he returned a broken man. As his post-traumatic stress disorder evolved, he became anxious, sleepless, and depressed. He experienced flashbacks of his combat experiences throughout the day and nightmares of them at night. He was driven to a suicide attempt. Fearful and unable to place the muzzle in his mouth or against his head or chest, he chose, with his knowledge of anatomy, to place it over his femoral artery in the groin, knowing that he would in short order bleed to death. He pulled the trigger and missed almost everything. Neither the femur (thigh bone) nor the femoral artery was damaged. The femoral nerve, however, was nicked resulting in weakness in the leg and numbness and pain over the anterior thigh.

Following surgical repair, his anxiety and flashbacks continued and became mixed with rapid mood shifts between tearful despondency and manic hyperactivity and rage. A diagnosis of bipolar disorder was made, and he was treated with anxiolytics and mood stabilizers and discharged from military service. His medications were supplied by Veterans Administration, but his mood swings were poorly controlled, and when he obtained his Medicare benefits, he consulted a private psychiatrist—an extraordinarily good one. Electroconvulsive treatments were given, and with these and the administration of Cymbalta, Abilify, Neurontin, and Hydrocodone for pain, he settled down at least a little bit. His restless mania and agitation were controlled, but he remained despondent and suicidal. After a few months of ongoing hopeless despair and another attempt at suicide, his psychiatrist elected to try a new and heroic form of therapy, the placement of a vagus nerve stimulator.

I have already written about the transcutaneous nerve stimulator and the dorsal column stimulator. Both of these forms of electrical stimulation create a counter stimulus, an electrical shock that overrides or distracts from pain (the same effect as rubbing the knee forcefully after it has been bumped against a hard object and is painful). The vagus nerve stimulator induces no tingling or buzzing. It works in quite a different manner. The vagus is the tenth of the twelve cranial nerves (arising from the brain itself rather than the spinal cord). They serve many functions including vision, taste, hearing, facial movement, and visceral activity. The vagus serves the latter. It is dedicated to cardiovascular and intestinal functions. Curiously, the right (the vagus nerves are paired) carries messages from the brain to the viscera, and the left carries messages from the viscera to the brain. If the right vagus nerve is stimulated, the heart rate slows, sometimes drastically, and for that reason the vagus nerve stimulator is always applied to the left. The nerve can be surgically approached in the neck, and the electrodes and battery pack placed in a manner not dissimilar to a cardiac pacemaker. We can suppose that the stimulator floods the lower brain with energy and activates the neurotransmitter system housed there (serotonin and noradrenaline and probably GABA). It has been FDA approved for the treatment of refractory depression and epilepsy and is being studied experimentally for the treatment of migraine.

"The stimulator helped me a lot, Doctor. I am sure I would have committed suicide by now. But I have a lot of pain in my leg, and I am still depressed. Can you help me?"

"Well, maybe," I said almost breathlessly. I have seen a lots of tough clinical problems, but this was one of the most remarkable I had ever seen. It was also my first exposure to the vagus nerve stimulator. "What are you taking for your pain now, Antonio?"

"Hydrocodone, and it is not doing anything."

Antonio's psychiatrist had performed admirably. I wasn't about to intrude on his pharmacy, but I was willing to introduce a stronger opiate. I wrote a prescription for Oxycontin 20 mg. every eight hours. I patted Antonio on the back as he left and crossed my fingers. I had no idea how this was going to turn out.

When I see a new patient, I use the initial consultation to analyze the problem and employ whatever abilities I possess to begin treatment. I enjoy that exercise greatly, but I enjoy even more the second visit, the first return, because when I enter the room, I can tell right away whether or not my patient is better.

On Antonio's next visit, there was a calmness and eye contact that I had not seen before. I knew my drug was hitting the mark, and he told me so.

"My pain is a lot better, Doc. It is a whole lot better."

"How about your mood? How is that?"

"That is the same thing Dr. Smith asked me. You two are a lot alike. My mood is a better taking the Oxycontin. I am not as depressed as I used to be."

"Keep taking Dr. Smith's medicine just as you have been, and I will see you again in a month."

I received a call from a pharmacist a few days later. She expressed concern. Antonio had presented her a prescription for ninety Oxycontin tablets. He told her that he wanted to pay cash for it rather than submitting it to Medicare. This is an alarm signal for pharmacists, and she did some investigation. She discovered that he had received a month's supply of Oxycontin under my signature the same day at another pharmacy. I asked her to fax the prescription to me, and it was a blatant forgery. Antonio had either found a blank prescription in my office or had photocopied and altered the one I had given him (it is not hard to do). My prescriptions, indeed most doctors' prescriptions, have two lines for signatures on the bottom. One is inscribed with *substitution allowed* and the other *dispense as written*. I routinely sign mine on the *substitution allowed* side. This allows the administration of generic (and cheaper) medication. Antonio (or somebody else?) had forged my name on the right-hand side, *dispense as written*. I guess he wanted the good stuff.

> *Opiate overuse*
> *is the most*
> *vexing issue*
> *in the field of*
> *pain management.*

I told the pharmacist to not honor the forged prescription and to have Antonio call me. I heard nothing. And then he returned, to my surprise, for his scheduled appointment a month later. I confronted him with a copy of the forged prescription and told him that I wanted to work with him (and I truly meant that), but that I needed some explanation for what had happened.

He denied that he had done it. He expressed no remorse and exhibited no particular anxiety about the matter. I told him that unless he was more forthcoming with me, I would have to terminate his care. With no emotional display whatsoever, he got up and walked out of the examining room.

This is, indeed, the saddest chapter. Antonio's psychiatrist had treated him with great energy and diligence. His vagus nerve stimulator cost Medicare many thousands of dollars, and it had helped him, or at least it seemed. My contribution was modest, but I had done my best, I am afraid, to no avail. Early in this book I wrote that I could substantially help 80 percent of my patients, and that when I failed, I usually knew why. Lucas, Troy, and Antonio occupy most of that 20 percent.

I hope that you, reader, have the same sense of frustration reading this that I had in writing it. These three men offered me no closure, no resolution, no understanding. I have, unfortunately, seen many—too many—such patients, and I have learned almost nothing from the experiences. (I will admit that Antonio's vagus nerve stimulator and his Oxycontin-induced mood stabilization—if indeed he was telling me the truth, and I believe he was—certainly got my attention.)

Opiate overuse is the most vexing issue in the field of pain management. And it is one not given to simplistic solutions. Were my patients truly
addicted? Were they craving their medicine for a sense of well-being? Or
did they simply need more to control their pain? Were they just hoarding
the drugs in anticipation of being deprived of them somewhere along the
way? Were they diverting, that is, selling their drugs? Were they giving
them to a friend or family member who suffered pain and was unable to
receive appropriate therapy? Or were they using their drugs to treat not
their pain, but their mental illness? (Remember bipolar Will from chapter
nine. He was using drugs of abuse to control his erratic mood swings.) I
never find out. And that is what is so frustrating. No closure, no resolution,
no understanding.

CHAPTER ELEVEN

Analgesic Rebound

C indy was thirty-three years old and the mother of two. I would come to know her well, but on this first visit, her mother would do most of the talking. She presented me with a strangely bifurcated question. Should Cindy submit to my care or should she go to a famous headache clinic in the Midwest?

I responded that the decision must rest with Cindy. If they wished, I would certainly review the case history.

Her mother said, "We are prepared for that. Here is a copy of Cindy's medical records."

She handed me several pages of notes from the neurologist who had attended her the past three years. I quickly scanned them and saw that Cindy had been given a remarkable number of drugs.

I commented, knowing that I would strike a nerve, "Cindy, you have been taking an awful lot of medicine, haven't you?"

She answered with the lament I hear so often from those who suffer chronic pain. "Yes, I've taken a lot of medicines, and I hate it. They are not doing me any good, and I want to get off of them. I just want to get well."

I responded, as I almost always do to that declamation, by telling Cindy that the problem was not that she was taking a lot of medicines. The problem was that they weren't working.

"No, they are not working at all. I have been with that doctor for three years, and I am not one bit better."

"Let's go back to the beginning. When did your headaches start?"

"Cindy had her first headache when she was eighteen years old. I knew what it was. I have migraine myself."

I directed my voice to Cindy and asked when she first sought medical attention. It did no good. Mother kept on talking.

"I took her to my internist. He had helped me with my headaches, and I thought he might help Cindy. He prescribed Amitriptyline. He said Cindy was depressed, and that the drug might help both the depression and the migraines."

"Cindy, did it help?"

"Yes, I remember that I felt better on the drug, and the headaches kind of settled down. I had them only occasionally."

"How long did you take the Amitriptyline?"

"I am still on it."

"Here is a list of the medicines that Cindy has taken for her headaches. I've typed it out for you. The ones with the asterisk are the ones she is taking now."

Drugs for migraine. Drugs for pain. Drugs for sleep. Drugs for depression. Drugs for anxiety. And none, it seemed, had really worked. The neurologist had shot virtually every arrow in the quiver but had not hit the mark.

I have been guilty many times of searching hopefully and perhaps carelessly for the perfect drug, the one that will cure everything. Such is the allure of the new pharmacy. I have learned, however, that the scatter-shot approach rarely works. Most of the time when I hit the mark, it is the product of thoughtful study and deduction and not chance.

In most patients with chronic pain, there is more than meets the eye. I was sure that would be the case with Cindy. I knew it would be tough, very tough, but I really wanted to treat her. A few days in a headache clinic wouldn't cure her, just as a few days with me wouldn't. It would take time, lots of it, to somehow trace the evolution of her painfulness by studying the life events which dictated its behavior.

"Cindy, I see that you have two children. Are you married now?"

"Yes, I am married."

"Your first?"

"No, this is my second marriage."

"Tell me about it."

"I got married when I was twenty-two. I left him after eight years."

Mother, who seemed expert in such matters, said, "He was a very controlling person."

"Did he abuse you, Cindy? Did he beat you?"

"No, he never struck me. The abuse was verbal and emotional. He tried to dictate everything I did, even the clothes I wore."

"Was he the father of your children?"

"Yes, I have two girls. They are six and eight years old."

"What happened to your migraines when you were pregnant?"

"At first they were really bad, and I know why. When I got pregnant, my obstetrician told me to stop taking the Amitriptyline. Whenever I had done that before, the headaches always got much worse. So I had a rough time for a few weeks, but then the headaches went away. I was free of headache for the rest of my pregnancies. Months without a headache—that hasn't happened very much."

A curious feature of migraine is its behavior during pregnancy. It tends to flare with increased frequency of attacks during the first trimester and then, almost always, it goes away although in some women, as they approach term, migraine erupts again. The influence of hormonal shifts on migraine is well known, but why they should express themselves in such a strange temporal pattern is really beyond understanding.

I cannot contest the internist's choice of Amitriptyline for the treatment of Cindy's migraines and depression. It did help, and I probably would have done the same thing myself. However, at age eighteen, Cindy's young mind was still developing and building an infrastructure that would provide, hopefully, a life of wellness. The introduction of Amitriptyline (and I am not picking on

In most patients with chronic pain, there is more than meets the eye.

that particular drug—it could happen with many others) into such a brain will, in a sense, alter the infrastructure. Over the short term, this is good—relief of migraine and depression. Over the long term, however, Amitriptyline is incorporated into the cerebral machinery, and it becomes a necessary ingredient in that organ's function. In the absence of that ingredient, the disorder it was given to control (migraine) reappeared full force—a rebound effect, if you will.

It was time now for another question, one I routinely ask of the female patient with chronic pain. "Cindy, did you have a problem with postpartum depression?"

She responded, as in reaction to most of my questions, tersely and without emotion. "Yes, I had a deep depression both times."

"How long did they last?"

"Three or four weeks."

"And then they went away?"

"Yes, I started back on the Amitriptyline, and they went away."

"What happened with the headaches after your pregnancies?"

"They came back about like before."

"What were they like? Tell me about them."

"I'd have a sense of nausea and sometimes sparkles across my vision, and then I would have pain, usually on one side of my head, sometimes both, and it was pounding. I could feel my pulse in my head, and I would have to go to a dark, quiet room. Light and sound, particularly sound, would make the headache much worse."

"How long would they last?"

"Oh, a day, sometimes less."

"That certainly sounds like migraine."

"I know."

"How often did you have them?"

"Well, looking back on it, I can see that they were becoming more frequent. After my last pregnancy, I was having two or three a week."

"Do you have any idea why?"

Mother again. "The marriage was coming apart. He started running around."

"Tell me about it, Cindy."

"He had lots of girlfriends. I divorced him three years ago, but even after he left, he stalked me a lot. He's a real pest."

"Three years ago? That is when you started seeing the neurologist, isn't it?"

"Yes, the headaches were really bad then."

"Tell me about them."

"Well, I still had the migraines, but I had another kind of headache also. It wasn't like a migraine. It didn't come and go. It was a constant pain, like my head was in a vise."

"Did the headache keep you awake at night? Were you able to sleep?"

"I slept pretty well, but it was a heavy sleep. By then I was taking lots of different medicines. You've got the list."

"How did you feel when you woke up in the morning?"

"Drugged."

"Why are you leaving the neurologist, Cindy? Is it because you are doing poorly, or did he suggest that maybe a second opinion was in order?"

Mother again. "It was my decision. On our last visit there, he said something that sounded very strange to me. He said that Cindy had analgesic rebound headache, and he told us that she would have to stop the Hydrocodone that she is taking for pain. He even said that stopping the medicine would probably make the headache go away. He told us he was not going to write any more prescriptions for pain killers."

"And that bothered you?"

"You are darn right it bothered us. He was the one who prescribed Hydrocodone in the first place, and of all the medicines she has been given, that is the only one that really helps her. She couldn't get by without it."

"Is that right, Cindy?"

"Yes, I don't see how I could get by without it."

"Cindy, are you depressed?"

"Yes, very depressed. It is this pain. I have had it three years, every day. I don't think it is ever going away. I don't have much to look forward to."

"Let's go back and talk about the headaches some more. Your records indicate that chocolate and alcohol are triggers for your migraines. Is there any kind of trigger for the constant headache? Is there anything that makes it worse, or is there anything that makes it better?"

"No, I just can't figure that out. All I know is that I have a headache all the time and that it gets worse every afternoon."

"About what time?"

"About two o'clock in the afternoon. I wish you could explain to me just why this happens."

"I won't try to explain it because I don't know why it happens. But I think you will be interested to know this kind of appearance of pain at a certain hour is very common. If it is any comfort to you, you are not alone. You have lots of company."

For the first time, I saw a hint of a smile in thin-lipped Cindy.

"You mean other people have this? Their pain gets worse at a certain time of the day—at the same time every day?"

"They certainly do."

"It all seems so unnatural. I have been afraid to tell people about it. I was afraid they would think I was crazy."

The science of chronobiology is the study of variations in the body's behavior along the dimension of time. Many of our physiologic and emotional activities, and very clearly some of our diseases, are dictated by rhythms, the body's clock, if you will. The most fundamental and inviolate rhythm, because it is life-giving, is the beating of the heart. Most of the other body rhythms are dictated by the mind, and the most important of these is the diurnal or circadian rhythm, a twenty-four-hour cycle commanded by the earth's rotation on its axis. The single most meaningful attribute of existence, consciousness, is altered along this dimension of time with, give or take, sixteen hours of wakefulness and eight of sleep. During this sleep-awake cycle, there are enormous variations in hormonal release and visceral function—and the perception of pain. We have already seen that many pains appear exclusively at night. Even the very act of thought may be profoundly influenced by circadian rhythms. How often have you awakened in the morning with a good idea, one derived while the brain was supposed to be resting?

Another important biologic rhythm is dictated by the moon's orbit around the earth. This is, of course, the twenty-eight-day menstrual cycle.

> *Many of our physiologic and emotional activities, and very clearly some of our diseases, are dictated by rhythms.*

During the fluctuations in hormonal activity that occur in the female according to this rhythm, there are also certainly changes in mood, and probably in the perception of pain. Many women with chronic pain of any type will report that it worsens during menstruation.

A third major rhythm is that commanded by the earth's rotation around the sun. This annual rhythm gives us seasonal and day length changes and certainly influences us in many ways. I have already written of the appearance of pain or depression (or both) according to the dictates of the calendar.

Annual rhythms also impose command on us by their influence on cultural habits, religious faiths, or personal experiences. The annual Holy Days for which some cultures fast and others feast certainly alter our mood (the Christmas blues). Anniversaries, whether they mark birthdays, weddings, or most especially the death of loved ones, are a much under-appreciated influence on our emotional and physical health, and I have already written about that subject. Thus, in addition to celestial rhythms, there are experiential or personal rhythms that are individual to each of us.

It has been suggested that many periodic diseases, those which recur, either regularly or randomly along the dimension of time—examples are depression, mania, migraine, multiple sclerosis, and as we have seen, pain —occur not by chance but rather by the influence of one body rhythm upon another. Their appearance may be created by the intersections of several different rhythms, both natural and experience derived. These intersections create, just as do musical instruments, a harmonic, a new rhythm derived from but independent of its origins. Was it some harmonic that dictated that Cindy's headache worsened every day at 2:00 PM? We can't be sure, but we know it wasn't by accident. It will be a long time before we figure out just how and why this happens, but it does.

Cindy's pain was the product of a complex constellation of her genetic heritage (migraine—and perhaps depression also), a series of life experiences, and very certainly celestial forces. It was a vastly complex, indeed unfathomably complex, derivation of all of these. On top of this, her physicians only made the matter more complex by introducing, over the course of several years, drugs that could alter her body's rhythms and harmonics.

Yes, there are drugs that can change the body's rhythms. Think of sleeping pills and birth control pills.

I didn't share these ponderous thoughts with Cindy. I only told her that we would go back to square one, removing her from as many drugs as possible. That done, we could start over, adding one at a time, and waiting a while to observe their response. I prescribed a step-wise reduction in most of her medicines but told her to continue the Amitriptyline. She had been on it for fifteen years, and it was part of her cerebral machinery. It didn't appear to be helping her much at this time, but I was rather sure that stopping it would create some problems.

When I saw her next, there was a quickness in her step and brightness in her eyes. The headache had disappeared.

She remained on Amitriptyline at night and Hydrocodone during the day, taking two or three pills beginning in the afternoon when her headaches became severe. I added Clonazepam to be taken at bedtime. Cindy, now removed from several of her sedating drugs, had become quite sleepless, and Clonazepam is helpful for sleep. Strangely, it was one of the few drugs that she had not taken before.

On follow-up a couple of weeks later, she reported that the drug was helpful. Her sleep was much improved.

"Do you feel better? Is your mood any better?"

"Yes, I believe so. Just getting a good night's sleep would help anyone's mood."

"Has your headache changed any?"

"Not at all. It is hurting just like before, and I need for you to give me some Hydrocodone."

"I will do that, and I am going to give you another medicine also. I am writing a prescription for Imipramine. It is a tricyclic drug, similar to the Amitriptyline you are taking now."

"Does that mean I can stop the Amitriptyline? I really want to get off of it. I've been on it so long."

"Once you get on three or four Imipramine pills, you can try to slowly reduce the Amitriptyline, but please go very slowly. I am not sure at all that you are going to be able to come off it."

I saw her next two weeks later.

"How are doing, Cindy? What do you have to report?"

"Not much. I did what you told me, and I tried reducing Amitriptyline. The very next day I had a terrible headache. I am afraid you are right, I suppose I am just stuck with the drug."

"What time of day was that headache?"

"In the morning. It hit me as soon as I woke up."

"So I suppose you got back on the Amitriptyline?"

"Yes, of course."

"What happened then?"

"The next day I had a headache just like before."

"At two o'clock in the afternoon?"

"Yes."

"Okay, Cindy, so far so good. It may not seem like we are getting anywhere, but we may be. You are sleeping better, and we know one thing that is very important. You are at least tolerating the Imipramine. We will push the dose up."

When I saw her next, I thought there was more spontaneity than I had seen before. She was a little more expressive and animated. Her features seemed less frozen and her behaviors less strict.

"You look better, Cindy. I hope you are feeling better."

"Maybe I am. The headache still bothers me, but it seems to be coming on later in the day. I still hurt, but you have given me a couple of extra hours a day with freedom from headache. It is hard to believe, but every time I add another Imipramine pill, and you told me to do it every five days, my headache would come on a little bit later, like twenty or thirty minutes. It is hitting me now about four o'clock in the afternoon."

"Cindy, we are doing great. You might be interested to know that your experience of the pain striking later in the day is really not unusual. Many of my patients express their improvement not only in the reduction of the severity of the pain but also the time of its appearance."

"That is interesting."

"Now, let's see—you have been taking a 10 mg. pill, and you are up to seven of them now. For your convenience, I am going to give you a larger pill, a 25 mg. size. You will start taking three of those each night and gradually increase to six. Understand?"

"I do."

She didn't. That night, she took seven of the 25 mg. pills, and she continued to do so until ten days or so later when, realizing her mistake, she called me.

"Are you having problems taking that many?"

"No, not at all. Actually, I am feeling much better. My headache is less severe, and it is not coming on until eight o'clock in the evening."

I told Cindy that probably no harm at all had been done. We were aiming for that dosage anyway, she just got there a little quicker than I wanted. I did suggest that she come in for blood levels because she was now taking two different tricyclic drugs in rather high dosages. The levels were acceptable, and Cindy was showing improvement. I told her to work her way up to ten of the 25 mg. pills. I also told her to be patient, that time was on her side. The medicines we were using were actually doing nothing less than rewiring the mind, and that enterprise often takes quite a while.

When I saw her next, there was quickness in her step and brightness in her eyes. The headache had disappeared, and she was experiencing no side effects at all. She told me that she was excited about a special event. Her husband was in the U.S. Air Force Reserve and had been called up for duty in Iraq. Friends were gathering at her house for a sendoff party.

The body's clock can certainly be influenced by drugs. It can also be influenced by life events, and saying good-bye to a husband going off to war is a life event of the first magnitude. I knew that Cindy's happiness at the prospect of gathering with friends would be short-lived, and I suspected that her recovery would be, also.

It was a month or so later when she showed up.

"Nothing is going right. I haven't heard from my husband. My father needs cancer surgery, and Mother is too busy with him to help with the children." She was fighting back the tears. "The headache is back. It is worse than ever, and I know what you are going to ask me. It is coming on now as soon as I wake up. Sometimes I even wake me up at three or four in the morning with a headache. What am I doing to do?"

Cindy, under the stress of a husband gone to war and a father ill with cancer, decompensated and recruited those maladaptations that had been a part of her life for three years—depression and pain. I was hopeful that Cindy's worsening was merely an adjustment reaction, and that with time it would go away. I was hopeful also because, with pharmacy, we had achieved restoration of wellness. For a short while her infrastructure had been healthful. Maybe that would sustain us.

"Cindy, we are going through a rough time here, but I believe you will get better soon. We are just going to have to endure some bumps on the road. I want you to increase your dose of Clonazepam and the Amitriptyline, and I will give you some more Hydrocodone for pain. Don't give up. There is light at the end of the tunnel."

She really opened up. We talked about her controlling mother, and she told me for the first time that she had entered counseling for depression and her relationship with her parents even before the headaches got so bad. She discovered that her husband had been very careless. She found a lot of unpaid and overdue bills, and she was strapped for money. She confessed to me that she was very unhappy in her new marriage. I gave her a hug and told her that I thought her backset was temporary. With time and a little more medicine, I held hope that she would get better.

It wasn't very long before I received her authorization to send her medical records to the famous headache clinic in the Midwest. They have forwarded their results of their examination and their progress notes, and it seems they are not doing very well with her at all.

I do not think that Cindy's headaches made her unique and somehow different from those who suffer other forms of chronic pain. But her disease is one of the more common states of painfulness and one that I believe is often misunderstood and mistreated, so I want to spend a little time discussing transformed migraine and analgesic rebound headache.

Migraine is a disease of episodic headache with a very distinct symptomology, well described by Cindy. It begins with a prodrome of a sense of unwellness, sometimes with mood change (depression) and sometimes with nausea. In its classic form, it is characterized by some disturbance of vision, most commonly scintillations (sparkles) in the visual field, and sometimes a loss of vision to one side. Then there appears a pounding headache, often with predominance on the left or right side and with it photosonophobia, a heightened sensitivity to light and sound. The victim seeks refuge in the dark quiet place, and if able to fall asleep often experiences relief of pain. There are many variations to this theme, and few victims experience all of these effects, but most experience some.

An important attribute of migraine headache, indeed its defining feature, is that with time, it goes away. Migraine, in its typical form, is a distressing disease but a self-limited one. It is a disease of periodic pain, not incessant pain. When the headache doesn't go away, be this in a matter of hours, days, or even a week or two, it is no longer migraine. It is something else, that which we recognize as transformed migraine. With the transformation of migraine into chronic pain, there comes a change in the defining features of what used to be migraine.

> *Migraine, in its typical form, is a distressing disease but a self-limited one.*

Visual effects diminish. The characteristic pounding pain is replaced by a constant squeezing or boring discomfort. Headache becomes generalized and no longer left or right side predominant. Sleep becomes disturbed and energy lost. With all of these comes depressed mood. Indeed, it is probably depression that is the actual agency of transforming migraine into chronic pain. As might be expected, transformed migraine does not respond to the triptans that can be so effective in the treatment of typical migraine. It does, however, respond to a host of drugs that we use in the treatment of chronic pain, including those that I used for Cindy.

I suspect that Cindy, under the stress of her divorce, entered depression. Typically, when the migraineur (one who suffers migraine) becomes depressed, there is an acceleration of migraines in both frequency and severity, and then comes the transformation into chronic headache.

Interestingly, treatment of transformed migraine often diminishes the incessant headache, but it sometimes restores migraine to its previous vitality. This strange scenario can play out many times in a person's life with their pain moving back and forth between typical migraine and the constantly painful transformed migraine. Indeed, the two can occur together—chronic headache punctuated by periodic attacks of migraine.

That which we now call transformed migraine was formerly identified as tension headache. I abhor that term and, fortunately, it is disappearing from the lexicon. Sure, the woman with chronic headache is tense, but she doesn't have headache because she is tense. She is tense because she has headache that nobody knows how to treat. Fortunately, as we come to better understanding of what chronic pain really means, all that is changing.

Cindy was told that she suffered analgesic rebound headaches. She was given Hydrocodone for the relief of pain by her neurologist, and then three years later was told that she must stop the Hydrocodone in order to get well. Before pursuing the issue of analgesic rebound headaches, I want to offer you another case study.

Dr. Cochran:

I am in the process of reading your book and am amazed that I am reading about myself. I have had to stop and cry several times, but I hope to finish it this weekend. I have been suffering for more than three years. It began with migraines during treatment for my endometriosis. Then, following a hysterectomy at age twenty-nine, I began experiencing a constant painful headache that is unrelenting. I have been to six or seven specialists (mostly neurologists), and I have had epidural injections and even acupuncture. I have tried dozens and dozens of medicine with little or no improvement. I am still experiencing migraines, which are responsive to Frova or Maxalt. This time I am being treated with Cymbalta, a Duragesic patch, and tons of various PRNs. I have been hospitalized three times in the past six months and have gone to clinics/ERs/Dr. offices dozens of times for a pain shot.

Your method of treatment sounds so promising, and perhaps that is what I need to restore some sort of quality of life. I live a couple of hours from Nashville and would be glad to travel for a consultation.

Thanks,
Judy Harbison

Judy was a registered nurse, and her husband was a school teacher. They had two children. She had, since her teen years, suffered typical migraine headaches, but they were quite infrequent, rarely occurring more than once or twice a year. Judy told me she more often suffered "sinus headaches." (I have written before that most sinus headaches, particularly those that recur, are in actuality migraine, albeit not in the typical or classical form.) She denied any issues of childhood trauma, and prior to her illness had never had a problem with anxiety or depression.

The evolution of her chronic pain unfolded with remarkable clarity. At age twenty-seven she developed painful menstruation due to endometriosis. In an effort to arrest her disease and to relieve her pain, she was given the hormone-altering drug Lupron. Her menstrual periods ceased, and her pelvic pain was greatly diminished. But, as often happens in the migraineur, hormonal manipulation made her headaches worse. Judy's migraines were no longer infrequent. They occurred two or three times a week. They were at least somewhat responsive to the triptans Frova and Maxalt, but they were such a bother that she elected to discontinue the Lupron therapy. When she did, her headaches diminished in both frequency and severity, but her pelvic pain returned full force. It was there all the time, not just during menstruation. Hysterectomy, the definitive treatment for endometriosis, was performed at age twenty-nine. Within but a few days, weeks at the most, there appeared in her words, "a constant painful headache that is unrelenting."

> *In my heart I believe that there is an answer out there for just about everybody.*

Judy had developed, with remarkable suddenness, depression and, with it, chronic pain in the form of transformed migraine. She was sleepless, fatigued, forgetful, and she began to crave sweets. Over the course of three years, she gained sixty pounds. Two years into her illness, she had to give up her job.

She presented me with a list of the medicines she had taken. It rivaled in length that of Cindy's. She was also currently on very aggressive opiate therapy including the use of Duragesic, a very powerful opiate applied as a skin patch. In spite of this, she required frequent hospitalizations and emergency room visits in an effort to at least temporarily relieve her suffering.

I thought that Judy's care (as well as Cindy's) had been well thought-out and appropriate. Both had been given most of the drugs that should have helped, and yet none of them did. I saw with Judy, as I did with Cindy, that there was not a lot of wiggle room for me, but I happily accepted her as a patient because in my heart I believe that there is an answer out there for just about everybody.

"Judy, how often do you have your migraines?"

"Oh, maybe two or three times a week. The Frova helps some of the time, and sometimes I use Maxalt, but neither one is working very well now."

"How about the constant headache, the unrelenting headache that you described?"

"It is always there, it never goes away. It is a squeezing pain all over my head like a vise."

"Tell me about your depression."

"Oh my God, am I depressed. I cry a lot, I see no hope for the future, and I have two young kids to raise."

"How is the marriage doing?"

"We are hanging on, but I know that I am a burden on him. He's been wonderful."

"Do you think about suicide?"

"Not yet."

"Judy, I want you to continue the Cymbalta that you are taking, and I will write a prescription for the Duragesic patches. I am also starting two new drugs, Imipramine and Clonazepam. I think we have a chance of helping you."

She returned a couple of weeks later reporting that she had a few days without headache, and she was grateful for that. I told her to increase the dose of the Imipramine and Clonazepam, and I prescribed the drug Actiq. It is the same drug that she was using as a skin patch, although it is administered as a lozenge on a stick (a lollipop) for her to place between her gum and her cheek when her pain was most severe. She requested something to take for her lesser headaches, and I prescribed some Hydrocodone. Judy would be on a lot of painkilling medicines.

I received a call a couple of weeks later from her husband telling me that the Actiq was working quite well, but Judy was taking a lot of it and needed a prescription for more. I saw her several days later. She was upbeat and positive and told me that she was sleeping better and feeling less depressed.

"That's good, Judy, I am happy for you, but let me ask you, any more emergency-room visits?"

She cast her eyes down and said, "Yes, a couple."

"What did they give you?"

"Demerol."

"How are you fixed on the Actiq and Hydrocodone?"

"I need more of them."

"Okay, I will write you a prescription for more, but Judy, you are a nurse and you know your way around. I am sure you know in your heart that you need to get off these painkillers."

"I know that, and I know I will never get well this way, but I want to tell you something that we didn't talk about before. One of my neurologists told me I had analgesic rebound headache. He told me that I absolutely had to come off the painkillers."

"What were you taking at the time?"

"Mostly Hydrocodone, but I was seeing lots of doctors, and I had a lot of different pain medicines. I was taking some Oxycodone and some Demerol also."

"How long had you been seeing that doctor when he made the diagnosis of analgesic rebound headaches?"

"Oh, six months or so, I suppose."

"Did you do what he said? Did you stop the medicines?"

"Yes, I did. He refused to give me anymore, and I went cold turkey."

"And then?"

"The worst six weeks of my life. My pain was excruciating. He finally put me back on the Hydrocodone, and then told me he had nothing more to offer. He suggested I consult with another neurologist."

"You have had lots of disappointments with this thing, haven't you?"

"Yes, lots of them. I am so frustrated. I want you to know something. I don't have a life. I used to be pretty. I was a homecoming queen, but now I am fat. I can't play with my children. I am so depressed, and I hurt so much, I don't even want to get out of bed in the morning."

"Judy, you know you have to come off this stuff, don't you?"

"Yes, I know I have to. I can't go on like this, but I am afraid. You understand, don't you? I am afraid."

Opiate addiction is difficult of definition. One of the best efforts I've heard, however, is that it occurs when more of the drug doesn't make the patient better. This certainly applied to Judy. Under my care she was taking more opiates than before, but her description of an occasional good day notwithstanding, she clearly was getting worse. Her visits to the emergency room had not diminished at all. We were six months into treatment, and my drugs were not working.

I don't believe that Judy was craving opiates for euphoria. She was craving them for relief of pain. She probably was suffering the disorder known as pseudoaddiction. She was hoarding the drugs and getting them from multiple sources—not to satisfy a craving, but to protect herself from pain.

She was hoarding the drugs and getting them from multiple sources—not to satisfy a craving, but to protect herself from pain.

We believe that the opiates are so commanding and dictatorial in their influence on the brain's function that they actually negate the influence of many other drugs. In the presence of opiates, Depakote, Topamax, Keppra, Imipramine, Clonazepam, and all the others that we use to prevent migraine simply don't work very well. Hopefully, with removal of opiates, they could start to exert their benevolence. It was time for consultation with an addictionologist.

Judy had something really important going for her. She had insight. She didn't tell me that she had a pain problem, not a drug problem. She knew in her heart that she had both, and she knew that she was never going to get well until she came off painkillers. Her commitment to see an addictionologist was an act of great courage. She had been through withdrawal once, and it had been a bitter experience. She was fearful of doing it again, but it had to be. She was admitted to the hospital and after a tearful, despondent first day, she achieved, under the sponsorship of Subutex, an uncomplicated withdrawal from her opiates.

Recovery from opiate addiction (or pseudoaddiction) is, we would like to think, a miraculous event, and it is. But the notion that with recovery from addiction the person will live happily ever after is naïve, and we have already seen examples of that. Judy's three years of opiate use had, in a very real sense, rewired her brain and altered the infrastructure. It takes a while, sometimes a long while, to rewire that organ back into wellness.

Judy did get better off the opiates. Her constant, unrelenting headache (transformed migraine) went away. She could play with her children again and, she told me, she awoke each morning hopeful for the new day. She had even taken a canoe trip with a church group, an activity unthinkable but a few weeks before. Unfortunately, however, her migraines began occurring with ever-greater frequency, and there were more emergency room visits for opiate injections. I didn't really expect her migraines to go away when we stopped the opiates. I did believe, however, that freed of opiates she would respond to one of the many splendid drugs we have for the prevention of migraine. I tried several of them again, (she had been on most of them before), but they simply didn't work. I had failed my patient, and I had no recourse but as an act of mercy to resume the Actiq lollipops, which had indeed been effective pain relievers. Maybe, at the least, I could keep her out of the emergency room. I had to tell her, and it broke my heart, that I had nothing more to offer. I suggested referral to a colleague at the university.

I was hopeful that the new neurologist, younger and more attuned to contemporary technology than I, would suggest placement of a vagus nerve stimulator. Experimental and dramatic therapy to be sure, but it just might have worked. It was not to be. He prescribed an anticonvulsant that Judy had taken before and told her it would be a long while before it started working. He also told her that if she had a severe migraine, she could come to the clinic for the administration of intravenous Depakote, a sometimes dramatically effective treatment for the acute migraine. Judy complied, and after a two-hour, head-splitting automobile trip, she was admitted to the hospital and given Depakote intravenously. It did not work at all.

I hate failure worse than God hates sin. I have written that when I fail, I usually know why, but I don't know why I failed with Judy. She had so many things going for her—a devoted husband, healthy children, and parental support. She had an education, and she had skills. Her depression and her transformed migraine had been lifted by withdrawal from opiates (at least most of them), but her migraine attacks have defied virtually every known form of pharmacy for that disease.

She is ever in my mind—and my heart. I keep in touch with her by periodic e-mail.

Her response to the most recent:

Dr. Cochran:

Thanks so much for contacting me. Things are a little different for me these days. I spent ten days at the Atlanta Headache Clinic, where I saw Dr. Harold Richardson. My headaches continue on a daily basis, but I am semi-functional, and I think I am heading in the right direction. His first step was to get me off narcotics . . . again! It went much easier this time than the last. He had a pic line in me and treated me with all kinds of concoctions. He used a "triple shot" to treat acute headaches—it is a combo of Ativan, Haldol, and Cogentin. It works at least 75 percent of the time—though I have to use it more often than I'd like. I'm also on Methergine for a few days, which is supposed to break the bad cycle I am in now. The biggest change is that I am on Nardil as a preventative. It hasn't had time to do much, but again, I am hopeful.

I will let you know how things progress. I will return to Atlanta in December, so we will see how it goes. I miss coming to see you, and it means the world that I am still in your thoughts.

Take care,
Judy

Both Cindy and Judy were told by their physicians that they had analgesic rebound headache. The fact that they were told this by the same physicians who prescribed the analgesics in the first place is, in the most favorable term I could use, ironic.

In my opinion, analgesic rebound headache is really not a disease. It is merely an expression of a very common effect of pharmacy. It is kindred to hundreds, if not thousands, of other rebound phenomena, and analgesic rebound headache does not deserve the importance it is given by identifying it as a disease. Nevertheless, this is what has happened, and the story of how it has happened, at least as I perceive it, is a sad one indeed.

Sure, people will rebound from analgesics. That is to say, symptoms reappear (often worsened) when the duration of the drug's activity ends. This will certainly happen with opiate analgesics (and disciples of the rebound headache school believe the same thing will happen with Tylenol, aspirin, and non-steroidals). It matters not, however, whether the analgesics are given for headache, or for painful neuritis, or for lumbar disc disease, or for irritable bowels, or whatever. Rebound pain will occur in all. There is no need to dignify the rebounding headache as something special, different, and unique from all of the others.

The rebound phenomenon occurs throughout all of pharmacy. If a person with hypertension does not take his medication at the appropriate time intervals, the blood pressure will rebound and rise, sometimes astronomically high. If the diabetic does not take her insulin in a timely manner, the blood sugar will rebound—again often quite high. People with depression rebound when they miss a few days of their antidepressant, and people with anxiety rebound when therapy is not taken appropriately. If the epileptic stops the anticonvulsant therapy that controls his seizures, he will, I assure you, rebound. There are many other examples—almost countless examples—but I think you see my point. The symptom or disease for which a drug is successfully administered will reappear if that drug is not taken appropriately and in a timely manner, sometimes extravagantly so.

Cindy got well, at least for a while, without stopping her Hydrocodone. I never gave any serious thought to terminating her analgesic therapy (her use of it was modest and appropriate, and it did give her some relief). I did feel that it was necessary to bring Judy off her analgesics. She had to be detoxed not because she had analgesic rebound, but because her use of opiates was dangerous and perhaps even life-threatening. Moreover, removal from the (usually) depressant opiates would correct that disease and free her from the transformed migraine that accompanied it. Lastly, there was the hope that off opiates, one of the many drugs we use for the prevention of migraine would work; but sadly, it was not to be.

Now let me present you with a very common clinical scenario. The drug Imitrex was the first of the triptans for the treatment of migraine. Drugs of more recent derivation have in some measure supplanted it for one reason. Many migraineurs report

The stress imposed on the physician by repeated failure becomes intolerable. The doctor, a human being like the rest of us, employs a defense mechanism.

that although Imitrex will relieve the migraine, the pain often returns after a matter of some four to six hours. This is recognized by all as a rebound effect, comparable, we would certainly surmise, to an analgesic rebound phenomenon. Now, would the physician tell his patient that if she simply stopped using the Imitrex, the migraines, for which it was given in the first place, would go away? No, of course not. But that is exactly what was told to Cindy and Judy. The disease for which the drug was given would go away if they simply quit using the drug that controlled their disease. Would we tell the hypertensive that his high blood pressure would go away if he stopped using drugs to control it? Or the diabetic his insulin? Or the arthritic his cortisone? I have never, in my entire career, seen a patient with headache get well simply by withdrawing from opiates—or Tylenol, aspirin, or non-steroidals. And I do see a lot of them getting well by the application of appropriate drug therapy for their chronic pain even while they are still on painkillers.

Cindy's and Judy's physicians (including me) were, and I can assure you of this, highly frustrated by their inability to get their patient well. As the office visits continue and the sense of failure pervades, the stress imposed on the physician by repeated failure becomes intolerable. The doctor, a human being like the rest of us, employs a defense mechanism. He exercises transference. He transfers his responsibility, his guilt, and his blame away from himself where it belongs, onto the patient. "If you will just quit taking those pain pills, your headache will go away." By this mechanism, the patient is forced to assume responsibility for recovery from her disease. It is not the doctor's problem anymore.

It hurts to write this, but I must. The analgesic rebound headache is well known to all neurologists. Indeed, it is probably the most common diagnosis in all neurology. Why, then, did it take Cindy's neurologist three years and Judy's six months to make the diagnosis and to initiate treatment? Do you not see it? Cindy and Judy did not have analgesic rebound headache until their physicians could think of no other form of treatment. Sadly, it is only when all else has failed that analgesic rebound raises its ugly head. Analgesic rebound headache is not a derivation of science. It is a derivation of physician frustration.

I have written harsh words, but I believe them to be true.

CHAPTER TWELVE

Childhood Abuse

E ve told me she had been painful and depressed for most of her life. She developed panic disorder and fibromyalgia in her twenties. Her pain was made worse by three automobile accidents in which she suffered whiplash injury. In her thirties, she had surgery for correction of temporomandibular joint disease and carpal tunnel syndrome, but she continued to hurt in the jaw and the hands.

The early-life onset of pain and panic is always suggestive of child-hood abuse. Eve did tell me that her father was alcoholic and that she was unhappy as a child. She denied any issues of abuse, however. She married, unwisely it turned out, at age eighteen. I asked, as I always do in an inter-view, how many times she had been married. Three, she told me, and three times divorced. Her marriages had all been brief, and she was for most of her life a single parent. She had one child, a daughter who had done well with a degree in pharmacy.

Along the way, she had seen many doctors and been given a variety of antidepressants, but it was only ten years before that she actually came under the care of a psychiatrist. That experience was terminated by her choice after just a couple of years. She had been seen briefly at a pain clinic and was given epidural steroid injections and was also prescribed morphine. She found the drug rather unhelpful and very constipating (a common side effect). She chose to leave the pain clinic and turned her care over to her primary care doctor. Hydrocodone was given for pain, but Eve felt that it wired her up and kept her from sleeping (it can), so she discontinued it. She preferred Darvocet.

"Eve, you've seen lots of different doctors. What brings you to me now?"

"For some reason my pain has been a lot worse the past three months. It is in my neck and shoulders. I can't sleep, and I am depressed. Dr. Jones thought you might be able to help me. No offense, I want you to understand, but I doubt it. Nobody else has."

"Okay, but I'll try. Let's talk a little bit about your sleep. Has it always been bad, or is this something that has just happened recently?"

"I have never been a good sleeper, but I don't sleep at all the past three months."

"Do you have restless legs?"

"Yes, I have restless legs. I've had it for a long time, but it has been a lot worse the past few months."

"Your appetite, has that changed?"

"Yes. I am eating lots of chocolate, and I have gained fifteen pounds."

"Has that ever happened before?"

"Yes, sometimes I will go on eating sprees and gain weight."

"How is your energy?"

"Very, very poor, but you would be tired if you had to go through what I've been through."

"How is your memory?"

"It is awful."

"And the depression, how is the depression now?"

"It is bad, too. Dr. Jones started me on Nortriptyline a few weeks ago. It is not doing anything."

"Nothing at all?"

"Well, it helps the sleep a little bit, but that is all. My pain is still terrible."

I then began my inquiries into medicines she had taken in the past and their effect, for good or bad. This is a necessary exercise before embarking on my own treatment program. She was given Clonazepam, but it caused, she said, bad thoughts and nightmares. Paxil had made her depressed, and Neurontin, Lyrica, and Cymbalta all changed her disposition and made her cross and angry.

I was beginning to get the picture. Nothing, absolutely nothing, except her daughter's successful career had gone right for Eve. She had never found a good man, and she had never found a helpful drug. Moreover, her reactions to my questions were, in the main, reflective of hopelessness and self-defeat. Nobody had ever helped her, and she thought it was unlikely that I would. Nonetheless, I would give it a try. I prescribed Lorazepam and told her to increase her dose of Nortriptyline.

On her return visit Eve was, as before, dour and distant. She had not been able to obtain the Lorazepam. It was not available under her Medicare insurance plan and was too expensive for her to purchase. I inquired if there was any benefit from the larger dose of Nortriptyline, and she told me there was perhaps some, but she didn't like to take it regularly. She just took it if she was having a particularly sleepless night.

"I would like for you to take it regularly, Eve. Why are you not doing that?"

"I don't have much money, and I really can't afford to take it regularly."

"Eve, I know you are having a rough time. I see clearly that you are not very hopeful for the future, but I do believe you can be helped. I believe almost everyone can be helped."

She looked me in the eye and said, "I don't think you are going to be able to help me."

Frustration is the lot of the pain doctor, but I try not to let it bother me.

"I want you to try a new drug. It is Lithium, and I want you to take one pill every night. I can assure you that it is quite inexpensive, and I want you to take it regularly."

I was not really surprised by what Eve told me on her return. I halfway expected it.

"My daughter, the pharmacist, told me not to take the Lithium. She said it was a dangerous drug."

"If you don't want to take the Lithium, that's your business, but you are tying my hands. You really are not taking any of the medicines I have prescribed."

"They are not going to help me. I know they are not going to help me."

"Eve, I want to ask you some personal questions. You seem very depressed, and if I may say so, very negative. I want to ask you, are there any pleasures in your life? Is there anything that gives you joy?"

"Only my daughter, and she is three hundred miles away."

"Do you have family or church or friends?"

"No, I really don't. I am separated from my family. They don't like me. I think it is because of the trouble I've caused them with my divorces and my need for financial assistance. I've had to borrow a lot of money from them, and I haven't been able to pay it back. They really don't want me around."

"There is no one for you to turn to?"

"No, no one."

Never give up. I've learned that lesson well. Most of the time there is an answer, but with Eve it didn't look particularly good. Beat down, self-defeating, hopeless, joyless, depressed, and poor as well. Keep on trying. Sooner or later something good will happen. I prescribed Effexor, one of the few drugs she had not taken before, and told her again that I thought a trial of the Lithium was worth while. Whether she took it was up to her, but I told her that there was hope.

She returned a few weeks later to tell me that she had taken a Lithium pill one night, and the next morning awoke with tremors in her hands, so she discarded it. The Effexor had done nothing. I told her to double the dose and to return in a month. I was hanging on by my fingernails.

Nobody had ever helped her, and she thought it was unlikely that I would.

She was different person when I saw her next. For the first time she had a smile on her face, and there was sense of animus and energy, features I had not seen before. Effexor is good, but it is not that good. Something had happened in this woman's life—of that I was sure.

"You look better, Eve. This is the best I have seen you. Is the Effexor helping you?"

"No, I am not taking the Effexor, but I want to tell you something. My sisters invited me to spend Thanksgiving with them, the first time in five years. It was bittersweet, but it was wonderful. We talked about lots of things, and I want to share them with you. You remember we talked about my childhood. I wasn't as open as I should have been. I need to tell you that my father sexually molested me throughout my teen years. That is the reason I got married when I was eighteen. I had to get away. You need to know also that my first marriage was terrible. I was physically and sexually abused. Many times, my husband tied me to a bedpost and held a gun to my head. He threatened to kill me if I didn't perform for him. And I want to tell you something else. I was raped. A man entered my home at night, cut me with a knife, and raped me."

"Do you know who it was?"

"No, we never found out. I had to move out of my apartment. I couldn't bear to stay there."

"When did this happen, Eve?"

"Eighteen years ago; I was thirty-two."

"Was your daughter with you at that time?"

"No, thank God. She was spending the night with my sister. I am so grateful for that."

"Thank you, Eve. Thank you for sharing all this with me. I think it will help us. Let me ask you this, do you ever flashback or have nightmares about all that has happened to you?"

"Yes, nightmares a lot and flashbacks some."

"What makes you flashback?"

"It is always when I am alone. Sometimes when I am alone in a big room, I become fearful, and it's strange, sometimes in a small room, like an elevator, I am afraid."

"God bless you, Eve. Would you like to get into counseling concerning this? Would you like to see a psychiatrist?"

"No! No more psychiatrists."

"Okay, if that is what you want, but let me ask you—did you ever tell your psychiatrist about your abuse?"

"No, I was too ashamed. I didn't want to talk about it until now. When I was with my sisters, the subject finally came up. Both of them had been abused also. We all knew it, but we never talked about it with each other—at least until now."

"How are your sisters doing?"

"Fibromyalgia and depression."

"I'm sorry, Eve, I am truly sorry, but unfortunately that is the way it often goes. Let me ask you, has your pain or your sleep or your depression changed any?"

"I really don't know, but somehow in some strange way, I feel better. I feel like I have confronted a demon. I really do feel better about myself. I am more hopeful. I would like to try the Hydrocodone again. I am not sure it really bothered me like I told you it did. I would like to have some pain relief."

"Very well, I am going to write a prescription for Hydrocodone, and I would like to try a new drug, Seroquel. I will give you some samples, and I want you to take it at bedtime. It should help your sleep."

"I will take it. I promise you."

She returned at the appointed time and reported that the Hydrocodone, which she had taken before with difficulty, was now helping her pain. The Seroquel, however, had produced sedation, and she did not wish to continue it.

> *The simple act of reaching out, touching, consoling, and sharing can be very therapeutic.*

The pharmacy is good, even splendid, but it is not always the answer. The simple act of reaching out, touching, consoling, and sharing can be very therapeutic. It had been with Eve, and I suspect that as we go along, in the months and years ahead, pharmacy that had been so ineffective, even disturbing to her, just might start working. She had become, through the agency of sharing and touching, at least hopeful of getting better.

In *Understanding Chronic Pain*, I devoted considerable attention to the frequency of childhood abuse in those who suffer pain. I felt then, and still do, that it is the root cause of many, and very probably most forms of chronic pain—and for that matter, very probably most forms of psychiatric illness.

The young mind, say from birth to age twenty-five, is a work in progress. It is hoped that our minds continue to be a work of progress throughout our lives, but it will never approach the velocity of that achieved in youth. During that formative period, the neurotransmitter systems—serotonin, noradrenaline, and all the rest—are being assembled and integrated into an infrastructure with all the necessary checks and balances to *control* mood, sleep, appetite, energy, thought, impulse, and yes, the perception of pain.

This infrastructure can be altered in many ways. There may be inherent faults due to genetics. Brain injury, such as meningitis or epilepsy, can do it, and so can the introduction in youth of drugs of abuse—false neurotransmitters, as it were. Trauma in the form of emotional, physical, or sexual abuse can also disassemble the evolving and fragile infrastructure of a child. When this happens, the victim is at risk for a life of emotional and biologic disorder. In the worst case, she (I employ the feminine but certainly males are abused also) suffers disordered mood with the appearance of depression and anxiety early in life. Sleep is disordered with insomnia and nightmares. Appetite is disturbed with the appearance of anorexia/bulimia or obesity. Cognition, memory, mental focus, and learning skills can be impaired. There is proclivity to impulse and disordered gratification and reward, this manifesting as recreational drug abuse and self-destructive, risk-seeking behavior including promiscuity. Lastly, the mind's ability to control the perception of pain is deranged, and chronic pain in one or several of its many forms appears early in life.

I will call to the reader's attention, as we move into further discussion of childhood abuse and also bipolar disorder, that the templates that dictate the behaviors of both are well nigh interchangeable.

Maureen left her husband after twelve years of unhappy marriage. She restarted her life as an elementary school teacher. This occurred some ten years before she came to me. She told me that she seemed to catch every infection the kids brought in—bronchitis, strep throat, and mononucleosis. She was started on Effexor, and found that it helped her fatigue and also perhaps her mood, for she acknowledged intervals of depression through her life, particularly in the winter months. As time went by, her appetite changed, with food cravings on some occasions and no desire for food on others. A year before she came to me, she developed mid-back and shoulder pain and increasing depression and insomnia. Her primary care doctor diagnosed fibromyalgia and prescribed Lexapro. She became, as so many painful people do, climatic sensitive with worsening pain in cold, damp weather.

I inquired about her childhood, and she told me quite candidly that she had been sexually abused from age nine to eleven by her mother's boyfriend. I then asked as to whether, along with her interludes of depression, she experienced episodes of high-energy well-being. She acknowledged that she did, and in response to my next question said she did indeed have a problem with disinhibited spending. So destructive was this activity that she forbade herself to carry a credit card. She also volunteered that she made a suicide attempt, overdosing with pills, during the time she was unhappily married.

"Do you think I have bipolar disease?"

"You well may, but we are certainly not going to jump to that conclusion."

"Well, I have often wondered if I have bipolar disease or maybe attention deficit disorder."

"Does anyone in your family have manic-depressive illness or attention deficit disorder?"

"Well, I am pretty sure that my father had bipolar disease, but I really don't know for certain."

"Okay, Maureen, I see you are taking Alprazolam and Trazodone at bedtime. I suppose they have been given to help you sleep. Are they working?"

"No, I am really having trouble sleeping."

"For the time being, keep taking those medicines, but I am going to add some more. They are called Clonazepam and Imipramine. Have you ever taken either of those before?"

"No, I don't believe so."

"I want you to be back in ten days, Maureen. I want to follow this thing very closely. If you have any problem with the new medicine, if it makes you feel bad or gives you strange thoughts, I want you to stop them and call me immediately."

I did indeed have a high suspicion that my patient was bipolar. The periodic depressions, the occasional energized euphoria, the wanton spending, the pain, and a possible family history all suggested it. It is well known that bipolars often suffer bizarre reactions to pharmacy. This can happen with absolutely any psychiatric drug in use today, but it is probably most common with the tricyclics. It turns out that my concerns were appropriate.

On her return she did look better, but the evolution over ten days was really bizarre. She told me that the first night she took one each of the new medicines and had very restless sleep with greatly increased pain. The next night she took two of each. Pain immediately diminished and sleep was restored. As she pushed the dose up, she began to experience sweats and a sensation of shortness of breath. And then she had a huge mood swing—dropping down into a tearful despair that lasted four days and then remitted.

"What you have experienced bothers me, Maureen. I wish you had called me. Mood swings like you had can be caused by medication, and I have real concerns that the Imipramine is giving you trouble. I want us to stop it."

"But I am feeling better now, I really am. I think the medicine is helping me."

"Well, it may be, but frankly, I am worried. Let me ask you, have you ever had mood swings like this before?"

"Yes, I have had them occasionally. They will just strike me suddenly, but I haven't had any of those recently, and I have never had one as bad as the one I told you about."

She was a time bomb ready to explode, and I was fearful that my pharmacy just might be setting the clock.

"Okay, Maureen, until proved otherwise I am presuming it is due to the Imipramine. I want you to stop it, and I am writing you a prescription for Effexor."

I really was concerned about my patient. I felt that she was time bomb ready to explode, and I was fearful that my pharmacy just might be setting the clock.

"I did what you told me. I started the Effexor, and I stopped the Imipramine, and I have to tell you what happened. The next morning my pain all came back. It was intense."

"What did you do then?"

"I got back on the Imipramine, and as soon as I did, the pain went away. It was just unbelievable."

"How much are you taking?"

"One pill each night."

"How about the others?"

"I am taking them just as you instructed, and I want to tell you I really feel quite well. This is the best I have been in a long time. My sleep is good, my mood is good, and my pain is gone."

It was six weeks before I saw her again, and she did look quite well. She was nattily dressed and talkative, rapidly talkative. It was a behavior I had not seen before, and although she seemed quite happy, I was still bothered.

"Maureen, I am glad you are doing so well. Are you still taking the same medicines?"

"No, I had to stop the Imipramine. It took me down again. I was suicidal."

"How long did it last?"

"Just a few days. It went away as soon as I stopped the Imipramine."

"I am glad you stopped it. The Effexor should take its place. They are similar drugs. By the way, are you having any side effects from the Effexor?"

"Yes, just like I did before—sexual dysfunction."

"I am sorry about that. It certainly can happen. I hope it is not too much of a bother to you. You are doing so well, I am reluctant to make any changes in your therapy."

"Doesn't bother me at all. I have had plenty of sex. I don't need any more."

"What do you mean you have had plenty of sex?"

"Oh, I used to be very active. If I saw a good-looking man, I would go get him."

"One-night stands?"

"Yes, many. More than I can count."

There was excitement in her voice as she related all this to me. She clearly was speeded up and manic. What to do? I decided very little. A state of low-grade mania is not a bad state at all. She was happy and free of pain. Don't intrude when the human machine is working well, but I did tell her that I was rather sure she had bipolar disease, and she should certainly be in touch with me if dramatic mood swings, either up or down, should occur.

"I am glad you told me. I have always wondered. Now I know, and I feel a lot better knowing it."

Coleen had suffered pain for most of her life. The most pressing issue, however, was persistent pain in the back and legs unrelieved by two operations, the first to remove a ruptured disc and the second, a fusion to correct spinal instability. When she came to me, she was taking Oxycodone and Neurontin from her internist and Lorazepam and Wellbutrin prescribed by her psychiatrist. I added Cymbalta. On the occasion of her first return visit, she reported that her pain and depression were somewhat improved on my therapy. She also told me that she had read my book, and she presented me with this letter.

Dear Dr. Cochran:

Your book was most helpful to me, and I want to offer you a time-line on my history and ask you to address some of my concerns.

1964: Born, fourth of five siblings.

1973–77: Molested by father (four years, nine to thirteen years old). Mother did not believe me. Took me to counseling but stopped after one session because mother said I wouldn't talk.

1977: Periods began (thirteen years old) and they were debilitating. Father physically and emotionally abused all five children. Oldest brother beaten more than others. Two sisters sexually abused to a lesser degree than me.

1982: Graduated high school at seventeen years old. Moved out the following day to live with my oldest sister.

1983: Married (age eighteen) a man twelve years my senior. After one year, I knew I had made a mistake, but my husband refused to give me a divorce ("We have a house and two cars; I am not giving that up.").

1985: Gave birth to daughter at age twenty-one.

1988: Gave birth to son at age twenty-four.

1988: After my son was born and my daughter was four, I began to have nightmares that my father was chasing me around my childhood bed trying to rape me. I connected that with my daughter getting older and at risk of being molested by my father. Although my mother begged me to let my daughter spend the night with my parents, I never left my children alone with my mother or father. My sisters and I were planning to confront our father together, but my mother sabotaged that plan by having my father call me. He said, "What's going on, kid? Mom says we have a problem." I confronted my father alone and told him unless he received professional help, I will be forced to sever my relationship with him. He told me, jokingly, that if I was going to worry about anything, I should wait until my daughter was nine (the same age I was when he began molesting me). He ended our conversation by saying, "It was nice knowing you, kid." I did not have any contact with my parents until ten years later, when my sister committed suicide.

1995: Divorced at age thirty. Right great toe bunionectomy. It was so painful that I never had the left done. Began having back pain and seeing a chiropractor. The treatments usually made it worse.

2001: Married again. Husband is workaholic, alcoholic, and puts his work, alcohol, children, and grandchildren above me.

2002: Due to all-over body pain, my primary care doctor referred me to a rheumatologist, who diagnosed me with fibromyalgia.

2003: (age thirty-nine). Got out of bed one morning, felt something odd in my back (not pain); ten minutes later I literally fell out of the shower with severe pain in back and right leg. On medical advice, I lay on the floor for three weeks, unable to stand more than ten to fifteen seconds. Laminectomy L5, S1. Back improved for a while, then worsened, moving to include my left leg.

2004: Spinal fusion L4, L5, and S1. Back and leg pain worsened significantly. Began Oxycodone, Neurontin (it does help).

2004: Began seeing psychiatrist for depression and treated with, in turn, Zoloft, Lexapro, Effexor, Amitriptyline (weight gain), Wellbutrin (now), Lorazepam (it does help chronic insomnia).

2005: While visiting my sister in Pennsylvania, I saw my father for the first time in many years. That evening I had an attack of severe abdominal pain. Doctor in the emergency room did a CAT scan and told me I had an enlarged pancreas. A few months later, my primary care doctor ordered a follow-up CAT scan, which showed no problem in the liver or pancreas.

2006: I met you.

Symptoms/Complaints:
- *Fidget, move around, constantly repositioning myself when I try to lie down and watch TV. Not necessarily associated with pain.*
- *Sometimes worse than others, have joint pain in the fingers.*
- *If I take less than five Oxycodone a day, it feels like my spine is in a vise.*

- *If I do not take Neurontin, I have severe pain and throbbing in my right leg. My right great toe feels "possessed" and on fire. Neurontin also reduces my back pain.*
- *Very poor memory and lack of ability to focus or stay on track. Have always been a problem for me. My son is ADD and on Ritalin. Could I have ADD?*

After three weeks on the Cymbalta you prescribed, depression and pain may be slightly improved, but problems with weight gain and beginning to have difficulty with urination.

I read her letter with care and expressed my appreciation for her candor. We chatted about several issues. I asked about her father, and she told me that he was always "hyper" and "manic" and subject to attacks of rage.

"That's a pretty good description for bipolar disease. Was that diagnosis ever made?"

"No, I don't think so, but you understand that I had no contact with him for many years. He died just last year—unmourned by his children."

"Your siblings' health?"

"All of them were depressed. One was a suicide, and my other sister has fibromyalgia."

"You began seeing a psychiatrist just a couple of years ago. Had you had problems with depression before that?"

"Oh, I have been depressed all my life. It is just when my back started hurting I realized that I really needed some help."

"You have been on several different antidepressants. Why so many?"

"Sexual side effects mostly. Wellbutrin has been the best in that regard."

"How is the depression doing now?"

"Poorly."

"And sleep?"

"Not bad since I have been on the Lorazepam."

"And the Cymbalta that I started three weeks ago—that hasn't been a world beater it seems."

"That is correct, I'm sorry to tell you, but it really hasn't done much at all."

"Okay, let's talk about this ADD thing. How long have you had a problem with mental focus and memory?"

"I can't really date it except to say it has been there a long time, maybe all my life."

"Did you have problems with your academic work? Did you have learning problems or hyperactivity?"

"Well no, no real hyperactivity—as least as well as I can remember. But learning has been a problem for me. I made good grades, but I felt like I had to work a whole lot harder than my friends to get them."

Coleen had told me enough. She was chronically painful and depressed and treatment resistant on both fronts. She had symptoms that were at least suggestive of attention deficit disorder, and—I believe this is very important—she had a family history of probable paternal bipolar disease and a child with attention deficit disorder. More than sufficient grounds for initiating therapy with a psychostimulant. Besides, I couldn't think of a whole lot else to do.

She had symptoms that were at least suggestive of attention deficit disorder.

"I am writing you a prescription for Adderall, Coleen, 10 mg. size. Start out taking one a day for the first week, and if there are no problems, you can increase it to twice daily. I will see you again in three weeks."

On her next visit, she reported improvement in her mental focus on the Adderall, and that her psychiatrist was comfortable with her taking Wellbutrin and Adderall together. She told me that he said he had pretty good luck with that particular combination. I increased the dose of Adderall.

"I can see definite improvement with the bigger dose of Adderall. It is remarkable how much my ability to think is improved and my depression also. I really do feel better."

"How about the pain?"

"Really no better at all. I still have to take the Oxycodone and the Neurontin, and I don't like doing it because they do sedate me a bit, but I guess I am stuck with them for the rest of my life."

"Okay, we are going to start a new drug. It is called Imipramine. I want you to start on a low dose and build it up gradually until your next visit here."

"Imipramine, huh? That is a tricyclic drug, isn't it?"

"Yes, it is a tricyclic. It is akin to the Amitriptyline you have taken before."

"I don't want to take it. I am really fearful of weight gain with these drugs, and I am fearful of sexual side effects too. I think I would rather go without it."

"That is your choice, Coleen, but you must understand, I don't have much else to offer—at least at this juncture."

"Okay, I'll think about it, but I am not ready yet."

"I'll see you in two months, Coleen."

She finally consented to take the Imipramine, but with much hesitation and fear of side effects. I don't think she really gave it an honest try. She thought it made her too hung over in the morning, so we have elected simply to maintain her Oxycodone, Neurontin, Wellbutrin, Lorazepam, and Adderall. We have been at it over a year now and without any real change in her therapy over the course of that time, she has progressively improved. Her pain has diminished and her depression also. With pharmacy, her infrastructure has been restored and in doing so has given the mind the resources to heal itself.

Shelly was physically and sexually abused by her father. She got married at age seventeen, while still in high school, to get away from the torture. Given the circumstances, one would anticipate that her marriage had little chance of survival, but survive it did and happily so for sixteen years until her husband died in an automobile accident, leaving her with four children. With that event, her lifelong, smoldering depressive mood erupted, and she required antidepressant therapy. Her adolescent problem with bulimia erupted also, and within a couple of years, she had gained weight from one hundred fifty to two hundred twenty-five pounds.

Also about this time, at age thirty-three, she required surgery for the removal of a ruptured disc in the neck. Her pain diminished significantly and was not to be a problem for several years. She did, however, evolve into a cycling disorder of mood with periodic depressions and a disorder of appetite with periodic weight loss and weight gain (more often the latter) and sleep with intervals of mind racing and the total inability to sleep at night—these lasting a week or two at a time. She also had another cycling disorder. She could always anticipate the coming of menstruation, she told me, by a real change in her disposition with irritability and fractiousness beginning ten days before the onset of her period. Nonetheless, she was able to continue working and raising her children. After six years of single motherhood she remarried, happily, she told me. Her strange periodic symptoms continued, and she endured them until a second cervical disc ruptured, and an operation to fuse the cervical spine was performed. Her pain did not abate.

"Tell me about your father, Shelly."

"He was bipolar. He had to be bipolar. He was always erratic, and he was subject to fits of rage. It was during those times that the abuse occurred."

"Do you ever see him now? Have you ever confronted him or have either of you attempted some kind of reconciliation?"

"No, I left him when I was seventeen years old, and I haven't spoken with him since."

"And you suffered depression from early on?"

"Yes, but it really wasn't that bad. I got by quite well. I loved my husband, and I was happy taking care of my children. I didn't have time to be depressed."

"Any problem with anxiety, flashbacks, or nightmares?"

"No, really none at all. I have heard of that kind of thing happening, but it really was never an issue for me. I don't know why."

"Nor I, but I am happy you don't."

I continued my interrogations searching for, among other things, some clue to bipolarity. After all, she had a probable family history of it. Aside from intervals of mind racing, sleeplessness, and periodic depression, I found none. I elected to treat her with Imipramine and Clonazepam. She called in a few days to report that she was quite unable to sleep at all and was actually beginning to experience visual hallucinations during the night. I was alarmed and told her to discontinue the medicine and come in to see me as soon as possible.

She was back within a week, and she opened the conversation by saying, "Dr. Cochran, I am desperate for sleep. I haven't slept for over two weeks now. I am still having hallucinations. Can you please give me something to help me sleep?"

"I will certainly do that, but you tell me you are still having hallucinations after you have been off my medicines for a week?"

"Yes, I've had these before. If I go several days without sleep, I will hallucinate, but this is the worst it has ever been."

I asked myself, were Shelly's hallucinations a product of my pharmacy or the product of the progressive worsening of her disease? Did she need less pharmacy or more of it? I split the difference. I gave her the sleeping pill Ambien, and told her to resume the Clonazepam. We would leave the Imipramine alone for the time being. Reflecting on it all, I was less alarmed by the hallucinations after talking with her. Two weeks of sleeplessness, after all, can generate virtually any psychiatric symptoms and mimic any psychiatric disease.

It was a month before I saw her again, a far longer interval than I had requested, but she did indeed look better. She told me she had tried the Ambien for a couple of nights, but she slept no better with it, and she felt hyperactive and nervous during the day. Then, contrary to my instructions, she resumed the Imipramine and actually increased the dose as I had originally instructed. She reported that she was beginning to sleep better, but she was aware of increasing fatigue during the day. She would wake up in the morning feeling rested but by 3:00 or 4:00 PM would often have to lie down and take naps. She told me also that her appetite was definitely diminished and that she was losing weight.

What a curious disease is chronic pain—cycling mood, cycling sleep, cycling appetite, and bizarre reactions to medicines. The Ambien kept her from sleeping and made her hyperactive and anxious, exactly the opposite of what it is supposed to do. And the strange nocturnal hallucinations. Were they a product of pharmacy or were they, with her fatigue and daytime somnolence an indicator of some form of narcolepsy?

I chose Adderall. I prescribed in my customary manner 10 mg. daily, taken in the morning for a week and then 20 mg. I knew I was playing with fire with this one. I needed to follow it closely, and I told her— indeed I demanded that she return to see me in ten days.

"I am better, I am a lot better. My mental focus is so much better, and I have more energy. My sleep is continuing to improve, and I am very happy about my progress."

"How about the pain in your neck?"

"I don't think it has changed much, but I feel so much better in every other way that it doesn't bother me. I will let you in on a little secret. I don't have an appetite anymore. I am losing weight rapidly, and I am proud of that. You know that always makes a woman proud."

"Let's increase the Adderall and come back in one month. I am very happy for you, Shelly."

"Dr. Cochran, I can't believe how much better I feel. I have been sick for many years, and most of the bad things have gone away. Really, all of the bad things have gone away."

"Tell me about it."

"I sleep well at night, and I don't get tired during the day. My mood is so much better. My disposition has changed, and I am more positive. I've talked with my husband about this. He says I am more even—that I am more tolerant than I used to be."

I continued my interrogations, searching for, among other things, some clue to bipolarity. After all, she had a probable family history of it.

"And the pain? How about the pain? That is what started all this business in the first place."

"A lot better. And I will tell you something that is really amazing. You know we talked about my problem with my period, which has just been terrible. Last month I couldn't even tell my period was coming. I usually know at least ten days before. And let me tell you something else. I have lost forty pounds since I started seeing you. That was three months ago."

"Forty pounds in three months. Shelly, that concerns me. That is too much weight loss too quickly."

"No, it has happened to me before. I've lost weight like that several times. You know, my husband has always been concerned about my weight. It bothers him a lot. I have told him several times that most people have a chemical in their brain that tells them to stop eating. I don't have that chemical. I've got it now, thanks to you, and I don't sense any need for food. I have noticed something very strange, though. After I have gone many hours without food, I will get a headache. I've learned that the headache tells me when I need to eat. As soon as I eat, my headache goes away."

Aside from an occasional hunger headache relieved by eating, Shelly was doing splendidly. Her pain was relieved, her sleep restored, her mood stabilized, her premenstrual maldisposition arrested, and her pathologic lust for food terminated. There was one more thing to get better, though.

It was three months later when she returned for a checkup and routine prescription refills.

"Dr. Cochran, I want to share something with you. I want you to know that I called my father. That is the first contact I have had with him in twenty-three years. I want you to know it was wonderful. He thanked me for calling him, and he apologized. He told me he was ashamed of what happened. He was crying, Dr. Cochran. He was crying through most of the conversation. I feel like I have the father I always wanted now. I am going to take the children and my husband up to Ohio to meet him next weekend. I thought you would want to know about this."

"That's remarkable, Shelly. I am happy for you, and I am very proud of you for what you have done."

When the right drug kicks in, *everything* gets better.

Betty was thirty-four years old when she came to me. She told me she had back pain all of her life but had just put up with it. About six months before, the pain had spread all over her body and was, she told me, "a hundred times worse than before." Her physician told her she had fibromyalgia. He prescribed Hydrocodone for pain, and by the time she came to me, she was taking it in astonishing quantities, up to twenty-four pills daily.

I inquired about her personal history, and she told me she suffered sexual abuse at the hands of her father and also a date rape at age fifteen. She got married at age seventeen. During this time she experimented pretty aggressively with alcohol and marijuana—a practice she gave up after a couple of years. After divorcing her husband at age twenty-eight, she entered depression. A psychiatrist treated her with Effexor. She recovered and in time was weaned off the drug. She told me that through her life she had intervals of depression, some with suicidal ideation, but she denied ever making an attempt. In response to my questions, she acknowledged that she was very dangerous with a credit card.

"Okay, Betty, I think we have a pretty good handle on the situation. But you must understand that if I am going to treat you, you are going to have to be compliant and take the painkillers as I prescribe. You are taking way too many of them."

"I understand. I will try to do better."

"Let me ask you, what was going on in your life when you started having this pain? Were you troubled in any way? Had you experienced any kind of disturbing life event?"

She turned her head down and said, "Yes, something terrible. My eight-year-old nephew hung himself. I am pretty sure he had been sexually abused."

"I am sorry, Betty, I am truly sorry. I am sure that broke your heart."

"Yes, it did. My own son was the same age, and they were best friends."

"What happened to you after that?"

"I got very panicky and depressed. I went back to the psychiatrist, and she prescribed Effexor and Lorazepam."

"Did they help?"

"Yes, they helped a lot, but I am afraid of the Lorazepam. I don't want to get addicted."

"You are afraid of one milligram of Lorazepam, and yet you are taking 240 mg. of Hydrocodone? That just doesn't make sense to me."

"I know, I know, but there are lots of times when my life doesn't make sense to me."

"What do you mean by that?"

"I can't really tell you. I don't know what it is, but things just never seem to work out for me. I can't keep a job, and I have a lot of trouble keeping friends."

"Why?"

"Maybe I am just too erratic and unpredictable. That is all I can say."

"You can take the Hydrocodone at the rate of six a day and no more. I want you to increase the dose of the Lorazepam. I think it will help your sleep. I am also giving you a prescription for Imipramine. Start with one pill and try to get up to four, taken each night."

She returned to see me three weeks later.

"I like the new medicine. I am sleeping better, and my pain has lessened a great deal. But something queer is happening to me. I am more emotional, and I find that I cry a lot. I don't really know why. It is strange that I am happier than I have been for quite a while, but I just am more emotional."

"Did this begin as soon as you started the medicines?"

"Yes."

"Have you ever had spells like this before when you cried so much?"

"No, never. You see, I haven't been able to cry for years, and now I am crying all the time. I am crying at the least little thing."

Curious indeed. Less pain, better mood, but more emotional. Was this something good that was happening or something bad that was happening? Crying and the display of emotion in one who has not done so for a while can indicate that the drugs are working. They can also indicate that the drugs themselves are creating the change. I elected to wait it out. More good things than bad things were happening.

"Betty, I want you to increase the Imipramine. Continue the others as before, and I hope you are taking them like I have told you to."

"I am, and I will do as you say. I am afraid you caught me on a bad day today. I got fired again."

"Sorry, thanks for telling me."

Through the next few visits, Betty's pain and her mood was bouncing up and down. She got her Imipramine dose up to 80 mg. and then started thinking of suicide. On her own she reduced the Imipramine, and her pain came back. She was also taking more Hydrocodone than I prescribed. I told her to stop the Imipramine, and I prescribed Cymbalta.

"The Cymbalta really does work. My pain settled down almost as soon as I started it. I did think it was making my legs jerk at night, so I stopped it just to see, and the pain came back. So I am taking it now as you prescribed."

"Still crying, still emotional?"

"Yes, but it is not like it was with the Imipramine. It is not nearly that bad, but I still cry pretty easily, and I still feel like I go up and down."

"Betty, don't be alarmed by this question, but I want you to tell me if you have any family members who have manic-depressive illness."

"I am pretty sure my sister does. She is the mother of the child who committed suicide."

"I am going to give you a new medicine. It is called Lithium. Have you ever heard of it?"

"Yes, I have. That is for bipolar disease, isn't it?"

"Yes."

"Do you think I am bipolar?"

"We are going to find out real soon, Betty."

"I need to tell you something. I asked my psychiatrist the same question, and she told me that I am not bipolar. What do you think of that?"

Many of my patients, familiar with my writings, react to my interrogation with the statement, "You are trying to make me bipolar, aren't you?" My typical response is, "I am not trying to make you bipolar, I am trying to make you well." A common rejoinder is, "My psychiatrist tells me that I am not bipolar." (We have already seen that scenario play out with Pat in chapter one.) My unstated response to that declamation is that no psychiatrist in the world can say with certainty that his patient does not have bipolar disease. As I have already written, bipolarity is a great imitator. It can mimic and appear as virtually any psychiatric disorder, and I believe that statement is incontestable. This is to say that the mere suspicion of bipolarity is sufficient for me to initiate treatment for the disorder.

I took a phone call from Betty only a week later.

"I'm sorry, Dr. Cochran, I really like the Lithium. When I took it I wasn't crying anymore, and my mood was much better, but it is very sedating to me, and I am unsteady. I almost had an automobile accident yesterday. I really wish I could continue the Lithium, but I just can't. What are we going to do now?"

"Come in to see me as soon as possible."

She came in just a few days, telling me she was having suicidal thoughts again.

"Betty, don't do anything foolish. We have a diagnosis, and we are going to get well. I don't know if it is going to be sooner or later, but we are going to get well."

Lamictal is a relatively new drug. It is an anticonvulsant helpful in the treatment of epilepsy but also in the treatment of migraine and bipolar disease. Like most mind drugs, it has potential side effects of sedation and unsteadiness, but it also has a fearsome side effect in the form of a severe, life-threatening skin rash. We have learned, however, that the rash can be avoided by starting Lamictal at a low dosage, only 25 mg. daily. Over the course of a few months, this can be slowly increased.

What is the relationship of childhood abuse to bipolarity? We would like a simple answer.

One of the downsides of Lamictal therapy, therefore, is that it may take two months or more to reach a therapeutic dose. Fortunately, it didn't take nearly that long with Betty.

"You cured me. I am well. My moods are even now, and my pain is gone. I have never felt this well. You have found the perfect drug."

"That's wonderful, Betty. I am so happy for you. It is remarkable to me that you feel so much better on such a small dose. We may have to increase it as time goes by, but for now we will stay where we are."

"You know something really strange is happening. I don't feel the need to spend money anymore. When I go to the convenience store to get gas for my car, I don't feel like I have to go in and buy a lottery ticket. That is odd, isn't it?"

"Not really, Betty. These drugs can do remarkable things. I am not surprised at all by what you have told me."

"Well, I will tell you something else that I feel like I don't have to do now."

"What's that?"

"Pick up men."

What is the relationship of childhood abuse to bipolarity? We would like a simple answer. We would like to be able to say that childhood abuse, which is so destructive to the brain's infrastructure, can actually generate bipolar disease. The issue, however, is quite complicated. Recall that several of the women I have presented had a family history of bipolar disease. Was their bipolar disease a product of genetics or of malnurture? We don't really know, but it is sure worth thinking about.

Now, what is the relationship of childhood trauma to pain? Do we have any evidence that the two are related? Yes, at a statistical level, the evidence is most impressive. Some 50 percent of painful women (and a lot of men also) that I see carry the heritage of childhood abuse, and I do not believe the relationship can be ignored.

Before closing this chapter, I want to present the story of someone I met only once and briefly at that. It was at a book signing in a neighboring state. I had a good crowd, and the discussion was spirited. A man, and I would put his age about forty, sat on the back row but involved himself with some intensity in the conversation. I knew right away that he had read my book, and his comments suggested strongly that he was challenging my thesis that chronic pain is a disease of the mind. He told the group that his problem was interstitial cystitis, or inflammation of the bladder. He had with him photographs of his bladder obtained during a urologic procedure. They showed ulceration and hemorrhage throughout the bladder wall. He passed the photographs around and recounted to the group that his suffering dated many years and that he had to leave a six-figure income with a manufacturing company because of his bladder pain. He was telling me and the group that his pain was coming from his bladder and not from his mind. The photographs showing ulcers and hemorrhage were graphic testimony to that fact.

I elected to not pursue the issue or to ask him, in the presence of others, any potentially embarrassing questions. I only offered my sympathy and told him that he was not alone, that I had seen many people whose lives had been destroyed by chronic pain.

At the conclusion of the discussion, he came forward and asked that I sign his book, which I did. He thanked me, looked me in the eye, and as his eyes reddened, he whispered to me, "He was a member of my father's congregation." And then he turned and left.

CHAPTER THIRTEEN

The Bipolar Spectrum

Ruth suffered bipolar disorder and with it, painfully arthritic knees. Her therapist suggested she take a look at *Understanding Chronic Pain*. She made an appointment in short order.

"I was very taken by your discussions about the relationship between bipolar disease and chronic pain. I would never have thought that my bipolar illness had anything to do with my arthritis."

"Well, I am really not sure bipolar disease has much to do with arthritis, but it may have a lot to do with your pain. Tell me about it."

"My knees have hurt for many years. I have had several arthroscopies and steroid injections. They helped at first, but they are not working now. I am told that I am bone-on-bone and will need knee replacements pretty soon."

"What are you taking for pain?"

"Mostly over-the-counter stuff—Aleve and Ibuprofen."

"Has anyone prescribed opiates for you?"

"No, they are reluctant to do that because of my bipolar disease. My psychiatrist tells me that I am in a very delicate balance, and he is afraid that painkillers might aggravate my emotional state."

"Tell me about your bipolar disease."

"I have had mood swings all my life. It seems that most of my family has the same kind of problem, always up or down."

"Did you seek any kind of professional help for it?"

"Not for a long time. I grew up on a ranch in Colorado and going to doctors just wasn't our thing."

"Keep going."

"I went to the University of Colorado and graduated with a major in communications. I moved to Chicago and got a job with a public relations firm there."

"And the mood swings?"

"They were always there, but I was successful with my career. Most of the time I had lots of energy, and I was very creative. My trouble began after my divorce. I got very depressed and attempted suicide. That was when I was diagnosed with bipolar disease."

"Did you have spells of mania with hyperactivity?"

"Yes, lots of them. And terrible depression also."

"Did you remain under psychiatric care?"

"You bet I did. My psychiatrist was really great. He tried lots of different medicines, and with each of them I would seem to get better for a while, and then I would lose it. We would then move on to another drug."

"Can you give me the names of some of the medicines you took?"

"Well, I remember some of them. I have taken Depakote, Tegretol, and Effexor, and there were others."

"How about Lithium?"

"Oh yes, I did take Lithium for a while, and now I remember. I took Neurontin and Prozac also."

"Ruth, let me ask you a question. Have you ever taken a medicine that actually made you worse?"

"Yes, I remember it well. Dr. Reynolds gave me Lamictal. It was supposed to be a mood stabilizer, but it destabilized me. I became very depressed, and I had to go into the hospital for a week."

"And then what?"

"He put me on Lexapro and Clonazepam. That has been the best combination ever. That was five years ago, and I am still on those drugs.

"What brought you to this city?"

"I remarried and moved here. We have been here three years. Except for my knees, things have been going very well. My husband and I are planning to start up a new business."

"Do you have a psychiatrist locally?"

"Yes, I do. I see him every two months, and he has maintained the Lexapro and the Clonazepam. I still have some mood swings, but they are not nearly as bad as they used to be."

"What does your current psychiatrist say about your condition?"

"He says that I am a rapid-cycling bipolar, and that under no circumstances should I deviate from my treatment with Lexapro and Clonazepam."

Ruth suffered Bipolar I disorder, the most severe expression of the disease. Not only that, she was a rapid cycler with mood swings occurring not at intervals of days or weeks, but of hours. Ruth had been a very sick woman for a long time. Her recovery, or at least something approaching recovery, was really remarkable. She was indeed in a delicate balance, and I was aware that almost anything I did might upset it.

She was indeed in a delicate balance, and I was aware that almost anything I did might upset it.

"How bad is your pain now, Ruth?"

"I would grade it a six or seven on a scale of ten. I am getting by, but barely. You must understand, it is important that I am able to be on my feet. Our new business will entail a lot of traveling to Europe and maybe even the Orient."

"How are you sleeping?"

"I am not. The pain seems to get worse at night. The sleep problem is new. I slept pretty well up until about six months ago, and now I can hardly sleep at all."

"How is your energy?"

"Oh, it is terrible. I have a problem with fatigue, and I get sleepy during the day. I suppose it is because I can't sleep at night."

"Anything else?"

"Yes, and this really bothers me a lot. I can't seem to remember very well. I just can't think like I used to be able to. I am in a fog all the time—and I don't need that while starting up a new business."

"Did you ever have any problems like this back years ago when you were so ill with your bipolar disease?"

"Yes, I remember times when fatigue and memory loss were a problem, but these usually happened when I was depressed. Right now I am really not depressed. If anything, I am a little bit manic. I am excited over the prospects for our business."

Oh boy, I had to think about this one. I didn't want to go to antidepressants or mood stabilizers. Ruth had already been on most of them, and one of them, Lamictal, actually threw her into depression. Maybe opiate therapy? I chose not, but looking back on it, had I seen her but six months past the time I did, I would probably have done that. I am glad I didn't, though, for I was about to learn something very important.

It may seem counterintuitive to use a stimulant for the treatment of manic-depressive illness because of the risk of inciting mania. However, there was the prospect that it would benefit her fatigue, forgetfulness, and possibly even her pain. So the risk must be accepted. Remember, there is risk with all drugs.

"Ruth, I am prescribing Adderall. It is like Ritalin, and I am sure you have heard of that drug. I really don't know whether it will work or not, but I want you to try it. If it fails, we can move into opiate therapy, but I don't want to introduce any more antidepressants or mood stabilizers. I am fearful of doing that."

"Ritalin, huh? Do you think it will make me manic? Decongestants really make me hyper, and I avoid them."

"Honestly, I don't know, but we will have to be very vigilant to that possibility. Nonetheless, my instincts tell me it just might help you, maybe a lot."

"You are saying this medicine might actually relieve my pain?"

"It could, it really could."

"You know, I remember Dr. Reynolds suggesting many years ago that we might try Ritalin. He was pretty high up on the food chain among psychiatric pharmacologists. I respected him enormously, but I told him I was afraid of it. However, if that is what you want, I am willing to take it."

"Okay, Ruth, I want you to clear this with your psychiatrist. It is very important that he knows what we are doing. Adderall, 10 mg. daily, and call me immediately if you develop any signs of mania. Come back in ten days."

It was two months before I saw her again.

"My pain is worse, it is a lot worse. I hurt all the time, and I can't sleep, I can't think, and I am fatigued. Can you help me?"

"Did you take the Adderall, Ruth?"

"No, Dr. Rich told me not to take your medicine. He thought it was too risky. He told me I should increase the dose of the Lexapro."

"Did you do that?"

"Yes, but it has done no good at all. I'm ready to try the Adderall. Please write a prescription for the lowest possible dose. Dr. Rich frightened me, but I have nowhere to turn, and I want to try it."

"Okay, let's try Adderall, 5 mg. Start out taking one a day, and after a week or so, if you are not having trouble, you can go up to two. I want you to increase your Clonazepam also. Another thing, Ruth. I appreciate your coming back, and I appreciate the opportunity to treat you. I know how concerned and perplexed you are, but I want you to be hopeful."

She was wearing a beautiful smile when she returned, and she was eager to tell me what had happened.

"I am elated. Within just an hour or so of taking my first Adderall, I could feel the pain leaving my knees. Since that first day, they have hardly hurt me at all."

"And your sleep, fatigue, and all the rest?"

"Unbelievable! I sleep through the night. I wake up refreshed, and I don't get sleepy during the day. There is something else, and we didn't talk about this, but I was having some really weird nightmares. They have gone away now."

"How about your memory and your mental focus?"

"Much better, I can stay focused now. I wasn't able to do that before. I must tell you that I feel so good, I am euphoric."

"Ruth, I am happy for your improvement, but you have me worried now. That word, euphoria, coming from a bipolar scares me. Are you getting manic?"

"No, I have been manic hundreds, maybe thousands of times. This is not mania. This is pain relief. This is recovery. This is happiness. This is euphoria."

My concerns about Ruth's euphoria were certainly appropriate. Victims of bipolarity can express their illness in many ways, including a feeling of energized well-being. Hearing the bipolar utter the word "euphoria" no longer bothers me because I have heard it so much. It is an expression of the flight to health and the achievement of wellness in people who have not known that experience for a long time.

"Any down side to the medicine?"

"Almost none at all. The first few days I felt a little nervous and jittery, but that has all gone away."

"Ruth, have you seen your psychiatrist since you started the Adderall?"

"Yes, he told me to keep taking it. He said he was glad you tried it. Let me tell you something interesting. I have seen my orthopedist. He told me has seen a number of people with very painful arthritis get better with drugs like Ritalin and Adderall."

"I do find that interesting. He must be a very observant doctor. You can tell him I said that. Let me ask you another question. If I recall correctly, you told me your moods were still shifting even with the Lexapro and Clonazepam. Has that changed any since you have been on the Adderall?"

"Yes, that has been truly remarkable. I really feel very even—no highs and no lows. That may be the most remarkable thing of all, except for one other thing that I really don't understand."

"What's that?"

"Within a day of starting the Adderall, I lost all craving for cigarettes. I was a pack-a-day smoker, and I have not had a cigarette the past month. I don't miss them at all. Can you possibly explain that to me?"

"Well, perhaps yes. You have had bipolar disease for a long time. I suppose you know something about neurotransmitters."

"Yes, quite a lot."

"You may have heard of the smoking cessation drug, the antidepressant Wellbutrin. It stimulates the release of dopamine, and that seems to diminish the pleasure derived from smoking cigarettes. The Adderall you are taking is a different drug, but it also stimulates dopamine. That may be why it helped you stop smoking. Amazing stuff, isn't it, Ruth?"

"Yes, amazing."

Okay, reader, I did take a chance giving a stimulant to a bipolar, but I feel like I am taking a chance anytime I prescribe a drug, especially to a bipolar. Fortunately, though, Ruth and I were greatly rewarded. She got well, and I learned something important. I was sure that Ruth would not be the last painful bipolar that I would treat with a stimulant.

I need to emphasize the suddenness of Ruth's recovery (she was better in hours), and most important, the totality. Her many and varied symptoms—knee pain, fatigue, sleeplessness, daytime somnolence, nightmares, want of mental focus, mood shifting, and cigarette addiction, to boot—went away virtually simultaneously under the sponsorship of a single drug, and that administered at a very low dose! It was a clinical miracle, and thanks to Ruth and several other painful people who submitted to my take-a-chance therapies, I see compa-rable miracles with remarkable frequency now. I will explore these in the chapters that follow, and I can't wait to get there, but first we must discuss the bipolar spectrum.

> *It was a clinical miracle, and thanks to Ruth . . . I see comparable miracles with remarkable frequency now.*

Psychiatrists now believe that bipolar disorder is a spectrum of diseases. It encom-passes the classic mood-swinging Bipolar I and also Bipolar II, in which the amplitude of the swings (they might better be called shifts) is less dramatic. Another part of the spectrum is attention deficit disorder. The other is narcolepsy. To review that subject briefly, it is a disorder characterized by daytime sleepfulness, sometimes coming in sudden attacks. It is associated with hypnagogic hallucinations, sleep paral-ysis, and also the curious phenomenon of cataplexy, which describes a sudden loss of muscular tone, often in response to startle or emotion. It is a brief interval of paralysis, sometimes causing the victim to fall to the floor. Recovery, however, is almost immediate.

Learning that bipolarity was, at least in theory, a spectrum of diseases, or perhaps better, a single core illness with multiple expressions, was a revela-tory—and comforting—discovery to me. It fit my recent experience with Ruth like a hand in a glove. She had features of the entire spectrum, narcolepsy, attention deficit disorder, and Bipolar I. And all the bad things went away with the administration of the stimulant Adderall. It was beginning to make sense. Bipolarity is a broad spectrum indeed, and its expressions are many and varied. Nonetheless, there is a single core disease, and that is why everything got better with the administration of a single drug. I was begin-ning to understand why, when the right drug kicks in, everything gets better.

I will suggest that we can extend the bipolar spectrum to include chronic fatigue and chronic pain, and I will explore this thesis in the case histories that follow.

Dear Dr. Cochran:

Your book was a great help to me, and I am taking some time to seriously consider its relevance and applicability to my challenges. I will see my MD tomorrow to talk to him about your book. Then we will send my medical records. I am very interested in pursuing this—just some general information.

Fifty-two-year-old Caucasian female.
History: Fibromyalgia, degenerative disc disease, bilateral carpal tunnel (one surgically corrected), restless legs syndrome, history of dysmenorrhea.
Married twenty-eight years; one daughter, age twenty-three.
Early childhood sexual abuse victim.
Alcoholic mother; mother and brother are bipolar.
Positive attitude despite life challenges.
No history of clinical depression but take Effexor (75 mg. a day, ostensibly for pain).
Successful business person before painfulness took over.

Between my age and the history of early childhood sexual abuse, I may not be the best candidate, but I found your book thought-provoking and a very logical extension of some of my life's experiences. I have done extensive psychotherapy and physical therapy to try to help myself. I currently use Lyrica, Requip, and Hydrocodone as well as Effexor. I hope your polypharmaceutical approach will help. Obviously I am already a walking cocktail.

Sincerely,
Janet Sugahara

She was an ebullient brunette charmer, graceful in movement and speech. Her pain began when she was in her twenties, and a diagnosis of fibromyalgia was made about her age thirty. She suffered disordered sleep at night and sleepiness during the day. Along the way, she was treated with Alprazolam and then Prozac and Paxil, but they were without benefit. Until she became painful, she had been lean and athletic, but since then she had experienced uncontrollable sweet cravings and progressive weight gain. Her challenges (as she so nicely put it) notwithstanding, she was quite successful in her endeavors, both in business and community affairs. Her marriage had been happy, and her daughter had recently graduated with a degree in architecture.

I enjoyed my conversation with Janet. I judged her to have a keen intelligence. There was a sense of command and confidence about her, and there was a sense of energy with none of it wasted. She spoke quickly and well with little pause for reflection.

"Janet, it does look as though my book was written for you, doesn't it?"

"Yes, very much so."

"I'd like to pursue some issues you mentioned in your e-mail. You wrote that you had been sexually abused in your youth. Could you tell me a little bit about that?"

"It began when I was five."

"Was it repetitive, did it go on a long time?"

"Yes, several years."

"At the hands of?"

"My mother."

"What was she like?"

"Alcoholic and bipolar. That was diagnosed about the time I left for college."

"Is she still living?"

"Yes."

"And your relationship with her now?"

"I work real hard on that, really hard. By no means are we best friends, but there has been some closure. I am more comfortable with her, and I am more comfortable with myself."

"Janet, many people who have endured the kind of experience you did have had a problem with depression and anxiety. Did you ever have anything like that?"

"Well, yes and no. Several doctors have given me antidepressant medications, but I have never really felt depressed. I did, however, have a problem with anxiety. It began when my daughter was five, and I am sure you can see the connection. When she turned that age, the same age at which my abuse began, I started to flashback, and I was very anxious. I became very protective of my daughter, perhaps too much so. I began psychotherapy, and after five years I was able to put it behind me. I have had no problem at all with anxiety since then."

"Flashbacks stopped?"

"Yes, no more flashbacks."

"Janet, you have been given several different medicines along the way. Have you ever had bizarre reactions to any of them? Have any of them made you feel depressed or have any of them energized you or wired you up?"

"Yes, about two years ago I was given some Oxycodone for my pain. That drug gave me the most wonderful feeling I have ever known. I felt empowered and energized. My doctor was alarmed when I told him this. He stopped the Oxycodone and gave me the Hydrocodone that I am taking now."

"Have there been other instances when you felt that way?"

"Yes, occasionally I get a sense of empowerment. When that happens I become hyperactive, and my mind races. I know what you are thinking. After I read your book, I wondered if I might be bipolar. What do you think?"

"I don't know yet, Janet, but before we get through, I think we will find out."

A curious problem relating to the treatment of the bipolar relates to the fact that a state of hypomania (low-grade mania) can be a wonderful condition to be in. It can be a state of happiness, hopefulness, and high-energy quick-wittedness. If I had been a psychiatrist attending Janet, I would have done absolutely nothing. She was in good emotional order, and who would want to change that with pharmacy? The problem, however, is that I am not a psychiatrist, and I was not called upon to address her mood. Rather, I was called upon to address her pain, her insomnia, her fatigue, and daytime sleepiness.

After a month of therapy with Clonazepam and Nortriptyline, Janet returned to report that her sleep was restored. She would have a couple of awakenings to void, but this was an improvement over the four to five times she had had before. She described a certain sense of refreshment when she woke up. It was easier, she said, to get going in the morning, and her fibromyalgia pain was actually diminishing a bit, but her sleepiness and fatigue had not improved.

Perhaps I should have left well enough alone because with relatively modest pharmacy, she had clearly improved. But I couldn't resist. I prescribed Adderall 10 mg. one to two daily. A month later, she reported somewhat to my surprise that the Adderall had given her a bit more energy but not much else. Moreover, she was having a little more pain and a little less sleep.

She told me that her pain had diminished from a seven to a three, and that she was thrilled with her progress.

Janet's report of worsening symptoms did not indicate to me that we were on the wrong track, perhaps only that we needed more medicine. I increased the dose of Nortriptyline and Clonazepam and doubled the Adderall to 20 mg. twice daily. A month later, she reported dramatic improvement. Her sleepiness and fatigue were just about gone. She told me that her pain had diminished from a seven to a three, and that she was thrilled with her progress. The whole evolution had taken a matter of only four months.

We had a nice chat, and I released her back to her primary care doctor. As we said our good-byes, I asked her what she thought of our experience together—her recovery, or at least near recovery, from thirty years of pain. She replied, "I am a Bipolar II, aren't I?"

"Yes, something like that."

"I have one last question for you."

"Okay."

"Could you see my daughter? She has a problem with fatigue, and I think you might be able to help her."

"Janet, I would be privileged to see your daughter."

Margaret was a stunning young Asian American. Her complaint was sleepiness and fatigue. She required nearly ten hours sleep each night but nevertheless, would awaken in the morning tired and unrestored. She often fell asleep during the day and for many years had a terrible problem dozing off in class. She developed panic disorder when she was a teenager and was given Effexor with good control of her symptoms. The year before she came to me, she developed a sudden tachycardia with a heart rate of one hundred eighty beats per minute. She was evaluated by a cardiologist and started on Metoprolol, a beta-blocker drug which lowers the heart rate and prevents tachycardia. The reader may recall the story of Frank from chapter six. The parallels between he and Margaret are quite remarkable.

She told me that sleepiness and fatigue had bothered her most of her life. She was sleep-needful. If she went without her usual complement of ten hours, she would get very achy and uncomfortable. In the main, however, pain was not an issue. She did report, in response to my question, that she was subject to very vivid nightmares, and after some of them she would be quite unable to move.

I suspected she had narcolepsy, and I thought stimulant therapy was appropriate. I was concerned, however, about her history of tachycardia and panic. Both could be worsened by stimulant therapy. Therefore, I erred on the side of caution and prescribed Nortriptyline and Clonazepam, the very same drugs that had been helpful to her mother.

Her nightmares did diminish, but little else was happening. It was time to take a chance. I told her we were going to start the drug Adderall in a very low dosage—5 mg. once or twice a day. She accepted the prescription and told me that her mother had reminded her that a few years before she had been given the drug Provigil for daytime sleepiness. She said she didn't tolerate it because of nausea.

She called me in a short while to tell me that she had taken the Adderall and experienced splendid improvement. Her fatigue was diminished, and she no longer felt the need for naps during the day. She was concerned, however, because a close family friend, a pharmacist, had told her that she should not take the Adderall because it would be bad for her heart. She consulted with her cardiologist, and he told her the same thing.

I had taken a double hit. Not just the other doctor saying no, the pharmacist also. Such is the lot of the pain doctor—always being told what he shouldn't do.

"Margaret, I understand where your doctors are coming from, but let me ask you—did you tell either of them how much better you felt taking the medicine?"

"No, come to think of it, I really didn't. They didn't even ask me."

I told her that her narcolepsy was as worthy of treatment as her tachy-cardia and panic. She faced the prospect of being somnolent and fatigued for the rest of her life. I was quite impressed by her response to Adderall, and I thought it invited continuance of therapy—not discarding it. She expressed confusion and fear that the drug would damage her heart. Understandable emotions to be sure, but I had the feeling that they were getting in the way of her recovery. I offered her a consultation with another cardiologist. She accepted and told me, "I am glad to do it, I really don't like my cardiologist. He has been pretty insensitive to me."

I received the consultation note in short order. He found no evidence of heart disease. The tachycardia was unexplained but could very likely be controlled quite easily with Metoprolol. He thought the use of Adderall was quite reasonable.

Margaret resumed her Adderall and reported ongoing improvement in her sleepiness and nightmares. Her fatigue, however, continued to bother her.

Then, a few months later, a reverse. Margaret asked the cardiologist if she might reduce the dose of Metoprolol. She felt it might be causing some of her fatigue. He concurred and reduced the dose by one-half. Within weeks, she had another spell of tachycardia requiring an emer-gency room visit for treatment. Adderall was discontinued, and the Metoprolol dose increased. Margaret's sleepiness and fatigue returned. She had lost all that she had gained.

This story will have a happy ending, though. I keep in touch with Margaret and her cardiologist. He is committed to getting her back on the stimulant therapy that had been so helpful. He may even proceed with the procedure that had so successfully corrected Frank's tachycardia (and the need for fatigue-producing beta-blocker therapy). The ablation procedure may have been somewhat experimental in 1994 when Frank underwent it, but it is widely performed now, and there is a very good prospect that Margaret can resume her Adderall and with it, control of her narcolepsy and fatigue.

I need to remind the reader that Margaret was quite a young woman, only twenty-three years of age, and in the span of that time had experienced several expressions of the bipolar spectrum—narcolepsy, fatigue, and on top of that, panic. Few would contest that panic may be an expression of bipolarity (there is almost nothing that cannot be an expression of bipolarity!). What does her future hold? Will her core illness (bipolar spectrum) remain in remission under the influence of therapy with Effexor, Clonazepam, and Adderall? Or, is it possible that she will break through with one or several other expressions of her bipolarity— be this mania, depression, attention deficit, or even pain? It is not a question of if, it is a question of when. Recall Ruth from earlier in this chapter. After a lifetime of struggle with mood swings, she finally achieved control with the drugs Lexapro and Clonazepam. Nonetheless, her underlying bipolarity found expression in the form of fatigue, forgetfulness, nightmares, and pain. The same sort of thing will almost certainly happen to Margaret. She has a long life ahead of her, and lots of things are going to happen. Even so, it will still have a happy ending because we have marvelous pharmacy with which to attack the many-headed monster that is bipolar disease.

> *We have marvelous pharmacy with which to attack the many-headed monster that is bipolar disease.*

Ellen had her mastectomy in 1994, some ten years before coming to me. Her cancer was aggressive, and she required chemotherapy. She became depressed and was treated with Zoloft. After a couple of years of disability, she abandoned her antidepressant and returned to employment as a social worker. Then, in 2001, she ruptured a cervical disc and required surgery to relieve her severe neck and arm pain. She told me that within a few days of her operation, she knew something was different. She felt depressed and fatigued. She started aching all over her body and began to experience frequent nightmares. Her mental focus became blurred, and she was very forgetful. Her treatments included Hydrocodone, Trazodone, Neurontin, and finally the opiate Duragesic, which only made her nightmares worse. She was also given Strattera after being told that she suffered attention deficit disorder. She found that drug somewhat helpful in restoring mental focus, but little else was happening. After two years of unsuccessful treatment of her pain and depression, she presented for my consultation.

"Have you ever had a case like mine? Have you ever had a case where somebody wakes up after surgery and is suddenly a different person? That is what happened to me. Have you ever seen anything like it?"

"Well, Ellen, I have. It does happen occasionally. I certainly have seen it happen after childbirth."

"Can you help me?"

I reviewed her history. She described good health before her breast cancer, and even after that she had been restored to a very satisfactory level of emotional and physical stability. I inquired about childhood trauma, and she denied any but commented that her mother was bipolar and very unstable.

"She was a Bipolar I, and I know what I am talking about. I am a social worker."

"Any other family members with bipolar disease, or have you ever been suspected of having it?"

"No."

"Let's talk about your childhood. You tell me your mother was bipolar. Many of my patients with chronic pain give me the same family history of bipolarity. A lot of them tell me that they were subject to abuse during childhood. I think there may be a connection. You know, I am sure, that the bipolar may become mean and destructive during intervals of mania, or for that matter, when they are depressed. Did you feel that you were abused?"

"Yes, I know well just how mean and hateful a bipolar can become. Fortunately, my abuse was only emotional and verbal—never physical or sexual, and I am very grateful for that. Looking back on it. I realize I came out of my childhood and a very dysfunctional family rather well."

"Any problem with depression, anxiety, or panic?"

"No, not at all. No problem with depression until my breast cancer."

"I am writing you a prescription for Imipramine and Clonazepam. I want you to continue the Strattera. Have you found that helpful?"

"Yes, I do find it helpful. I am more focused when I take the drug, but as far as the rest of it, the nightmares, the fatigue, and the pain, nothing has helped."

For some reason, Ellen and I had trouble getting together. She was not diligent in her appointment keeping, and I sensed a certain lack of commitment on her part. She was ambivalent about the Imipramine, concerned about its affect on libido and also the sense of dryness that she felt when she took it (a common complaint). It was a few months into her treatment before she finally addressed the reality of her situation. She was getting progressively more painful and depressed. Her nightmares were ever worsening, and some of them, she told me, were attended by a state of paralysis.

I had heard enough. "Ellen, I am prescribing a stimulant known as Adderall. There is some redundancy using it with Strattera, so I want you to taper that drug as we increase the dose of Adderall. Let me see you again in three weeks."

She returned at the appointed time to tell me that the nightmares were gone, and that her sleep was much improved. Her memory was better, and her pain was diminishing.

Was it because her brain, under duress, was hungry for a false neurotransmitter that it had become accustomed to?

"I am happy for you, Ellen. It looks like we have hit the nail on the head."

"Indeed we have, but there is something I must talk to you about. When I was younger, in college and for several years afterward, I abused amphetamine. I used it to keep my weight down. I had always wanted to be an entertainer, and my appearance was important to me. I am fearful of getting back into abusing amphetamine, but I must admit this is the best I have felt in three years. What do you think I should do?"

"Ellen, the drug has been marvelous for you. I want you to continue it, but we must monitor this very closely. You must keep your appointments and take the medicine exactly as I have prescribed."

"That I will do."

Ellen had given me a lot to think about. Stimulant therapy was certainly appropriate because her pain was accompanied by features of both attention deficit disorder and narcolepsy. So far, so good. But what is the relevance of her long-ago abuse of amphetamines? Could they have so altered her brain's infrastructure that although that organ was capable of compensating for a long time, it finally collapsed under the provocation of breast cancer, depression, and an operation on her neck that rendered her almost immediately depressed, sleepless, nightmare-ridden, and painful? And her response to Adderall, which is amphetamine. Did that happen because she suffered fragments of the bipolar spectrum? Or was it because her brain, under duress, was hungry for a false neurotransmitter that it had become accustomed to so many years ago? I really don't know, but it is worth thinking about.

Rhoda was an attractive thirty-six-year-old nurse with interstitial cystitis. She also suffered fibromyalgia, migraine, and carpal tunnel syndrome. Remarkably, all of these had appeared in her teens.

Faced with so many painful disorders appearing at such an early age, I directed my interrogations toward the issue of childhood abuse. She told me that her parents divorced at her age seven, and this was very distressing to her. She denied any issues of physical or sexual abuse. I inquired about her family history. Her mother was a chronic depressive, she said, and an older brother had just been diagnosed with bipolar disease.

"Did you have a problem with depression when you were young, Rhoda?"

"No, not when I was young. That came with my divorces."

"How many divorces?"

"Three."

"And you are married now?"

"Yes, and to a really good man. He is the father of my children."

"You have been married four times, Rhoda?"

"Yes, four times."

"All to different men?"

"Yes, four times to different men."

"Why so many?"

"I don't really know. I wish I did. I guess I just expect too much."

"But you are happy with your marriage now?"

"Yes, very happy."

I have learned to routinely ask how many times my patients have been married. Multiple marriages and divorces can be a clue to bipolarity, and Rhoda's record was pretty impressive.

"How are you sleeping, Rhoda?"

"Poorly. I have to get up several times at night to empty my bladder, and I still hurt in my pelvis and back. I roll over in bed at night and awaken with pain."

"Fatigue?"

"Of course."

"Are you subject to mind racing? Do you have periods of high energy? Do you have trouble handling your money? Do you go out and spend foolishly?"

"No, none of those."

"Are you depressed?"

"You know, not really. I was depressed after my divorces, and I took drugs like Paxil and Prozac, and I guess they helped. But no, I am not depressed. I know what that is like, and that is not the way I feel now."

Rhoda, it seemed, was a young woman who had an inordinate number of problems with pain and maybe inordinate problems in finding the right husband. Perhaps she was bipolar, but I saw little to really suggest it. I elected to start with Clonazepam and Nortriptyline, knowing that the latter can often reduce the frequency of urinary voidings.

On her return, Rhoda seemed quite excited about her progress. She had a lot to tell me. She felt terribly sedated on the medicine but had experimented and discovered it was the Clonazepam that was giving her trouble. She discarded it and continued the single Nortriptyline pill each night. When she tried to increase the dose, she was very sleepy the next day, so she settled on 10 mg. each night. She told me excitedly that her bladder pain was diminished and her fibromyalgia also, and she was sleeping better than she had in years.

When it is too good to be true, it sometimes is. On the visits following, Rhoda reported reappearance of bladder problems and also fibromyalgia. I elected to add Cymbalta. It didn't go well at all. Within two or three days of starting the drug, Rhoda's bladder pain flared, and she began passing bloody urine. On my instructions she stopped the Cymbalta, and her symptoms gradually improved.

Coincidence or drug effect? I have faced that dilemma thousands of times. I hadn't been able to do as much as I had wanted for Rhoda, and I was hopeful that the Cymbalta might help us turn the corner. Weeks later, I told her to try it again. She did with the same result. And that is just the way it goes. We give drugs to relieve pain, and in some cases the pain actually worsens. We should expect that. There is no reason to believe that every person will respond the same way to every drug.

As time went by, Rhoda and I became very fond of each other. We enjoyed our visits, but in the end game, I really had achieved but little. She was sleeping better, and her bladder pain had diminished a bit, but I did not sense anything approaching a resurrection, and that is what I am aiming for when I treat the painful. I told her that I was sorry that we weren't doing better, but I would keep trying.

"You have helped me! I don't know how to say it, but I feel better since I have been with you."

I didn't think my pharmacy was doing much for Rhoda. Whatever benefit she achieved was, I believed, due simply to having someone to talk to, someone who liked her, and who was not dismissive of her many complaints. It wasn't the outcome I really wanted, but it was better than nothing. Then she said something that startled me.

"Can you give me something to help me think and remember? Do you think I could have attention deficit disorder? After my first child was born a couple of years ago, I suddenly couldn't remember. I lost my mental focus, and I couldn't seem to keep my mind on any one thing for any length of time. I have to write notes. I write down every time I take a medicine or I give the kids medicine, because I literally cannot remember if I gave it or not."

I'll take any clue I can get, even if my patient has to beat me over the head with it to get my attention. I prescribed Adderall. The effect was maybe not miraculous, but it was close.

"It is really helping me, it really is. I can actually remember things. I can take care of my home, my children, and my husband much better. I am organized, and I haven't been that way in two years."

"How about your pain?"

"Well, it is still there, but I don't know how to say this—it just doesn't bother me as much. I find that there are times when I don't even think about my pain, and I haven't been that way in a long, long time."

"Anything else to tell me, Rhoda?"

"Yes, since I have been on the Adderall I feel more even. I realize that my moods were swinging up and down, and I don't have that anymore."

When I hear the word "even" from a patient on my pharmacy, I can be rather sure I am dealing with a bipolar. Let me suggest, and this is important, that Rhoda's newfound emotional evenness did not happen because her pain was relieved. It happened because Adderall can actually be mood stabilizing.

Let's review the stories of the women I have presented in this chapter. They all had a family history of bipolar disease (Ruth, a probable, the rest more certain). Ruth, she of the rapid-cycling Bipolar I, experienced pain, fatigue, nightmare-disturbed sleep, and forgetfulness. Janet was Bipolar II and painful, insomniac, and daytime sleepy. Her daughter, Margaret, suffered panic disorder and narcolepsy. Ellen awoke from a surgical operation with the sudden appearance of fatigue, painfulness, narcolepsy, and attention deficit disorder. Lastly, Rhoda, multiply married, painful, and following the birth of her child, attention deprived. Can you not see the continuum? Can you appreciate that there may not be much difference between bipolar disease, narcolepsy, attention deficit disorder, chronic pain, and fatigue? Can you not see that these five women all suffered expressions of a single core illness, and that all were benefited by the treatment of that illness with the stimulant Adderall?

Remember Ruth's "high up on the food chain among psychiatric pharmacologists" doctor suggesting the use of stimulants many years before she came to me. Psychiatrists have long known that stimulants can occasionally be helpful in mood stabilization. They have been little used for that purpose, however. The reasons for this are several. First of all, stimulant therapy for the bipolar is, as I have written, counterintuitive. Exciting a bipolar brain with stimulants can indeed induce mania, and I will describe such a case shortly. Moreover, we already have many reasonably effective mood stabilizers. Lastly, stimulants are potentially addictive and therefore, in the minds of many (perhaps most), should be avoided.

In the chapters that follow, I will present the case histories of people who have been cured by potentially addictive drugs. They are resurrections beyond almost any that I ever dreamt I would witness.

CHAPTER FOURTEEN

The Opiate Cure

Roy weighed more than three hundred pounds. He was afflicted with that condition known cruelly as morbid obesity. He was six feet tall, and he carried most of his weight in a massive upper body. He had no neck at all. It was just a mass of corpulence fixed to his huge shoulders. He moved about slowly as he settled himself ungracefully onto the oak examining table that had many times before borne the weight of the obese painful patient.

"You don't know me, Doc, but I remember you very well. You took care of my father many years ago. He died of lung cancer. I am sure you don't remember."

The mind of a physician is a strange place. It has an almost preternatural ability to recall patients seen in the past. It took a few moments for the recall to register, but it did. I said, "I think I do remember. Your father had brown eyes and dark black hair just like you, didn't he?"

"Yes, that's right."

"But I remember your father as a lean and wiry man."

"That's right. That's the way I looked before I got sick. I have gained one hundred sixty pounds since then."

Roy began his story and has he did, his eyes reddened and tears began to flow. He was forty, a mechanic, married, and the father of two boys. About age thirty he developed panic disorder and required treatment with Zoloft. Two years before he came to me, he hurt his back in an industrial accident. A ruptured disc was surgically excised, and his back and right leg pain disappeared, but only for a few months. They recurred, worse than before, and Roy underwent a much bigger operation, the fusion of one lumbar vertebra to another to restore stability. His pain did not abate at all, and in short order he experienced intense sweet cravings and gained weight rapidly.

Then, as occasionally happens in thick-necked people, particularly painful ones, he developed sleep apnea with heavy snoring at night and frequent attacks of somnolence during the day. An operation was performed on his throat to open up the upper airway. His snoring and daytime sleepiness improved but nothing else did. His pain continued, and he became progressively depressed, speaking often of suicide. He was subject to attacks of agitation and occasionally of violence, striking his wife and children. His bipolar disease evolved rapidly, and he required several hospitalizations, some for extended periods of time. Only after the employ of several different drugs was his psychiatrist able to achieve any control over his irascibility and mood swings. When he came to me he was on Effexor, Clonazepam, Provigil, and the mood-stabilizers Zyprexa, Risperdal, and Trileptal. He was also taking the opiate Hydrocodone four times a day.

Drugs were hardly touching either his depression or his pain.

Roy must have been a very sick man to require that much pharmacy. However, the drugs were hardly touching either his depression or his pain. I had to ask an important question. "Did any of your doctors ever suggest electroconvulsive therapy?"

"Yes, they did, but I was afraid of it. I refused shock treatments."

"How are you feeling now, Roy?"

"I feel horrible. I can't do anything. I can't drive a car. I can't sleep. I can't go see my kids play ball. All I do is sit around and eat, and I am still gaining weight. The doctors say it is due to the cortisone I have taken, and they tell me that some of the medicine I'm on causes people to gain weight."

"Well, Roy, that is probably partly correct, but I suspect there is more to it than drug effect. I think your weight gain is part of your illness."

"Nobody has ever told me that before."

My treatment options with Roy were limited. He was at best in precarious balance, and even his pathetic state of being was achieved only by the administration of many different drugs. I elected to consult with the psychiatrist and to introduce no drugs without her consent. She was available and happy to take my call. She recounted the history much as

Roy had given me. She commented that both she and her consultants very much wanted to do electroshock treatments, but Roy refused.

"Why so many drugs?" I asked.

"That is what it took to control his mood swings. He really has been a difficult management problem. Do you have any ideas about what we might do?"

"Only one. He is on Hydrocodone for pain now. I wonder what would happen if we added morphine?"

"You know, that is really not a bad idea. We have tried to avoid using much opiate because we had enough problems without introducing them, but I am in agreement. You go ahead and prescribe it, and I will help you keep a close watch on him."

I told Roy to continue taking the medicines as he has been, including the Hydrocodone, but that I was going to add morphine in the form of MS Contin. I wrote a prescription for a 15 mg. pill and told him to take one every twelve hours. If he found it helpful and wanted more, he could go up to two every twelve hours. The prescribed dosage, a minimum of 30 mg. or a maximum of 60 mg., is not really small doses of morphine, but by no means truly large. I thought the risk was low and the potential for gain was significant, although I had no idea it would work nearly as well as it did.

On his return, he told me he was taking 60 mg. a day and feeling much better, at least until a couple of days before. The drug had allowed him to be more active. He went into his garage, and for the first time in two years actually sat down on his motorcycle.

"When I did that, the pain all came back. It got a lot worse. I am afraid we are not getting anywhere at all."

Again, the physician must expect and be prepared for reverses in the painful. They are almost inevitable. He must also be ever-hopeful and must share that faith with the patient because it is the lack of hope that most defines chronic pain. It was highly unlikely that the simple act of lifting a leg, no matter how big it is, over a motorcycle and fantasizing about riding it would destroy a fused spine. It is much more likely that it would do nothing more than sprain muscles unaccustomed to that kind of movement. I told Roy that I thought we were just suffering a temporary backset. I gave him a shot of cortisone. I was not sure it would help, but at least I was doing something. I told him to maintain his opiate therapy as before and come back to see me in a couple of weeks.

He returned with a big smile on his face. "Doc, I could just hug you."

I said, "Please don't do that, Roy. You would kill me!"

He laughed, maybe the first time he had really laughed in two years.

"I can't tell you how much better I feel. I even got back on the bike, and it didn't bother me at all this time."

"Roy, you are smiling and you are laughing. It looks like the depression may be going away."

"Yeah, Doc, it really is. My moods aren't swinging like they used to. I don't feel angry and agitated anymore, and my pain has almost gone away. I think I can start getting off some of the other medicines. I am not sure I need them anymore."

"Let the psychiatrist call the shots on that one."

"I saw her just a few days ago. She was really impressed with how well I was doing. She said we would probably come off the drugs, but we would have to do it very slowly. She wants to wait a while."

"I agree with that."

"Doc, there is something really amazing that is happening to me. I am very proud of it, and I want you to know about it. Since I started the morphine, I don't crave food the way I used to. I have been on it a month now, and I have lost twenty pounds!"

I have written before and will continue to write that when the right drug kicks in, everything gets better. The morphine relieved Roy's pain, and that is what I hopefully expected to happen. It also relieved his depression. I didn't expect that, but I had heard of similar cases. I never anticipated, however, that morphine would arrest his violent bipolar mood swings and certainly not his pathologic appetite. (Was that a symptom of his bipolar disease? I wouldn't bet against it.)

I have seen my share of clinical miracles, but Roy was unique in that the totality of his recovery was so unexpected. It was an exercise in serendipity, which means discovery by accident. It was an eye-opener for me. Opiates for the treatment of mental illness! I had never entertained the notion. I had dedicated my professional life to relieving pain by treating, with psychiatric drugs, the mental illness that so often is its root cause. I had never seriously thought about the converse, that by treating pain with opiates, I could cure mental illness!

A brief digression here. I began my medical studies in 1955 and entered practice in 1963. That span of eight years witnessed the birth of modern psychiatric pharmacy. It still boggles my mind when I think back to it. When I began, we had virtually no effective drugs for the treatment of mental illness. When I completed my training, we had the first tranquilizers in the form of Meprobamate (older readers may recall the proprietary names Equanil and Miltown) and Librium, the first benzodiazepine. We had the

When the right drug kicks in, everything gets better.

first antipsychotics, Reserpine and Thorazine. Also the first antidepressants, the tricyclics Imipramine and Amitriptyline. And a new anticonvulsant, Tegretol, for many years to remain the bedrock in the treatment of nerve injury pain and bipolar disease. So great was the enthusiasm for the new drugs, my mentors, as best I can remember, never told me that before they came on the scene, morphine was sometimes used in the treatment of psychosis and mania and was occasionally quite successful—an effect that was called the *opiate cure.*

A year or so ago I was attending Joan, a woman with severe spinal pain. I was treating her with morphine in the extravagant dose of 300 mg. daily. Nonetheless, her pain, she told me, was insufferable, and she requested something—anything—to give her relief. I elected to add a second opiate, and I chose Methadone. I don't know why I did it. It had never been one of my favorites; indeed I had used it but rarely. Nonetheless, something, Providence perhaps, directed me to try the drug. I prescribed it at the rate of 10 mg. three times daily, a test dose to see if she could tolerate the drug.

She returned at the appointed time and said, "It is working. It is really working. I am almost free of pain. I can't tell you how much better I feel."

"I am astonished, Joan, I am truly astonished. I certainly didn't expect that kind of response, but I am happy that you are better."

"I am astonished, too."

"Are you taking it as I prescribed, three times a day?"

"No, I am taking it only once a day. That is all I need. I haven't even tried to go up on that dose."

"Say what?"

"I am only taking one pill a day. That is all I need."

"You are taking only 10 mg. of Methadone. That on top of 300 mg. of morphine, and you are better, you are a lot better?"

"Yes, absolutely. I don't hurt anymore, and there is a certain calmness that I feel. I guess relaxed is the word. Before I started the Methadone, I always felt frustrated and irritable with my pain. That has all gone. I am grateful to you."

"Joan, let me hear this again. You took one pill, and you felt so much better that you didn't feel the need to even try a second one?"

"That is correct. One pill a day is quite enough."

Oh, my God! A woman's bitterly painful life had been transfigured suddenly and totally by taking one Methadone pill a day.

Joan's response to Methadone was by any measure unexpected, atypical, and bizarre. But I feed on the atypical and bizarre. They are my sustenance. I had learned something that might turn out to be very important, and I stashed it away, certain that when the right time came, I would try the morphine and Methadone combination again.

A word now about Methadone. It was synthesized—that is, made from scratch—in Germany in 1937. Unlike Hydrocodone and Oxycodone, which are semi-synthetic, the opium poppy is not necessary for its manufacture. Methadone has the most erratic metabolism of all the opiates, and its clinical effect is sometimes unpredictable. Nonetheless, it is an effective painkiller, easy to manufacture, and relatively speaking, dirt cheap. It has several curious features, and the best known is its capacity to diminish cravings for heroin. It is widely employed for that purpose, and there are Methadone maintenance clinics in every major city in this country that administer Methadone to heroin addicts in recovery. Another curious feature of Methadone, referenced early in this book, is that in addition to being opioid agonist, it is a glutamine antagonist. And remember,

> *I feed on the atypical and bizarre. They are my sustenance.*

glutamine is the neurotransmitter that we believe is responsible for mania, panic, pain, and almost certainly many other bad things.

Alice walked into the examining room with excruciating slowness. She was wearing a thick collar about her neck and a stocking cap pulled over her head so low that her face was hardly visible. She was helped onto the examining table, an activity associated with grimacing, wincing, and an occasional cry in pain. She was exhibiting her suffering. I asked her to remove her collar and her cap. She did so slowly, protecting herself from painful movements. I took the opportunity to scan the referring doctor's brief letter.

Dear Dr. Cochran:

I am referring Alice Driver to you for consultation regarding (1) neck pain, (2) depression, (3) anxiety syndrome, (4) post-traumatic stress disorder, (5) fibromyalgia, and (6) headache. I am not comfortable prescribing controlled substances for her, and she is requesting pain medicine. I am willing to release her to your care. When you have completed your evaluation, I would be interested in your impressions and recommendations.

Sincerely,
Roy Conner, MD

Well, it turned out he had missed a couple, but it was a pretty good start. I looked at my patient, her face and head now exposed. She had a large surgical scar on the right side of her neck, and her scalp was adorned with electrodes attached by wires to a miniaturized electroencephalograph (EEG) for recording brainwave activity. I knew I was in for an interesting visit, and I asked her to tell me about her pain.

"There is a bullet in my neck. They say they can't remove it. I would be paralyzed if they did. I am in constant pain."

"How did it happen?"

"My ex-husband shot me."

"Was it an accident?"

"No, he was trying to kill me."

She told me that her carotid artery had been damaged and that she required emergency surgery. The artery was successfully repaired, but the bullet had lodged deep in the neck in the vertebral column and could not be surgically removed. This had happened some seven years before. Remarkably, she had been able to go back to work on an automobile assembly line.

"Wasn't that painful?"

"Yes, but I had to work. I had to have some income, and it was really a good job."

"You can't work now, can you?" I asked, stating the obvious.

"No, I had to retire two years ago."

"Because of the pain?"

"Well, that was part of it, but I had another problem. I became very nervous, and I started dreaming about being shot. Sometimes the memory of it would come back to me out of the blue."

"Flashbacks?"

"Yes, flashbacks. They told me I had post-traumatic stress disorder. I got very depressed, and I tried to commit suicide."

Stress disorder need not appear immediately following the stressor. It may, and often does find expression years removed. Alice told me that her anxiety and depression came on when she started talking to friends about her assault. She had kept those thoughts and memories to herself for several years, but then when she started sharing them with others, she became very ill and increasingly painful.

> *Stress disorder need not appear immediately following the stressor.*

"What are taking for pain?"

"Nothing, I am on so many medicines already the doctors are afraid to give me pain drugs."

I looked at her intake history and saw the drugs listed—Effexor, Abilify, Lamictal, Seroquel, Diazepam, and most recently Lyrica. Aggressive psychiatric polypharmacy for sure. The employ of four mood stabilizers suggested there might be something more than stress disorder.

"Did any of your doctors tell you that you had bipolar disease?"

"Yes."

"When was that diagnosis made?"

"After I attempted suicide."

"When was that?"

"About six months ago."

"Have you always been moody, up and down?"

"Yes, for a long time."

"And the drugs—are they helping your moods?"

"Yes, they are helping some, but I am still up and down." And then she looked at her boyfriend.

"She sure is up and down. Sometimes she gets real angry, but I know it will pass away." He patted Alice on the shoulder.

"Alice, how is your pain now? Pretty bad?"

"Yes, it is really bad. It's the bullet in there. Can you help me? Can you give me something to relieve my pain?"

"Probably, Alice, but another question. Your doctors are doing brain wave tests on you even as we talk. Do they suspect that you have some kind of seizures?"

"Yes, they began when I was in the hospital. I started having passing-out spells. I would just go blank, and I wouldn't know what was going on around me."

I directed my attention to the boyfriend, because the victim of convulsive seizures usually is unable to recall the experience. Valuable information can be obtained, however, from an observer.

"Have you ever seen a seizure?"

"Yes, I have seen lots of them. She goes blank, and then she stares into space. Her eyelids kind of flutter, and then her eyes turn up."

"How long do they last?"

"A few minutes. I put a cold washcloth on her head, and that seems to help."

As I have written many times before, what a strange disease is chronic pain! There was so much more to Alice's discomfort than a bullet lodged in the neck. Equally important, perhaps even more important in the evolution of her pain was her bipolar disorder, post-traumatic stress disorder, and almost certainly pseudoseizures.

There are many types of convulsive seizures. All are attended by an alteration of consciousness and many by muscle jerkings that can be quite violent. In occasional cases, muscle contractions are less dramatic and consist of a few repetitive jerks or semi-purposeful movements of the extremities. Sometimes there is no abnormal movement at all but only a blank stare. Alice, perhaps, had the latter, but the appearance of epilepsy at this stage of her life was statistically improbable. Moreover, very few seizures are attended by fluttering eyelids, and very few seizures get better with the application of a cold washcloth to the forehead. I was quite sure that her EEG would turn out to be normal.

> *There was so much more to Alice's discomfort than a bullet lodged in the neck.*

Pseudoseizures, as the name suggests, mimic convulsions but are not real seizures at all. Rather, they are a psychologic reaction to stress appearing in the form of blackouts. As traditionally defined, the pseudoseizure is not a conversion reaction, but it is awfully close. The neurologic loss is not vision, or strength, or sensation. It is consciousness. I have already written about pain behavior and conversion as but another of the many expressions of chronic pain, and prognostically a good one at that.

As bad as it all seemed, I was very hopeful, even confident, that I could help Alice. I couldn't remove the bullet from her neck, but I am not sure that had all that much to do with the pain. Remember, after her injury, she was able to go back to work assembling automobiles. It was only when she quit trying to repress the experience and shared its dreadfulness with her friends that her bipolarity, post-traumatic stress disorder, and severe pain appeared. The reader is reminded of the story of Eve in chapter twelve. She started getting better when she finally began to talk about her past trauma. Alice got worse when she did. It is hard to understand, but that is the way it goes.

What to do? What options were available to me? Her bipolar disease, her depression, and anxiety were only marginally controlled with by the employ of *four* different mood stabilizers. I didn't want to toss another vegetable into that particular stew. It was time, I decided, to see what I could get out of opiate therapy in another unstable bipolar.

Alice replaced the collar around her neck and the stocking cap as I wrote a prescription for MS Contin. I gave her a low dose. One must always go slowly and carefully. As she left the examining room, her pain behaviors intensified, and she walked hesitantly with the assistance of her boyfriend, grimacing with each painful step.

I saw her two weeks later. She told me the brain wave test was normal (expected in pseudoseizures). She still exhibited her painfulness with hesitancy of movement and protective posturing, but there was a difference. It wasn't quite as striking as before, and her boyfriend had something approaching a smile on his face.

"How are we doing, Alice?"

"The medicine is helping. I am sleeping a little bit better, and I don't feel quite as nervous."

"She is better," the boyfriend said. "She is more even."

"The pain, Alice—how is the pain?"

"It is still pretty bad. The medicine takes the edge off, but it is still plenty bad. What can we do?"

Perhaps I should have simply increased the dose of morphine. It was helping her, and she was tolerating it. Why not just give more?

Let's look at the cards I was holding at that point in time. I had witnessed Roy's resurrection with morphine and Joan's with Methadone on top of morphine. Experience with two very atypical patients should hardly *dictate* treatment strategy, but it certainly could *influence* it. Besides, I had another card, a very good card. I knew, at least in theory, that bipolarity and probably pain are driven by the neurotransmitter glutamine. I also knew that Methadone antagonizes glutamine.

The time had come.

I prescribed Methadone 10 mg. every eight hours. The dosage I was employing, it should be emphasized, was really quite modest for a bullet-in-the-neck pain.

I saw her next a couple of weeks later. She came in with a huge smile on her face. She was free of her collar. Her gait was unencumbered, and she did not step up on to the examining table—she hopped onto it. She said her pain was gone, her sleep restored, and that her flashbacks had gone away.

"She is a lot nicer," the boyfriend said.

Alice laughed and said, "The medicines are the perfect combination, absolutely perfect. Everything is better."

"Tell me about it."

"Within a day of starting the Methadone, I could tell I was different. My pain was much better, and my mood was even. I didn't feel depressed at all. This is the best I have felt in a long time. And you know what? My seizures have gone away."

I re-wrote the prescription and watched in absolute astonishment as she walked out of the examining room quickly and gracefully, exhibiting no suffering, no pain behavior at all.

Please recall the referring doctor's note in which he wrote, "I am not comfortable prescribing controlled substances for her." Such is the fear engendered in physicians by the unstable mentally ill. And he was a pain doctor! Unlucky him. Lucky me.

I knew I had discovered a new weapon, perhaps an incredibly powerful weapon. I resolved to use it cautiously, and for the time being, only when all else had failed.

Michelle was sixty, and she had been fibromyalgia painful for at least fifteen years. She entered my life shortly after my epiphany with Alice. She told me that her childhood was rough, and she described emotional abuse as a child, an activity that continued into her first marriage. She told me she had been married four times and was twice a widow. Panic and agoraphobia appeared in her twenties, as did depression. She had seen many psychiatrists and psychologists, and she described the feature so common in the bipolar, bizarre reactions to medicines. Prozac made her homicidal, and Diazepam made her feel suicidal to the point of an actual attempt. She reported an automobile accident two years before in which her shoulder was damaged. Since that time she had become progressively fatigued and sleepless, and every afternoon overwhelmed with unaccountable feelings of anger. At the conclusion of the interview, I asked the inevitable question, "Michelle, have any of your doctors suggested that you had bipolar disease?"

"Yes, one of my psychiatrists thought I was bipolar."

"Did he or she give you medicine for it?"

"Oh, I have taken so many different medicines from so many doctors that I really can't remember for sure. I do know this, whatever he gave me didn't work. Nothing has ever worked very well for me."

"Well, Michelle, I think you may be bipolar. There is much of that disease in what you tell me—the strange reactions to Prozac and Diazepam, the anger, and the depression. I think you have a very complex biology going on in your brain, and I want us to be very careful with the medicines I will be prescribing. They may alter your mood in the right direction or in the wrong direction. They may give you feelings that make you uncomfortable. I want you to report anything like that to me right away. Understand?"

"Yes, I understand."

I prescribed Imipramine and Clonazepam. Two weeks later, she told me she was sleeping better than she had in quite a while, but she was feeling more depressed and also more angry.

"Michelle, we are going to stop the Imipramine, and I am going to start the drug, Lamictal. Again, I want you to call me if you have any unusual reaction to it, and I want to see you back here in three weeks."

"I want to tell you, I have read your book, and you have made me very hopeful. I know in my heart that you are going to find something to make me better."

"Thank you, I'm glad the book was helpful to you, and I promise you, if we don't find the right drug, it won't be for lack of effort."

Lamictal, she told me, did nothing the first week, but by the second she felt very restless and agitated and of her own accord discontinued the drug. She also told me something I had never heard before. Certain smells, particularly those of soaps and detergents, would incite severe generalized pain lasting several hours. Well, why not? If a migraineur had told me that the odor of soaps and detergents triggered a headache, I would accept it unequivocally. So I will accept the same stimulus can trigger a fibromyalgia flare.

"Michelle, we are going to try Ritalin. Have you ever taken any kind of stimulant drugs before? They can be helpful in treating the bipolar."

"No, I don't think I have ever taken a drug like that."

"Ritalin, Michelle—one pill daily for a week and then, if you are tolerating, up to two a day."

She told me the first couple of days she felt quite well on the Ritalin. She said she was energetic and happy and was her old self, and then she became cross and irritable. She had done some experimentation, and for a while tried taking the Ritalin every other day, but her efforts failed, and she discarded the drug. I prescribed Lithium 300 mg. nightly for a week, and if she tolerated it, up to 600. It went nowhere. She actually felt more depressed on the Lithium.

"Michelle, you have been a good patient. You have done everything I have asked you to, but we certainly haven't hit the right drug yet. There is another one that I want to try, though. It is called Methadone. It is a painkilling opiate, and I have seen one person with bipolar disease do very well with it."

"Methadone? That is for heroin addicts, isn't it? I don't want to take that drug."

"I am not giving it to you because you are a heroin addict. I am giving it to you because you are hurting, and it is a legitimate painkiller. I really want you to try it."

"As you say."

Within two days, she told me, she could tell a difference. Her pain had diminished markedly, and her mood was much improved. She no longer felt angry, and she was able to resume painting with oils, an activity that she formerly had enjoyed but was quite unable to pursue with her painfulness. A month later, she reported continued improvement. She told me everything was better.

Three months of failed trails with Imipramine, Lamictal, Ritalin, and Lithium and then recovery, or at least the beginning of recovery, within two days of starting the Methadone.

My God. What a weapon! My confidence in it and my willingness to employ it were growing rapidly.

Carol's bipolar disorder first manifested with a suicide attempt at age twelve. Her migraines began at age twenty; she was now thirty-two.

Migraine is rather common in the bipolar, and it can be a particularly virulent disease. It was in Carol. Her headaches occurred almost invariably at night, awakening her from her sleep. They were always right-sided, and they were intense. They were unresponsive to any of the triptans and to any of the opiates given orally. She suffered, she told me, an emergency room-level headache once a week, and a hospital headache once a month. She would require admission for a few days for intravenous Dilaudid therapy. In the month before she came to me, she began to experience increasing mood shifts with crossness and irritability and once or twice a week, intervals of intense anxiety lasting several hours.

As is often the case in the bipolar, she grew up in a destructive environment. Her father was alcoholic and physically abusive, and after her suicide attempt, she left home to live with an aunt. Over the course of twenty years, she had required four psychiatric admissions for treatment of suicidal depression, and she had been on a variety of drugs to control her mood swings. When she came to me she was taking the anticonvulsant Depakote from her internist in an attempt to control her headaches. From her psychiatrist, Prozac and Lamictal. We certainly have many treatment options in the bipolar migraineur— Depakote and Lamictal can be effective in both diseases. Neither was doing a terribly good job with Carol, however.

Her handicaps notwithstanding, Carol had led a busy and productive life. She was twice married, currently very happily. She had four children and a very responsible job with an insurance agency. Until her headaches had become so severe in recent months, she had been seeking a degree in accounting at night school. Such is the incredible capacity for achievement in the energized bipolar!

I prescribed Imipramine and Clonazepam. Her response was a flash in the pan. For a couple of weeks her headaches abated, but it was not to be sustained. A month into her treatment, I took a phone call from her obviously concerned and also frustrated internist.

"Can you think of *anything* that we can do for Carol? She is back in the hospital again. She has been here three days, and she is requiring intravenous Dilaudid."

"Yes, there are some possibilities. Try to see her through this siege with Dilaudid and get her back to me as soon as she is out of the hospital. I think I have a pretty good idea."

"She has taken a lot of opiates along the way. Do you think these are analgesic rebound headaches? Do you think we can get rid of the headaches by detoxing her?"

"Almost certainly not. This lady has migraine and bipolar disease, and there is no need to invoke any other diagnosis."

"Thanks, glad to hear you say that. I agree. Good luck."

Just out of the hospital, Carol was headachy and haggard when she came into my office. She cried when she told me that she was desperate for some kind of relief.

> *Carol was headachy and haggard. . . . She cried when she told me that she was desperate for some kind of relief.*

"We are going to get well, Carol. Somehow we are going to get well. I want you to believe in that."

I outlined my plan. She was to take Actiq as needed for the relief of severe pain. It is a very strong opiate and is administered as a lozenge to be placed between the cheek and gum. It is rapidly absorbed and very quick in action. Next, Lithium, occasionally an effective migraine prophylactic and also, conveniently, a mood stabilizer. And then, and surely you are expecting this, Methadone to be taken every eight hours as needed for pain. Only rarely will I initiate therapy with two different opiates simultaneously, but Carol was desperate, and I had a good feeling—a real good feeling.

On her return visit, I entered the examining room to find her in a migraine mode. She was lying on the examining table in a fetal position, her hands covering her eyes.

"I am sorry, Carol, I had hoped we would be doing better. Real bad headache?"

She sat up and, her pain notwithstanding, she gave me an absolutely gorgeous smile. "No, it is really not that bad, and guess what—my headache is on my left side! I have never had a left-sided headache before. Never in all my life. They have always been on the right. I need to talk to you because some really strange things are happening to me. I am sleeping better, and my headaches are definitely less severe. But I feel like I am getting more depressed, and I am also getting some swelling. Look how big my legs are!"

"How are you taking the medicine?"

"Just like you told me. I am taking two of the Lithium pills every night, and I take Methadone when the headache gets real bad."

"How often is that?"

"Maybe three or four times a week. On some days I have to take a couple of them."

I had placed myself in a fine pickle—which drug was doing what? Lithium and Methadone can certainly cause swelling. Both can improve sleep, and both can worsen depression. Both can diminish headache, and both can change a right-sided headache into a left-sided one.

I elected to discontinue the Lithium and increase the Methadone dosage to 10 mg. taken regularly, every eight hours, headache or not. I didn't know if my decision was correct, but I did know that I would find out pretty quickly.

She was radiant when I saw her next. "You have cured me. Everything is better!"

"Tell me about it."

"I hardly know where to begin. Let's see, my swelling has gone, and in the past two weeks I have only had a couple of headaches, and the Actiq took care of them real well."

"Which side?"

"The left."

"What else is good?"

"My mood. I feel even like I have never been before. It may be hard for you to understand this, but this is the best I have felt in twenty years. I have had no anxiety attacks, and my husband says I am not cross and irritable anymore."

"That's great, Carol, I am really happy for you. You are taking the Methadone three times daily, as I instructed?"

"Yes, exactly as you instructed me, but I am also using the Actiq every morning. Can you write me a prescription for more of them?"

"I'll have to think about that. What are you getting out of the Actiq? Have you tried going without it?"

"Well, the Methadone is the best drug I have ever taken. I am sure of that. But the Actiq just does something—it makes the Methadone work better."

"The Actiq has a very short duration of action. It should be gone within a couple of hours or so. Do you feel any different when the Actiq wears off?"

"Yes, maybe a little mood shifty in the afternoon and evenings, and there is just a certain sense of not being right when I wake up in the morning. That is when I take the Actiq."

What to do? Try to increase the Methadone so we can get off the Actiq, or conceivably even doing the reverse? Either would have been an attractive intellectual exercise for the doctor but not necessarily for the patient. Carol was nearly well, and her recovery had been achieved with the simultaneous use of two different opiates. Never discard that which is working. I did tweak it a little bit.

Fentanyl, which is the opiate in the Actiq lozenge, can also be administered in the form of a skin patch that requires replacement every three days. Thinking the patch would give more even and consistent blood levels than the lozenge ever could, I wrote her a prescription for the smallest size, telling Carol that she could keep the Actiq in reserve if she felt it was necessary. Or, if she wished, she could apply two of the Duragesic patches. I would see her again in two weeks.

"Almost perfect, almost perfect, but I think I need just a little bit more."

"Okay Carol, I am writing a prescription for the seventy-five size. That is equal to three of the ones you are taking now. Let me see you again in a month."

She was eager to talk. "It is not too big, it is not too little. It is just right. It is absolutely perfect. I don't want any more medicines. I am happy where I am right now. This dose is right for me. I just know it."

"I'm happy, Carol. We will just stay where we are. Any downside to the medicines?"

"Not really. I did have one pretty bad migraine, and I had to go to the emergency room, but it went away quickly with the Dilaudid."

"Well, I understand. There is no reason to think you are never going to have another headache the rest of your life."

"Now there is something I just have to tell you about that migraine. I was in Denver at a conference. I woke up about two o'clock in the morning with an intense headache. I passed out briefly, and that sometimes happens. Also, my vision was blurred, and it took me a while to see well enough to call hotel security. They called an ambulance, and I was taken to the emergency room. There were no other patients at that hour, and my doctor was really nice. I told him what I needed, intravenous Dilaudid, and that I knew my blood pressure was high, and that it always goes up when I have a migraine. I told him he could just watch the blood pressure come down when the Dilaudid started working. He did everything I asked, and I think he kind of enjoyed working with me. He was particularly interested in my treatment for bipolar disease and migraine with Methadone and Fentanyl. He told me he had never heard of anything like that. I said it was an incredible combination, the best ever. I told him to go to your Web site and check it out."

"Carol, I am finding this kind of funny. You are in an emergency room in Denver, Colorado, you are having a migraine, you are receiving intravenous Dilaudid, and you are chatting with your doctor about me. That is a mental image that I just find funny."

"Well, it was kind of funny, even with the headache. I was having a good time with my doctor. Do you know what he said about you?"

"I really have no idea. My first guess is that he would think I am some kind of kook."

"No, nothing like that at all. He spent about thirty minutes on your Web site and then came back to check on me. He was smiling, and he said, 'That guy is cutting edge.'"

Well, maybe I am cutting edge. But it is not exactly rocket science.

Casey was twenty-three and, until illness took command of her life, a college student. Her migraines began at age eighteen, and with one of the early ones, she experienced a stroke with weakness in her right leg. Yes, one can suffer a stroke with migraine. Fortunately, it happens only rarely. Casey required a cane to get about, and as time went by, her weak leg became progressively painful. She was requiring large quantities of Darvocet for relief. At age twenty-one, she crashed into a severe depression.

Wellbutrin was prescribed, but she reacted adversely, becoming suicidal. Hospitalization was necessary. Wellbutrin was withdrawn, and she then entered an agitated, manic state. Aggressive therapy with mood stabilizers was begun. She had to be removed from school and became not only homebound but also bed-bound. She was on occasion depressed to the point of immobilized catatonia (a waxy, plastic muscular rigidity). On others she experienced anxiety, agitation, and manic hyperactivity with these shifts in behavior occurring over intervals of a few hours. Casey was a crippled, painful, rapid-cycling bipolar. She was about as sick as a young woman can get.

> *Casey was a crippled, painful, rapid-cycling bipolar. She was about as sick as a young woman can get.*

On her first visit to me, she was on treatment with Neurontin, Geodon, Alprazolam, Cymbalta, and Zyprexa. She was untidy, and she appeared to me to be overmedicated, and in her few moments of speech, (her father had to do most of the talking) she acknowledged that she felt that way. I was sure her psychiatrist had loaded her up with medicines to control her mood swings, and that it was his intent to slowly reduce them as she tolerated.

I prescribed Oxycodone, and her pain was at least somewhat assuaged, but little else good was happening. Her bipolar shifts continued, and she was reduced to a state of near obtundation by the drugs necessary to obtain a semblance of emotional evenness. After a couple of months, I changed her over to Oxycontin, a longer-acting preparation, and that seemed to help a bit.

It was sometimes hard for me to look at Casey. She was always disheveled and sometimes unclean. Her eyes were always reddened and her matted hair moist with sweat. Most of the time she was apathetic and nearly mute. On others, she was restless, anxious, and tremulous. I was told by her parents that when she got that way, she was to be given an extra dose of Zyprexa. It seemed to help, they said.

Her psychiatrist worked diligently, constantly trying new drugs and new drug combinations. I assumed a secondary role. I would provide opiates but introduce no other drugs without his permission. I did suggest that a trial of Ritalin might be in order. He agreed and prescribed the drug. Casey went manic, requiring another hospitalization. Six months into my care of her and six months from the date of this writing, I elected to introduce my new weapon. I prescribed it in the usual manner, 10 mg. three times daily.

I was astonished by what I saw. She limped into the examining room with her cane but, for the first time, was smiling and reactive. She was neatly dressed and groomed. She was wearing makeup and for the first time ever, I was actually able to engage her in meaningful conversation.

"I can't believe how much better you look, Casey. Tell me what is happening."

"I don't know where to begin. My pain is a lot better, and my moods aren't swinging all over the place. My emotions are not running away with me. I am not nervous, and I am sleeping better. I feel calm. I guess that is the best thing. I feel calm. Can I please keep taking the Methadone? It has saved my life."

"It is a miracle, Dr. Cochran. I never dreamed I would see anything like this," her father said.

All was well. I told her to continue the Methadone three times daily and to come back in a month.

When I saw her next, she clearly had lost ground, a lot of it. She was back to square one—sweaty, red-eyed, unclean, mute, and agitated. I was disappointed, but I knew in my heart I was going to win this battle. I wrote another prescription for Methadone with the instructions to take two to three pills every eight hours. I wrote for two hundred seventy pills, nine daily—sufficient for a month. I was to learn later that no pharmacy in the area had that quantity in stock, so she received only one hundred eighty pills. Casey's diligent parents, and they were indeed diligent, rationed her supply of Methadone by giving her one pill every six hours. When she became agitated, as she did virtually every day, they administered the remaining two pills to calm her down. I was told that it worked much better than the Zyprexa.

At her next visit, she looked a little better, but barely. I asked why I had not been informed of the shortfall and her father said that he didn't want to bother me. How frustrating! I was passionately interested in Casey and the outcome of my therapy, and I was upset by not being told. I didn't scold, however. Instead, I had my nurse contact several pharmacies to see what quantity of Methadone they had available, and I wrote several prescriptions, each to be filled at the selected pharmacy. I wrote for three hundred sixty pills, up to four every eight hours—twelve a day. There was virtually no limit to the amount of the drug I would employ to get Casey well.

My efforts were rewarded. She carried a sweet smile and was actually wearing earrings. She really looked quite pretty, and her dress, I suspected, was brand new. Yes, she told me. She and her father had gone shopping in the mall the day before—for the first time in two years. After purchasing the dress, she was able to spend a couple of hours in the Borders bookstore. She enjoyed it enormously, she said, because she loved to read.

"How much of the Methadone are you taking, Casey?"

"Nine pills a day."

"I wrote that you could go up to twelve a day. Did you try to do that?"

"Didn't need to. Nine a day is just perfect. When I got to that dose, I knew I was just right. I am well now."

I had just witnessed a resurrection of biblical proportions. I had lifted a young woman from her living deathbed, and I had done it with a drug that has been around for seventy years and has never, as best I can tell, been knowingly employed for the treatment of bipolar disease. Knowingly is, indeed, the operative word. I want to tell you about another patient cured with Methadone. Most of the good work was done before she came to me, and my only real treatment decision was to resume the use of a drug that had been so helpful to her. Her story, however, is compelling, and I will share it with you because it will help me make an important point.

Linda was fifty-seven years old and arthritically painful for twenty of them. Two years before, she came under the care of a pain clinic and was prescribed Methadone. She told me she found the drug extraordinarily helpful—not just in controlling her pain but in stabilizing her erratic mood shifts. There were insurance issues, however, and she was forced to leave the pain clinic and seek another. To her surprise, the new clinic refused to provide Methadone. Instead, they offered her Hydrocodone. Dissatisfied with this, she sought my care.

She began seeing a psychiatrist at age nineteen after a suicide attempt. She required a several-week hospitalization and was told that she was a paranoid schizophrenic. Treatment with Thorazine and then Stelazine (precursors of the modern antipsychotics), however, made her "violent." Her disease was later recognized, appropriately, as bipolar disorder, and she was given many different drugs, among them Nortriptyline, Lithium, Depakote, Risperdal, and Topamax—all without any significant benefit in her mood swings.

She had never married and had no children. She was quite sleep disordered and carried a diagnosis of sleep apnea, but the treatment of that disease had been of modest benefit. She continued to be sleepless through the night, not falling asleep until 4:00 or 5:00 AM and then awakening in the mid-afternoon.

She told me quite explicitly that as soon as she got on the Methadone, she knew something was "different," and it was good. Her moods were more even, and she told me that no other drug had been so stabilizing to her emotions.

"I am perfectly willing to write the Methadone for you, Linda. You must understand that you have to take it exactly as I prescribe. How much Methadone were you taking?"

"20 mg. four times a day."

"That is a pretty big dose. You promise me that is exactly what you are taking?"

"Yes, I promise."

"Linda, I have to ask you—did your doctors at the pain clinic realize that Methadone was helping your mood swings?"

"No, I never told them about it. I didn't want them to know I was bipolar."

"Why not?"

"Dr. Cochran, do you have any idea how much bipolar disease scares most doctors? Some of the doctors I have been to for my pain actually refused to treat me because I was bipolar."

"But you told me you were bipolar. Why did you do that?"

"Because I read your book."

"Are you seeing a psychiatrist, Linda?"

"Yes, I go to a mental health clinic, and the doctor prescribes Zyprexa for me."

"Does it help any?"

"I don't really know. I have been reluctant to take it. I have had so much trouble with drugs before."

"Okay, here we go. Methadone 20 mg. four times daily. Whether you take the Zyprexa is your choice. Back in one month."

"Dr. Cochran, it just took a couple of days. I started sleeping through the night. My mood is stable, and my pain is a lot better. My psychiatrist saw it right away. He was really impressed and proud of himself. He thought the improvement was due to the Zyprexa."

> *Linda's life had, to put it cruelly but correctly, been wasted. A teenage suicide attempt, psychosis, and a psychiatric hospitalization. Unstable mood swings, unstable sleep, and pain—always pain.*

"Maybe it is. The improvement doesn't have to be due to the Methadone."

"Yes, it does. I get my Zyprexa prescriptions from him on every visit, but I never fill them. He thinks I am taking it, but I am not."

I saw her next a month later, and she continued to do well. She extolled the Methadone—reminding me again that she had never taken a drug that was so beneficial for her moods.

"Dr. Cochran, there is something I want you to do for me."

"What is that?"

"Could you send a letter to my parole officer? I have to check in with her, and she wants to know what medicine I am taking. Can you write her a letter?"

"Yes, I will certainly try to help you, but you are going to have to tell me why you are seeing a parole officer."

"I had an argument with a woman, and we began to fight. I ended up strangling her to death."

"And then?"

"I was convicted of second-degree murder and committed to the Kentucky Prison for Women, Special Needs Section."

"How long were you there?"

"From 1991 to 2002."

"Did you receive pain medicines or any kind of treatment for your bipolar disease while you were there?"

"Yes, I was given lots of different medicines, but the doctors finally figured out I was better off not taking anything. So many of them disagreed with me."

"I will write the letter, Linda."

Bipolar disease often begins in the teen years and may present as a hallucinatory psychosis. Thus the diagnosis of schizophrenia. We now recognize how common bipolar disease is, and that which a few years ago was diagnosed as schizophrenia is now correctly diagnosed as bipolar disease. The spectrum of the disease and its variety of symptoms beggars the imagination. Among them is a proclivity to aggressiveness, anger, violence, and yes, even murder.

Linda's life had, to put it cruelly but correctly, been wasted. A teenage suicide attempt, psychosis, and a psychiatric hospitalization. Unstable mood swings, unstable sleep, and pain—always pain. Years of abortive treatment at mental health clinics and then bipolar-induced rage, murder, and a ten-year incarceration in jail. Sadly, not until she was fifty-five years old, after nearly forty years of untreated illness, did she finally recover. It breaks my heart to think about it, but at least she is finally well. Her response to Methadone dates more than two years now without a hint of a relapse. And the doctor who had so miraculously cured her did not know nor, I suspect, even care to know that she was bipolar.

Some psychiatrists in my community whose bipolar patients I have helped with Methadone have reacted with incredulity. I do understand. It all seems so unlikely. Nonetheless, the effect is real and some, indeed, have become believers.

I received a phone call a few days ago from my favorite young psychiatrist.

"Bob, I have got a question for you about Methadone."

"Shoot."

"I have a bipolar patient. She has a terrible problem with pain after a mastectomy. I started seeing her a month ago and knowing what you have done with Methadone in one of my patients, I prescribed it for her. I am just seeing her for follow-up, and the reason I am calling you is that she has developed a lot of swelling. Is that some kind of reaction to the Methadone?"

"Yes, that is a Methadone effect. It is pretty common, and you will have to stop the drug."

"Well, I will do that, but I just have to tell you something. She told me the Methadone was the best drug she had ever taken for her bipolar disease. She had never felt so well. I wish there was some way to continue it, but the swelling is really bad."

"Okay, Susan, you have my attention. Here is what let's do. Stop the Methadone, and see if the swelling gets better. If it does, I suggest you start her back on a very low dose—maybe just 2.5 or 5 mg. a day. Let's see what we get out of that."

"Would you be willing to see her?"

"I can't wait."

It never happened. There was no need. My favorite young psychiatrist called me but a few weeks later to tell me that her patient was doing splendidly on 5 mg. of Methadone daily, and the swelling had gone away. Her patient was thrilled with her progress and saw no need to seek consultation with a new doctor.

I must emphasize to the reader that the most remarkable thing about the Methadone bipolar effect, other than perhaps the fact that it occurs at all, is the totality of the recovery. No other mood stabilizer, and we have many of them, has, in my experience, ever restored a patient to the level of wellness achieved by the opiate cure. The transfiguration that comes to these people is astonishing. They become attentive. They become engaging. They sleep better. They are calm, and they smile and laugh and employ wit in conversation. Posture improves and they acquire gracefulness of movement. They look younger. The women become pretty and the men become handsome.

I have been employing Methadone regularly for the treatment of the painful bipolar for several months now. I have prescribed the drug to dozens of people, and I judge that some 60 or 70 percent of them have been benefited, most remarkably so. The remainder has usually been intolerant because of nausea or itching, or sometimes by unusual psychic effects including depression (just about what we would expect in the bipolar). Be advised that a 60 or 70 percent recovery rate in people who were highly unstable *in spite of therapy with multiple mood stabilizers* is truly an astonishing number.

I have already emphasized the totality of recovery. Remarkable also is the suddenness of recovery, with the patients reporting a change in their emotions and pain within but days and sometimes hours of taking the first Methadone pill. Equally remarkable, and physician readers will certainly be interested in this, is the great variation in the dosage required. With no other neuropsychiatric drug that I have ever used has my patient been able to define for me with such precision that they are exactly on the right dose. Clark, of the knee and hip replacement in chapter four, needed 5 mg.—no more—taken each night to control his depression and pain. Anne, who stopped drinking on 9/11 in chapter nine, needed fifteen. Joan, in this chapter, knew that 10 mg. was the perfect dose. She never even attempted to take more. All the cases presented in this chapter followed this pattern as well. Bullet-in-the-neck Alice required thirty. Michelle, of the soap-and-detergent-induced pain, ended up requiring sixty. Carol, of the migraines, required 30 mg. of Methadone and seventy-five of Fentanyl. When she got there, she knew she was in the right place. Casey knew she was where she needed to be when she got to ninety, and Linda eighty.

Dick, like Linda, came to me already taking Methadone from a pain clinic. He was at the incredible dose of 240 mg. daily. He recounted that when he became painful he was severely and suicidally depressed. In response to my questioning, he acknowledged that before he started Methadone, he would often remain awake for days on end, talking incessantly. He told me that none of the painkillers worked until he started Methadone. As soon as he started on it, he knew that something was better. I asked why he was taking such a large dose, and he told me every time the dose was increased, he had a little less pain. I told him, and I truly believed this, that his doctor showed great courage in continuing to push the dose up so high, and I asked him how he felt when he got up to the big dose he was currently taking. When he finally got to 240 mg., he said, his pain was totally gone, and he had even called his doctor to tell him that he was on exactly the right dose. I asked him what happened to his mood when he got to that dose, and I will never forget his reaction. He extended his arm palm down and moved it from left to right parallel to the floor.

"Even, Dick?"

"Yes, even. Very even."

"Okay, Dick, you called your doctor and told him that you were free of pain on that dose. Is that correct?"

"Yes, exactly."

"Did you tell him that your moods were even when you got there? Did you tell him that you were no longer depressed and that your moods were not swinging up and down?"

> *The age of medical specialization has, I regret, deprived us of insights into the Methadone effect in the bipolar.*

"No, he never seemed very interested in my moods, only my pain."

Now let's discuss what is certainly the strangest aspect of the analgesic and mood-stabilizing effects of Methadone in the painful bipolar. Why has it not been discovered sooner? Methadone has been around for seventy years, and bipolar disease has been recognized for more than one hundred. Why did it take so long to find something that might turn out to be quite important?

Let's go back fifty years and see where we were at that time. The opiate cure, albeit rare, was recognized by all. And studies on the anti-depressant and mood-stabilizing effects of opiates were, in at least a limited way, being pursued. Even into the 1970s, there were reports on the subject from first-rank scientists. The pursuit petered out, however, because we were acquiring new drugs, hundreds of them, for the treatment of mental illness, and unlike the opiates, most of them are non-addictive.

Still, the question remains. Why was the mood-stabilizing effect of Methadone not discovered even by accident? That is how I discovered it, and over the course of the past six months, I have treated of dozens of bipolars, many quite unstable, with great effectiveness with Methadone. Let's explore why this wasn't discovered sooner.

One of the big reasons, and perhaps the most humbling one, is that we, scientists and everybody else, *simply don't see what we are not looking for.*

For example, ever since the emergence of microbiology and the ability to grow microscopic organisms on a gel in a Petri dish, microbiologists have been frustrated by the occasional unwanted entrance of the ubiquitous penicillium mold (that which turns bread blue) into the dish and its destruction of their beloved germs. Even Sir Alexander Fleming, who ultimately discovered penicillin (and won a Nobel prize) after witnessing the mold's ability to inhibit the growth of the streptococcal germ, sat on the observation for several years before doing anything about it.

The age of medical specialization has, I regret, deprived us of insights into the Methadone effect in the bipolar. Psychiatrists, those who treat bipolar disorder, are usually not terribly interested in chronic pain and, therefore, they have little involvement in the use of opiates, including Methadone. There are, however, doctors who do prescribe Methadone regularly. Many of them are pain doctors, almost all anesthesiologists with little knowledge or interest in psychiatric disease. (Remember, Linda was afraid to tell her doctor about her bipolarity, and Dick's doctor never even bothered to ask.) There are another group of doctors who prescribe Methadone regularly. They work in Methadone maintenance clinics and use it for the treatment of heroin addiction. They are beginning to report that after heroin cravings are diminished by high dose Methadone, the Methadone dosage is then slowly reduced, symptoms in the form of mood shifts, panic, and depression appear and then diminish when the Methadone dosage is increased.

I have found these reports to be interesting and comforting. Doctors at Methadone maintenance clinics are looking at the issue from the top down. Bipolarity appears when Methadone dosage is reduced and then disappears when the dosage is increased. I am looking at it from the bottom. Bipolar disease goes away when I begin Methadone therapy. We are both seeing the same thing, albeit through different prisms, so I am not alone.

Now let's look at addiction, an issue about which I am increasingly confused. Our society, our government, and our medical establishment all recognize that heroin addiction is an enormous and expensive public health problem. The intravenous use of the drug spreads HIV and Hepatitis C infections, both of which can be terribly expensive to treat. Therefore, the use of a drug, any drug, which can counteract that particular craving is worthy. The addiction for heroin, which is an uncontrolled behavior, is cured by the administration of Methadone, which can be controlled. We substitute an oral medication for an intravenous one, and the heroin addict is rendered dependent—but by no means necessarily addicted—to Methadone. The benefit to public monies and public health in preventing the spread of HIV and Hepatitis C is enormous.

Now let's look at another major public health issue and that is addiction to opiates other than heroin. Again, public monies and public health. Opiate addiction is costly. It spreads disease. It renders people incapable of work and paying taxes. It is the root cause of many crimes with all of the costs and sorrow that that recruits. Therefore, anything that we can do to prevent opiate addiction is worth exploring. Remarkably, we have discovered that Methadone diminishes the cravings not only for heroin but also for all of the other opiates. I have written in this book about the new drug Subutex, which is useful in relieving withdrawal effects from opiates and also for diminishing cravings for them. And yes, Subutex is increasingly being used for the treatment not only of opiate addiction but also chronic pain. However, it probably is no better in that regard than Methadone. Many drug treatment centers are now routinely employing Methadone for the treatment of opiate addiction.

This takes us to the potential utility of using an addictive drug, Methadone, in the treatment of bipolar disease. Don't believe for a moment that bipolar disease is not an important public health issue. Look at Linda. Bipolar from childhood, she was a ward of the state. She was unable to work and never contributed taxes. She only took them. She lived through years of futile care in public-supported mental health clinics, then a murder, and then ten years of incarceration in prison. Her story is played out thousands, if not millions, of times in this nation alone. If that is not a societal and public health issue, I don't know what is.

Methadone and the other opiates—and the stimulants also—have the known potential for addiction. They are, therefore, "bad" drugs. Because they are bad, they are feared. I have personally struggled with this fear myself, and my bias against opiates is evident in *Understanding Chronic Pain*. My bias is gone now. Opiates and stimulants are no longer bad drugs. They are good drugs—they are splendid drugs. They are curing and will in the future continue to cure many people with bipolar disease and pain and perhaps even bipolar disease without pain. That is my absolute conviction.

CHAPTER FIFTEEN

Anger and Pain

I have long known of the anger felt by those who suffer chronic pain, and I addressed the issue in my first book. An excerpt:

> I attend many people with cancer, stroke, and heart disease. These people, who know they are likely to die of their illness, are accepting, unquestioning, and trustful. They understand the nature of their disease and their behavior, most of the time, is one of quiet dignity. Patients with chronic pain, who do not understand the nature of their illness, exhibit quite a different behavior. They will live, rather than die, with their fibromyalgia, chronic headaches, or back pain, and they are unsettled, questioning, suspicious, and often angry. . . . Pain, more than any other chronic illness, produces a sort of mind warp in its victims. In their mental constructions, they present the physician not with their symptoms, but rather with their conclusions. "No, I don't sleep, but it is just because the pain keeps me awake." "Sure, I have gained weight, but it's because I can't do anything. It hurts too much." "Yes, I am tired all the time, but you would be too if you hurt like I do." The anger can be palpable, and it finds direction toward those who they feel are responsible for their condition, the driver of the other car, the employer who terminated them, the insurance company that denied them their just benefits, or the doctor who won't or can't cure them. "Why, that man even told me it was in my head. I am not crazy. I just hurt. This pain is real! Don't you understand?" The grimacing and wincing and protective postures, known as pain behaviors, imply exaggeration, and the demand for relief often becomes highly personal. "Doctor, you have got to give me something to relieve my pain." An unhappy interface, an angry, pain-filled patient, and an impotent physician.[1]

I can see now, four years removed from that writing, that this paragraph is an incredibly rich opportunity for exploration. There is so much in there that, at the time, I did not see.

Note that I did mention pain behaviors ([they] imply exaggeration), but I paid it little heed because I *presumed* that the behavior was merely an emotional reaction, albeit a somewhat unpleasant one, to the experience of pain. Now, a few years later, I have devoted an entire chapter to the subject of pain behavior and offered my belief that it is not simply an emotional reaction experienced by some people to their pain. Rather, it is inherent to the disease. It is just another expression of a very complex disorder along with disturbed sleep, appetite, and all the rest.

> *I have felt the need many times to address the issue of anger with patients.*

With that in mind, let's look at what I wrote about anger in the painful. I *presumed* (that word again) that anger was nothing more than an emotional reaction to the experience of pain. It was a very common one, though, and I have felt the need many times to address the issue of anger with patients in whom I felt it was excessive and maybe even self-destructive. My conversation would go along this line. "I am sorry you feel so angry. Let me tell you that I think it is probably justified considering your circumstances, but I want to remind you that anger is an unhealthy emotion, and I wish that somehow you could discard it. If you could, I think it would be quite helpful. In my experience, angry patients do poorly."

Angry patients indeed do poorly, but I recognize now, and this has been a revelatory experience to me, that they do poorly not because they are angry, but *because I have failed to recognize—and treat—their bipolar disorder.* With this in mind, I will in this chapter explore anger and other nuances of bipolar disease and illustrate just how often that disorder is comorbid with chronic pain.

Carolyn and I began our relationship with a very difficult interview. She was frequently tearful and expressive of her frustration and anger over the way she had been treated by her physicians. She had hurt her back at work a year before. Her workup revealed little, and surgery was not advised. She consulted a rheumatologist, and a diagnosis of fibromyalgia was made. She adamantly denied depression and told me quite forcefully that she was not going to take antidepressant pills. Other doctors had tried them and they didn't work. She acknowledged that her sleep was erratic, sometimes sleeping too much and some too little. She admitted to a lack of mental focus and distractibility. She also told me that she felt very irritable and, indeed, she demonstrated it to me many times—often snapping at me in response to my questions.

I prescribed Imipramine and Clonazepam. She demanded to know the exact purpose of each of the drugs. I did the best I could to explain, telling her that Imipramine was an antidepressant but was little used for that purpose now. Its primary usefulness was for the treatment of pain. She recoiled at my explanations, and told me that she didn't believe in medicines, and she wasn't going to take them. She was angrier when she left than when she came, and that is saying a lot.

To my surprise, she returned only ten days later, smiling and coyishly charming. She had decided, she told me, to give the medicine a try. Within a few days, she felt better. She admitted that she had been feeling depressed, and that was less of a problem now. Her pain was diminishing, and she said she would be quite happy to continue the medicine. It was not to be. A couple of weeks later she told me that the drugs were disagreeable to her and that she had discarded them.

As time went by, Carolyn and I evolved into a repetitive *pas de deux*. I would prescribe a drug, and after a couple of weeks she would discard it, telling me that it changed her disposition. This went on through some six months—and six different medicines. Her temper and explosiveness became ever more evident, and I realized that Carolyn could be a different person at different times—occasionally charming, but more often curt, hostile, angry, and confrontational. I prescribed Lithium, and she told me for the first time that her mother was bipolar, and that Lithium had disagreed with her. She refused to take it.

On one of her visits, she initiated conversation by saying, "I bought your book."

"Why, thank you, Carolyn. What do you think of it?"

"It is no good. I don't like it. It is too wordy."

"Well, Carolyn, I appreciate your candor. I can see how you might consider it too wordy."

I remember it all so well—how she looked at me with an air of smug defiance, as if she was glad she had hurt me.

Unable to control her pain or her very evident shifting in mood and behavior with psychopharmaceuticals, I prescribed the only thing I had left— opiates. She found the Hydrocodone quite disagreeable because it upset her stomach. She requested a different painkiller, and I gave her Oxycodone.

"I think I can tell a little difference now. My pain is not nearly so bad."

"How about your mood? I have always sensed that you have had a problem with shifting moods. Has that changed any?"

She smiled and said, "Yes, I do have mood shifts, and I think they are a little bit better. I want to keep taking the Oxycodone. It is helping me."

"Okay with me, Carolyn."

It was a month or so later when she returned to tell me, as she had so many times before, that her medicine was no longer working. We needed, she said, to make a change.

"Well, the Oxycodone worked for a while. I am going to give you some Oxycontin, which is actually the same drug, but I can give it in a bigger dose. We will try that for a month, and then I will see you again. By the way, Carolyn, you and I have talked several times about whether you might have bipolar disease. I don't know if you do, but it is a possibility, and I would like to explore some more medicine for that. You recall that I gave you the Lithium before, but you refused to take it. What do you think about trying a different kind of mood stabilizer?"

"No! I am not a manic-depressive, and I want you to quit talking about it. I just want you to give me some more pain medicine!"

"As you say, Carolyn."

She returned at the scheduled time to report a remarkable development. She said that with the Oxycontin she was back to her old self. Her mood swings were not nearly so bad, and she was getting splendid pain control, but that this had lasted only two weeks. She experimented, as she was want to do, and doubled the dose of Oxycontin without any additional benefit at all.

Never give up. Keep trying. Somehow there has got to be an answer.

"Carolyn, I am sorry you are not doing any better, but this kind of thing seems to come up over and over with you, doesn't it? You take medicine, and it works for a while, but then it quits working. All of them have quit working. Isn't that correct?"

"Yes, that is exactly what happens, and I wish I knew why."

"Let's talk about your mood swings."

"I'll admit that I do have mood swings, but I want you to know I am not bipolar! I don't have the big mood swings that real bipolars do. I have read about that. I know what that is like. That is not me."

"How are you sleeping now, Carolyn?"

"Pretty good. I slept real good the first two weeks on Oxycontin."

"Do you ever have dreams, really vivid dreams?"

"Why do you ask that?"

"It is because I am trying to help you."

"Well, I do. I have real vivid dreams. I have had them for a long time. I don't see what that has to do with my pain, though."

"Have you ever had a vivid dream from which you awoke feeling paralyzed and unable to move?"

"Well, yes, but it always goes away. I have never let it bother me."

"Do you feel sleepy through the day or do you have sleep attacks where you just doze off when you shouldn't?"

"No, I have nothing like that."

"Carolyn, there is a disorder called cataplexy. It is a sudden loss of muscle strength that people can experience just out of the blue or sometimes when they are startled or emotional. It can cause them to suddenly drop things they are holding, and sometimes their legs go out from under them, and they fall. Have you ever had anything like that?"

"Oh, my God. I sure do. It happens to me occasionally. It just comes on me suddenly, and I will find myself on the floor. Then I get up and go about my business. Dr. Cochran, you are beginning to kind of interest me."

"You are beginning to really interest me, too. I am prescribing Methadone. It is a painkiller, but it is different from the ones you have taken before. I want you to take it three times daily and check back with me in short order—something like two weeks."

"Methadone—that is what heroin addicts use, isn't it?"

"Yes, that is what heroin addicts use, but I am giving it to you for pain."

"I am not going to take it!"

"Carolyn, you are going to take it, and it is going to cure you."

"You really think so?"

"Yes, I really think so."

Carolyn had the full expression of the bipolar spectrum. She was mood labile and behavior erratic. She was ridden with anger, and she suffered narcolepsy and probably attention deficit disorder also.

"I couldn't believe it. Within an hour of taking that Methadone pill, I felt the pain leaving my body. I had the sense that something was coming over me, and I felt an evenness like I had never known. None of the other drugs affected me this quickly. I really think we are on to something."

Along with curing Carolyn's pain and mood swings, the Methadone seems to have cured her narcolepsy, her attention deficit disorder, and her anger.

"I am happy for you, Carolyn. My instincts tell me that this is not going to be a flash in the pan. I think this effect is for real, but I will have to follow you closely."

"I have to tell you something. Since I have been on the Methadone, my memory actually is improving. My mental focus is much better and I can concentrate. It is amazing what has happened to me."

"That's good, Carolyn. I forgot to ask you about that, but it is important information. That reminds me, how about your dreams and your falling spells? Have they changed any?"

"Yes, I am not dreaming as much, not nearly as much, and as far as those catty things that you talked about, I haven't had any, but it is too early to know about that. They happen only a few times a year. So I can't speak to that. Dr. Cochran, you've got me thinking—a lot. Everything is better now, and I want to know why. You told me you thought I was bipolar, and maybe I am, but what's that got to do with my dreams and my catty spells and my memory and mental focus?"

"They are part of your disease, just as are your mood swings and, if I may say so, also your anger."

"Okay, I don't want to accept it, but I will, and thank you for taking care of me. I want you to know something else. I am reading your book, and I really like it."

"Well, thank you, Carolyn, but just a few months ago you told me you didn't like my book. You said it was too wordy. I remember it well."

"This may be hard for you to understand, but back then I couldn't comprehend it. By the time I had finished a chapter, I had forgotten the first part. It was too wordy because I couldn't remember. I can remember now, and thanks for writing the book. It has helped me a lot."

"I do understand, Carolyn. Really I do."

Along with curing Carolyn's pain and mood swings, the Methadone seems to have cured her narcolepsy, her attention deficit disorder, and her anger. I would not but six months ago have imagined that possible.

Charles had endured two back operations in the span of a year. His back and leg pain was undiminished, and he acknowledged depression. He told me that since his injury his life had changed totally. Formerly he had been high-energy hyperactive and quite a good worker. Now he was fatigued, forgetful, and very frustrated.

I maintained his Hydrocodone therapy and added Clonazepam and Imipramine. I saw little to indicate bipolar disease, but in retrospect, that was probably because I didn't pursue my questioning aggressively enough. My first clue came quickly. Within days of starting the Imipramine, he told me, he had become very sleepless and ever more despondent. I discontinued the Imipramine, almost certainly the culprit, and wrote a prescription for Cymbalta.

"My depression got better when I stopped the Imipramine. I did what you told me. I started on 30 mg. of Cymbalta, and I immediately felt better. But when I went up to 60 mg., I started grinding my teeth at night, and I felt unwell."

"Anything else happen?"

"Yes, you may remember I have high blood pressure, and I am on medicine for that. I checked my pressure and found out that it had gone up a lot on the Cymbalta. I have reduced it to 30 mg., and I am feeling pretty good. My blood pressure is okay now, and my pain is better."

"That's good, Charles. Let's stay the course. I will write you some more Hydrocodone and continue the Clonazepam and Cymbalta at your current dosage. Let's take another look in three weeks."

So far, so good. We were but six weeks into therapy, and after some misfires, he was clearly better. I anticipated that he would continue to do well, but it was not to be.

"Dr. Cochran, I am really having trouble with the Cymbalta. It worked at first, but after a while it changed my disposition. I became very angry. I was mad at everybody. I was snapping at my wife and my children. They want me off the medicine. Do you have any idea about what else we could do?"

"Yes, there is always something else we can do. We will try Effexor, and hopefully you won't have the problems with it that you did with the other drugs."

On his next visit, he told me that Effexor was indeed helping him. He felt better emotionally on the drug, but his pain was still quite a bother and was not being controlled with the Hydrocodone. I added Methadone. I was giving it to him for analgesia, but I knew that Methadone can do some other truly remarkable things.

"Doc, I am 100 percent improved. My pain doesn't bother me at all. I was able to go to church with my family for the first time in a long while."

I was happy with his progress and interested that Methadone had made him feel so much better. It had not just diminished his pain but actually made it go away virtually entirely. When the pain goes away *entirely*, it is usually a clue to bipolarity. Clues also were his Imipramine-induced depression and his Cymbalta-induced anger. The reader may recall Chris, he of the bipolar demon in chapter five, who became angry when he was given morphine. I had some more questions for Charles.

"I am happy you are better, but I want to review some things with you that maybe we didn't talk about too much before. You told me you were angry when you took the Cymbalta. Have you had a problem with anger along the way? Have there been times when you reacted angrily when you really didn't need to?"

"Yes, I have had that problem for a long time, and I have had to struggle with it. There have been times when the least little thing would make me angry, and I would lash out at people."

"Have you ever had a problem with hyperactivity and not needing sleep, maybe staying up all night on a project or talking a lot?"

"How did you know that? Ever since I got hurt, I've have spells like that."

"Has the anger gone away now? Can you tell a difference in your feelings?"

"Yes, a lot. I don't feel angry like I used to."

"One last question, Charles. Have you ever had a problem handling your money? Do you sometimes go out and spend money needlessly? Do you buy things that you don't need?"

"I appreciate what you are doing for me, Doc, but you are really kind of scaring me. I don't know how in the world you know so much about me. Yes, I do have had a problem with my credit cards."

"Have you ever filed for bankruptcy, Charles?"

"Yes."

"How many times?"

"I am in my second one now."

I explained bipolar disease to my patient. I told him that it is unfortunate that he had the disorder, but that it was treatable and probably in this era even curable.

I met George at a book festival, and I liked him immediately. He was a lean, dark-complexioned, handsome man, and he exhibited a sense of powerful animal energy. He spoke rapidly and well and asked about my book and my work, telling me that he did indeed have a pain problem. We also discussed his forthcoming book about a revolutionary way to lose weight. As we parted, he asked for my card and in short order made an appointment.

He was forty-two years old and until his injury, a practicing podiatrist. Two years before, he suffered severe fractures of his ankle and lower leg. For several months during which time he required a total of five operations, he was in intense pain, requiring the rather large dose of 80 mg. of Hydrocodone daily for relief. He acknowledged that he was sleepless and depressed during that six-month interval. Then, following a successful surgical fusion of the ankle, his pain and depression went away. He remained well for about a year and then experienced sudden back pain going into his left leg, opposite the injured side. He sought out the opinion of several orthopedists and neurosurgeons. None found any evidence of spinal disease.

"What medicine are you taking for your pain, George?"

"Ibuprofen."

"Is that controlling it?"

"No, it is hardly touching it."

"You took a pretty high dose of opiate when your ankle was so badly damaged. Do you feel you need an opiate now?"

"I probably do, but you need to know something. I am being investigated by the Board of Medical Examiners now because of all of the opiates I took when my ankle was broken."

"Why in the world should that be? Your use of them certainly does not seem inappropriate to me."

"Well, the Board is investigating me because I was writing prescriptions for myself. They have revoked my license."

I betrayed no emotion, but I thought to myself, *Oh, my God, this man committed an imbecilic error of judgment—self-prescribing opiates! He has violated one of the most fundamental tenets of his licensure. What could he have been thinking?*

"Why did you do that, George?"

"My primary care doctor told me it was perfectly all right for me to do that. Now he denies ever having said that."

"George, I am truly sorry for your misfortune. What does the future hold for you?"

"I would like to practice again, but there are lots of other opportunities for me. There are several teaching positions open, and I know they are eager to have me. And I am sure my book is going to be a bestseller. I will probably make a lot of money on it. It is a self-help, inspirational book about how to lose weight. I will be fine."

Bipolar disease for sure. Six months of sleepless, painful despair and with it the profound disinhibition of prescribing opiates for himself. He was also exhibiting other, more subtle, expressions of his bipolarity in the form of insouciance, an expression almost of unconcern and guiltlessness—"My primary care doctor told me to do it"—and grandiosity—"I am sure my book is going to be a bestseller."

I elected Imipramine and Clonazepam. George reported that his sleep was restored, and he felt his pain was diminishing. Time went by, and he did not sustain his improvement. I tried the mood-stabilizing, pain-relieving anticonvulsant Topamax, but it only produced sedation. Next, Lithium, always worth a therapeutic trial, but it was without benefit. Then Lyrica—not a bad choice at all, but it was ineffective. I even offered opiates, telling him that I would do it with caution, and that close monitoring would be mandatory. He refused, telling me that his pain was a four to five on a scale of ten, and that it was tolerable.

George was exhibiting a curious feature that I sometimes see in painful bipolars. It is subtle, but it is there. They simply don't look very sick, and they don't act very sick. They are often energized and thought-busy, and they can exude an air of wellness. George was very likely in a mixed state. That is, he was simultaneously experiencing both manic well-being and pain. Probably only a minority of bipolars really experience mood shifts between high-energy euphoria and suicidal despair. Most of the time they exhibit some mix of different bipolar moods and behaviors.

Six months of sleepless, painful despair and with it the profound disinhibition of prescribing opiates for himself.

A year or so into treatment, George told me that he was satisfied with his progress. His sleep was satisfactory, and he was anxious to get on with his life, telling me that his book had just been published. At his request, I sent a letter to his primary care doctor asking him if he would provide George's medicine. I was not to see him again for nearly a year.

He returned then to request my assistance in getting his Social Security benefits. I filled out an impairment rating (a statement of his physical limitations), and we chatted a bit. He told me that a surgeon had performed an operation on his back, but that it was without benefit. He also told me his book was doing quite well. He was more talkative than I had ever seen him, and a sense of unease began to appear. He was more restless than usual, moving frequently about the room, unable to stay in one place for any time at all. I had the feeling that for the first time since I had started seeing him, he was, indeed, uncomfortable with his emotions.

He was speaking rapidly. "You are right. I am feeling very frustrated and edgy. I can't hold still. I feel driven. I can't slow down. I can't stop. There are times when I feel like I am an animal in a cage. But I want you to know I am having really good ideas. I am developing a new TENS unit. You know how they have three electrodes on them to apply to the area that hurts, don't you? I am building one that has twenty-two electrodes, and I am going to be able to relieve pain all over the body, not in just one area."

Grandiosity if there ever was. I was alarmed. George was clearly in bipolar mania, and I had to do something.

My choices? Methadone or a stimulant? By the time of that encounter with George, I had experience in their use for the painful bipolar, and I would have been quite willing to try either. But George, after his experience with the medical board, did not want to take addictive drugs. So I moved him to a more conventional mood stabilizer. Even though George had failed my attempts with three of them (Topamax, Lithium, and Lyrica), there were a lot more out there. I elected Lamictal, and, looking back on it, it might well have been a mistake. Because of its rash-inducing side effect, Lamictal must be administered initially in low dosage and increased gradually over the course of several weeks. In retrospect, Depakote or Tegretol would have probably been better choices, but I got lucky—or maybe God really is with me when I attend the painful.

I saw him three weeks later, and I could see a difference right away.

"I sat through church without a lot of shifting around, and I haven't been able to do that in a long time. I feel better—I guess the word is mellow. My pain is just not bothering me like it did."

"How much Lamictal are you taking now, George?"

"Just like you said, 50 mg."

"This is great, George. We can move up a little faster now. You can gradually get your Lamictal up to 100 mg. twice daily, but go slowly, and I will see you in three weeks."

He returned at the appointed time in company with his daughter, an exquisite, slender, long-limbed ten-year-old.

"I am doing a lot better. Lots of times I don't even think about my pain. I am taking 200 mg. of Lamictal now. Do you want to continue that dose?"

"That is fine with me, George."

"Honey, tell the doctor what has happened to me since I have been on this medicine."

She smiled and said, "Daddy doesn't get angry with us anymore."

Sherry suffered painful menstruation due to endometriosis. A hysterectomy was performed at her age forty-five. Six weeks later to the day, she experienced the sudden onset of pain in the vagina, the external genitalia, and the perineum (the area between the legs). Imaging studies were unremarkable, and her gynecologist was quite unable to explain the sudden appearance of pain. She received injection therapy in the form of nerve blocks, but these were unhelpful. A trial of therapy with Lyrica, the nerve pain fighting anticonvulsant, did little other than make her nauseated. She was given Hydrocodone for her pain. She told me it was extraordinarily helpful, but she discontinued it on the recommendation of her doctors. She said they made her feel guilty for taking such a painkilling drug. She denied any prior problems with depression but acknowledged that since she became painful, she would have intervals where she inexplicably went down and felt very despondent. I prescribed the usual, Imipramine and Clonazepam.

Ten days later I received a call from her telling me that her pain was unbearable, and that she needed Hydrocodone. This always bothers me. If my patient needs painkillers, I think it appropriate that they ask me when we are face to face. I have already written of the occasional reluctance of the patient to in general express their need for opiates and in specific to express their need for exactly how many. It is, I suppose, an embarrassment and perhaps reflection of guilt. Because of that, the act is better performed, I suspect, over the telephone than in person. It is my custom to deny such requests. When I do so, I tell my patient that if they really needed opiates, they should have told me at the time of my evaluation. I disobeyed my convention, however, with Sherry. I called the pharmacy and prescribed Hydrocodone (one can do that with Hydrocodone, not with the stronger opiates—they require a written prescription). Her request recalled to mind that she told me about the extraordinary benefit of the drug. Extraordinary benefit, I now believe, defines the patient as either drug addicted, or bipolar, or—and I will return to this subject—both.

When I saw her next, she clearly was agitated. She was talking rapidly and wringing her hands together as she did so.

"Something is happening here. I don't know what it is. Some days I feel well, very well. I feel energized, and my mind is full of good ideas. And then suddenly I will become depressed. I just want to stay in bed all day. You may not believe this, but lots of times I hold my urine in just because I don't feel like going to the toilet. I can't seem to remember anything. I feel like I am losing my mind. I am out of the Hydrocodone now. I have been this way before, and the Hydrocodone was the only thing that seemed to control it. Please give me some more Hydrocodone. I am losing it. I am really losing it. Can you give me more of the Hydrocodone?"

> *She looked me in the eye and said, "You cannot believe the anger that I feel."*

"Okay, Sherry, I am going to work with you, and I will give you more Hydrocodone, but I have a few more questions. You told me that when you took Hydrocodone, you said it was very effective. What was it effective for?"

"It was effective for pain, and I will admit, it was effective for my mood swings. I didn't tell you as much about them as I should have perhaps, but ever since I have been painful, my mood would swing up and down."

"How are you sleeping?"

"Sometimes I can't sleep at all, and sometimes all I do is sleep. I will stay in bed and sleep off and on all day."

"Mind racing?"

"Yes, mind racing, a lot of mind racing."

"Sherry, another question. Do you feel angry?"

She looked me in the eye and said, "You cannot believe the anger that I feel."

"At whom?"

"Mostly at my husband. And there is no need for it. He is a wonderful man, and he is very kind to me. I don't know why I feel so angry."

"How is your pain?"

"My pain is terrible. It is excruciating. I can't bear it."

"Okay, Sherry, here we go. I am going to give you the Hydrocodone at a dose you are accustomed, one four times daily, but I am going to add another drug. It is called Methadone, and it is a painkiller similar to Hydrocodone. I want to take a single 10 mg. pill every eight hours, and I want you to continue the others. Do you understand that?"

"Yes, I do."

Sherry's bipolar disease was unfolding pretty dramatically. Bipolar disease can often be precipitated by emotional or biologic trauma, and its appearance after a surgical operation is by no means unheard of. And yes, pain—and anger—can be presenting symptoms of bipolar disease.

Sherry's mood shifts and her pain were partially controlled by Hydrocodone. Why was I not satisfied with simply prescribing that drug and, in addition, a mood stabilizer? The answer is that I believe Methadone to be the best mood stabilizer there is for the painful bipolar, and also the quickest. I wrote her a prescription.

My nurse took her call the next day. She had taken but a couple of Methadone pills and then experienced intense nausea and vomiting and itching, a common side effect of opiates, particularly Methadone. I instructed my nurse to tell her to discontinue the drug and follow up with me at the earliest possible time.

"Sherry, I am sorry you had trouble with the Methadone. It happens sometimes. We just have to rethink this thing and go back to square one."

She hesitated for quite a while, staring at me with the look of a deer in the headlights and said, "No! No! I have to tell you about this. I took the first Methadone pill, and this was incredible. I could feel the pain leaving my body, and I had a sense of calmness, an evenness that I hadn't known since this pain struck me. After the second pill I felt even better. And then the nausea and vomiting and itching came on. I also had a real bad headache. I know you told me to stop the Methadone, and I did, but a few hours later, I guess it was twelve hours or so, the pain came back, and I felt terribly depressed. I went back to the Methadone, taking just one pill a day. My nausea, headache, and itching gradually went away, and now I feel much better. I have gotten up to one Methadone pill twice a day, and I can't tell you how much better I feel. My pain is gone—it is absolutely totally gone, and my mood is good. I feel positive and happy."

"How is your sleep?"

"Sleep is very good."

"You told me about your anger before. Do you still feel angry?"

"No, it is astonishing. I don't feel angry anymore. I don't feel angry toward my husband. Let me tell you something. I had sex with my husband for the first time in a long while. It didn't hurt, and it used to. The Methadone has cured me. It is the perfect drug."

Lean, athletic Grace tripped and fell down a flight of stairs. The fall compressed, accordion-like, a vertebra in the low back. It was an uncomplicated fracture; that is to say, there was no intrusion upon the nerve roots. Although her pain was severe, her recovery with time, about six weeks or so, was to be expected. Her pain, however, was to continue for a year. Her orthopedist could find no accountant and referred her to me. She acknowledged that she was somewhat depressed and fatigued. She offered the words that I hear so often from the painful—"this thing is getting me down," and "I am not the same person I used to be."

She told me that she had never experienced depression in the past. She described herself as energized, happy, and successful in all of her endeavors. She had actually graduated from law school, but in love with a very nice man, she elected to forego her career and become a homemaker. Her marriage was going well, and she had two healthy children. All this is to say that there was no reason, no reason at all for her pain to continue unremitting for a year—that is, unless a little something was happening in her cerebral infrastructure.

I prescribed the usual. The Imipramine, she told me, made her nauseated and jittery, and she had discontinued it. But with the Clonazepam she was sleeping better and reported that she was some 25 percent improved. I added Cymbalta, but she was unable to take it because of nausea. Nonetheless, she reported continued improvement. She was sleeping better and having fewer back spasms. She was quite happy with her progress. Then, as sometimes happens, a sudden reverse. The pain reappeared full force, and I pursued therapy with, in turn, Effexor, Doxepin, Topamax, and Lyrica. I even prescribed Adderall, but she became very speeded up and sleepless on the drug and chose to discontinue it. Reluctantly, more than a year into her failed treatment, I prescribed Oxycodone (had I seen her but six months later, it would have been Methadone).

"I really like that drug. That has been the best one yet."

"Tell me about it."

"I don't know how to say this, but I just feel better. My mood is better and my pain also. The Oxycodone seems almost like a perfect drug, but there is something I need to tell you. About three or four hours after I take it and the effect wears off, the pain comes back and I feel very angry and cross. It is just like something comes over me. I don't know what it is, but when my pain comes back, I feel angry. I feel mean."

"Have you ever felt that way before?"

"No, never. Can you tell me what is happening to me?"

"Well, I am not exactly sure, but I think we have some options here. I am going to let you continue the Oxycodone, but I am going to give you more of the drug in the form of Oxycontin. It is a long-acting preparation, and it may prevent some of the breakthrough pain. I will be interested in seeing what happens with this."

"I will certainly take it. I want to tell you that we are getting awfully close to getting me well."

"Thanks for telling me that, Grace."

On her return, she told me that she was not just better, she was cured. Her pain had gone away totally. "It is remarkable," she said. "Ever since my pain has gone away, I don't feel angry at my children. I was always shouting at them when I hurt. I am not that way anymore. Can you tell me just what is happening to me?"

Grace was, I believe, bipolar. Her symptoms of that disorder were pain, anger, and—"this thing is getting me down," and "I am not the same person I used to be." It was her pain that brought her to me. All the other things, she thought, were peripheral and secondary only to her discomfort. She was wrong. They were an integral part of her disease, and all of them were cured by Oxycontin. Her anger, "this thing is getting me down," and all the rest did not go away because her pain was relieved. They went away as her pain was relieved.

Yes, I believe all of the opiates can be helpful in the treatment of the bipolar. Oxycodone helped Grace. Hydrocodone helped Sherry, but its benefit paled next to that of Methadone, which almost certainly is the best opiate for the treatment of bipolarity and pain. George, however, got better without opiate therapy. Lamictal did the trick with him. We do have marvelous pharmacy for the treatment of bipolarity. Where does stimulant therapy fit in? We need all the weapons we can get, and stimulants can be very good ones.

Jeremy was terribly depressed. I saw him in company of his wife, who helped me with the history-taking; Jeremy told me that he was having a bad problem with his memory. He had suffered back pain for many years and had used Hydrocodone regularly. Two years before, his pain became much more severe, and an operation to fuse his lumbar vertebrae was performed. It was unsuccessful. His pain progressively worsened, and he became very depressed, speaking often of suicide.

"Have you ever been depressed before?"

"I don't think so."

"Honey, don't you remember—you took Prozac many years ago. You were depressed back then."

"Oh yes, I remember now. I did take Prozac for a while."

"Did it help?"

"I guess so."

His wife said, "It helped a lot, and he was able to quit taking it after just a few months."

"What are you taking for depression now?"

"I can't remember the names."

"Honey, you are taking Trazodone and Cymbalta."

"What are you taking for pain?"

"My doctor gave me morphine. He told me that was a strong painkiller, but it is not helping me at all."

"Any other pain medicines?"

He started crying. "Yes, I am taking Hydrocodone, and I am addicted to it."

His wife put her hand on his shoulder and said, "You are not addicted to that drug. You just take a little bit extra every now and then."

I could see right away that addiction was not our problem, and for that matter (at least for now) pain was not our problem. His depression, however, was a huge problem. I learned that he had been admitted to a psychiatric hospital on two occasions over the past two years. On his last one some six months before, he received electroconvulsive therapy.

He was weeping. "I am not going to have any more shock treatments. It was horrible. I will never do that again."

Which drug to choose? Pain and treatment-resistant depression. Neither pharmacy, and Jeremy had been given a great number of antidepressants, nor even electroconvulsive therapy gave him any relief from a demonic depression. I will advise the reader that electroshock treatment is the absolute gold standard for the treatment of depression. Nothing works as well, but it didn't work at all with Jeremy. What was going on?

Every time I enter the care of a victim of chronic pain, I carry with me into the enterprise the belief that there is a drug or drugs that can help almost anyone. It is my conviction that if I am given a level playing field, if my patient will stick with me through trial and error and give me his trust, he will be rewarded. I will admit I do fail sometimes, but I am quite often, indeed most of the time, successful—and getting ever more so. I know that if I keep trying I will find the right drug.

Every time I enter the care of a victim of chronic pain, I carry with me into the enterprise the belief that there is a drug or drugs that can help almost anyone.

I didn't have many choices with Jeremy, however. He had already been on most of the antidepressants and also most of the opiates. As I reviewed his medical records, I was happily surprised to see that he had never been given any form of stimulant therapy. Well, why not? There was nothing much to lose, and the use of stimulants in treatment-resistant depression is well accepted. I decided on Adderall and asked Jeremy to come back to me in three weeks.

Another miracle. He was smiling when he came in, and even before I could begin conversation, he said "I am at least 30 percent better."

"Honey, you are not 30 percent better, you are 90 percent better. You went to church for the first time in three years. You went to watch the grandkids play tennis. You are 90 percent better, maybe 100 percent."

"Yes, she is right. Everything is better."

"Even your pain?"

"Even my pain. It is just about gone. I'll take the Hydrocodone every now and then, but I rarely hurt at all."

I can't congratulate myself too much on this one. I prescribed Adderall simply because he had never been given any form of stimulant therapy, and I will try any drug—any drug—that might make my patient better.

As is often the case, at least up till now, I didn't make a correct diagnosis until I had cured my patient. I have been seeing Jeremy for some eight months now, and I enjoy the visits. He is a charming and attractive man. He wears red suspenders and laughs easily—a vast difference from the man I first encountered.

Wiser now than before, I made a few inquiries.

"Jeremy, let's talk about what you were like when you got sick. I know you were depressed. We talked about that. But was anything else going on? Were you hyperactive or did you have mind racing? Were you spending your money foolishly? Were you feeling irritable and angry?"

He looked me in the eye and said, "You've got it. That last thing. I was very irritable and very angry. The least little thing would make me flare up. I remember there were times when I felt so hateful that I would call my wife just to talk mean to her. I did that a lot. I would call her just to curse at her. I am ashamed of myself when I think about it now. I remember so well how she would say, 'I am not going to talk to you when you are angry like this. It hurts me when you are angry.'"

Anger is a common symptom of bipolar disease, perhaps one of the most common. I ask you, reader, to reflect on all this. If pain, the most distressful physical experience, is the product of excessive glutamine, then could not anger, perhaps the most distressing emotional experience, not also be the product of excessive glutamine? And could this not be why pain and anger are such common companions in the bipolar?

---

[1] Cochran, Robert T. Jr., MD. *Understanding Chronic Pain: A Doctor Talks to His Patients* (Franklin, TN: Hillsboro Press, 2004), 6–7.

CHAPTER SIXTEEN

Dreams and Pain

T here are few feelings quite as good as the one I get when I meet with patients I have successfully treated. I often take the occasion to chat about their lives and their families and sometimes about certain medical issues that I may have overlooked or skirted on previous visits.

I was talking with Belinda, who was doing extraordinarily well on Methadone therapy for her daily headaches and her bipolar disease. I elected, out of the blue, to bring up a topic that is increasingly on my mind.

"By the way, Belinda, I don't think I have ever asked you this. Do you have vivid dreams?"

She gasped. Her eyes widened and began to tear up. Her hands trembled, and her body rocked back and forth in the chair. She looked at me with an anguish I have rarely seen, and as she did, she began to hyperventilate.

I told my nurse to get Belinda's husband from the waiting room and bring him back to help me comfort her. It was several minutes before we were able to get her calmed down.

"I'm sorry, Belinda. You must know I had no intention of hurting you so."

She nodded her head up and down slowly, and when speech returned, she said, "I understand, but hearing you say that word brought it all back to me. I have had nightmares for a long time. They are the most fearful things I have ever known. They have gone away with the Methadone, and I haven't had one for several months. But when you asked me about my dreams, the terror came back."

"Do you feel like talking about it some more? If you don't, I will certainly understand."

She was beginning to compose herself, and she said, "No, I am okay now. I am willing to talk about them."

"They must have been horrible."

"Yes, I dream I am in hell. It is the same kind of dream every time."

"What is hell like, Belinda?"

"I am surrounded by demons. There are demons in my bedroom, and I live with them. They are real."

"What is it like when you wake up?"

"I'm always crying, and many times I can't move. I am paralyzed. Sometimes in my dreams I am paralyzed, and I can't get away from the demons."

"Thanks for sharing that with me. Again, I am sorry I hurt you."

"That's all right, I am fine now. I know you didn't mean to."

Hypnagogic hallucinations can indeed be terrifying, and they can also be diagnostic of narcolepsy. Let's revisit the issue and talk once again about demons, ghosts, and the presence of evil and the incredible pharmacy with which we can attack them.

Reggie's headaches began on Friday evenings and didn't go away until Monday morning. The weekend headache phenomenon is not rare. Many people have migraines exclusively on weekends—the body's rhythms again. I must admit, however, that I had never before seen a person whose headaches invariably lasted sixty hours and struck with such regularity every weekend for a year.

"What happens to your mood and your feelings when you have the headache?"

"When the headache comes on, I suddenly feel fatigued, and I don't understand this, but I feel angry."

"Do you have anger at other times?"

"Yes, but the only person I am really angry at is my sister."

"Why so?"

"She is so erratic. Sometimes she can be pleasant, but sometimes she is just mean and hateful. I don't like to be around her because I never know which sister is going to show up."

"Are you depressed?"

"No, I don't think so, except when I am having my headache."

"How are you sleeping?"

"I've had trouble with that all my life. I go to sleep okay, but I wake up after really weird dreams."

"Are they vivid dreams? Do you sometimes feel like they are real?"

"Yes, a lot."

"Are they bad dreams?"

He chuckled and said, "They are not good."

"Do you ever have the sense that you are paralyzed, that you are unable to move when you awaken from a dream?"

"Yes, I have that some, but it goes away quickly."

"Do you have a problem with mental focus and memory?"

"Yes, that is getting to be a problem for me."

"Tell me about it."

"I've got a real good job at a manufacturing plant, but it is demanding, and I have a lot of responsibility. I am afraid I am just not performing very well. I always seem distracted. I can't focus on a project anymore."

"Are you subject to mind racing?"

"Yes, that is a problem. I have that a lot at night."

"Are you subject to mood shifts? Do you swing from high to low?"

"Not really, except on the weekend when I have my headaches. I do get down."

"Do you have sleep attacks during the day?"

"Yes, and that is beginning to bother me more and more."

"One more question, Reggie, and it may seem a strange one, but it is important to me. Do you have trouble with your money? Are you a spender?"

He laughed and said, "That has really been a problem for me. I don't let myself keep a credit card anymore. I have a tendency to spend money very foolishly."

Many people have migraines exclusively on weekends—the body's rhythms again.

What an amalgamation of so many fragments of the bipolar spectrum! Nightmares, sleep paralysis, mind racing, forgetfulness, financial disinhibition, and periodic (weekend) sieges of anger, fatigue, depression, and pain.

I prescribed Adderall.

"How are you doing on the new medicine, Reggie?"

He smiled and said, "Don't ever give me anything like that again. It was terrible. I had an out-of-body experience. I really felt sick on it."

"Well, it happens. I'm sorry."

"Dr. Cochran, I've been thinking a lot about our visit, and I have talked to several of my friends and people at work. They tell me that I really do seem to be moody to them and also that I am more angry than I should be. I believe I do have a mood disorder, and I have been thinking about this bipolar thing that you mentioned. I have researched it some, and I sure don't have the big mood swings, but there is an awful lot of me in what I have read about the disease."

"Did your research lead you to any information about how common narcolepsy and migraine are in the bipolar?"

"Yes, it sure did. I was amazed."

"Reggie, I don't think you are going to get better until we start restoring sleep, so I am going to prescribe Clonazepam for you. I am hopeful it will help you sleep, and I am hopeful it will help some other things also. We will just have to wait and see, and understand that it may take us a little while to wade through this thing, but I am pretty sure you are going to get well."

It didn't take long, he later told me. Within but a few days of starting the Clonazepam, he felt different, and he felt better.

"Headache, Reggie? I saw you two weeks ago, so you have had two weekends. Tell me about it."

"A little headache a weekend ago. None the past."

"Nightmares?"

"No, they have gone away."

"And mood swings and anger?"

"Gone away, too."

I saw him next a month later, and he told me he had lost some ground. He was still sleeping well through the night, and his mind racing had been arrested, but his moods continued to shift and his weekend headaches were recurring. I added Methadone.

When he returned a month later, he told that we had hit on the perfect combination. He felt calmer on the Methadone, but he raised an interesting issue.

"Dr. Cochran, my emotions are better than they have been in years. I see that clearly now. You have cured me, but you have not made me whole. I have had dark feelings about my sister for a long time. I think she may be bipolar and, for whatever reason, my thoughts toward her are very destructive. Could you refer me to a psychiatrist or psychologist? There are some things I need to talk about. There are some things I don't believe will ever go away with pills."

"I quite agree with you, Reggie. Medicines can't cure everything. I will be happy to make the referral."

Roy told me he had lower back pain for six years. It radiated into his right leg and, for the two years preceding, had been quite bad. He was having increasing problems in his work as a cable installer because it was difficult for him to climb ladders. His physicians could find no explanation for his pain, and one of them had given him Hydrocodone. He told me that he got good pain relief with that drug and also felt he had more energy. He said it was extraordinarily helpful to him (remember extraordinary benefit from opiates can equal bipolar disease), but his doctors were reluctant to maintain him on opiates.

"Are you depressed?"

"I don't think I am depressed, but I am worried about my job. I can't afford to lose that. I have a new son."

"How are you sleeping?"

"I have a lot of trouble with that, always have. I wake up frequently at night, and my mind races when I try to go to sleep. Sometimes I just can't slow it down."

"Do you dream?"

"Oh, I live my dreams. They are so vivid and real that sometimes I am not sure I am dreaming."

"Are your dreams frightening?"

"Yes, I am embarrassed to say this, but sometimes I am crying when I wake up."

"Do you ever awaken from a dream feeling you are paralyzed?"

"No, I don't. I do have that feeling sometimes—I will wake up paralyzed, but it doesn't necessarily occur with the dreams."

I prescribed Adderall, and on return he told me he felt a little bit jittery at first, but did feel like his energy was improving. The effect, he told me, was similar to the Hydrocodone he had taken. Unfortunately, there had been no change in his pain, sleep, mind racing, or dreams.

I added Clonazepam and Methadone, the latter to be taken in small doses at first and gradually increased. I've learned that a slow increase can diminish some of the distressing side effects of the drug.

"It's working, it's really working. My pain is a lot better, and emotionally I feel better."

"How about the sleep and the mind racing?"

"Much better. I just feel calm, and I feel even."

"That's great. How about the dreams?"

"Gone. No more strange dreams."

"Let me ask you, Roy, do you think you are at the right dose of the drugs? Are you where you want to be?"

"I think so."

"Roy, you are taking 10 mg. of Methadone three times a day now. I am going to give you the option of going up to 20 mg. three times a day. I want you to experiment. You can take more or you can take less. If you need more than I have prescribed, we will talk about it on your next visit, and I will probably allow an increase. I have strong feelings that your body will tell you when you are on the right dose. I'll see you in a month."

> *It is still hard for me to believe that I would actually tell him to pick out the dose of the drug that he wanted.*

It is still hard for me to believe that I would actually tell him to pick out the dose of the drug that he wanted. Physician readers will know what I am talking about. It is all so bizarre. I actually gave Roy more of the drug than he felt like he needed. Such is my confidence in the ability of the painful bipolar to decide just exactly how much Methadone he needs. It is uncanny.

Let's address an important issue straight up. I have treated Roy, a young man, with three potentially addictive drugs—Adderall, Clonazepam, and Methadone. Have I committed him to a life of addiction and wanton use of his drugs? Or have I cured his bipolar disorder and thereby prevented a lifetime of pain, disordered sleep, mind racing, and nightmares? I think the latter.

Heather was a petite beauty with migraine. Her headaches were infrequent but severe. She took Imitrex without benefit, but the kindred drug, Relpax, was helpful. A year before she came to me, she developed a urinary tract infection and was treated with an antibiotic. Within a week or so, she developed swelling, shortness of breath, and tremors severe enough to take her to the emergency room. Her illness was thought to be a reaction to the antibiotic, and she was referred to an allergist. He treated her with cortisone, which she took for several months. During this time, her headaches became progressively more frequent. They were occurring every three or four days, and they were debilitating.

"Are you depressed, Heather?"

"No, I am not depressed, but I will have to admit this thing is getting me down, and it is affecting my anxiety level. That has gone up a whole lot the past year."

"How are you sleeping?"

"I have always had trouble sleeping."

Had I seen Heather a year before, I would have concluded that she was entering depression and suffering sleeplessness, anxiety, and an accelerating frequency of migraine. I would have treated her with a tricyclic in combination with a benzodiazepine and perhaps, in addition, one of the many anticonvulsants that we possess for the prevention of migraine. I will never know whether that choice of therapy would have worked, because my interrogations took me on a dramatically different track. This is because I now routinely inquire about dreams when I interview the painful.

"Heather, you say you have a problem with your sleep. Do you dream a lot?"

"Oh, how I dream. I have the most vivid dreams. I feel like I am living them."

"What do you dream about?"

"Mostly about my children being sick. The dreams are frightful."

"Do you ever awaken from a dream with the belief that what has happened is real and not really a dream at all?"

"Yes, that happens a lot."

"Are you ever paralyzed when you awaken from a dream?"

"Yes, many times. How in the world did you know that?"

"We will talk about that in a minute. Do you have a problem getting sleepy during the daytime?"

"Yes, the past year I very easily go to sleep. Sometimes I'll just nod off. That is getting worse, and it bothers me a lot."

"Do you ever have spells where your arms or legs kind of give way with you—you fall or drop things for no reason at all?"

"Yes, I do have those. I am having more and more of them."

"Heather, we've got bad news and good news. The bad news is that you not only have migraine, but you also have narcolepsy. The good news is that you are almost certainly going to get well."

"You are giving me a lot to think about."

"I know, but I am really looking forward to treating you. I'm going to prescribe Ritalin for you. I am going to treat your narcolepsy first and hopefully the migraine will get better when we get your sleep problem under control."

That was about as counterintuitive a drug choice as one could imagine. Ritalin for migraine. It makes no sense at all. Migraine is a disease of abnormal reactivity of the blood vessels of the head, and Ritalin is a drug that certainly can increase vascular reactivity. It can raise blood pressure, and yes, some people are unable to tolerate Ritalin because it gives them headaches. Nonetheless, the neuropsychiatric disorder must be treated if we want the pain to go away, so Ritalin it was. I will admit this was certainly one of my bolder choices, but I had a feeling, and I couldn't wait for her return visit.

It was another deer-in-the-headlights moment. She simply stared at me, her features frozen, and then she said, as if in wonder, "I cannot believe how much better I am."

"Tell me about it."

"Everything is better. I've only had one little headache, and my anxiety level has gone down a lot. I didn't realize how anxious I really had been."

"And your sleep?"

"Much better, and I am not having dreams. I would have them most every night, but two weeks and no bad dreams. And there is something else that is happening. My mental focus is a lot better. I had become very distracted and forgetful. All that has gone away. And my energy is good. I don't get sleepy during the day anymore. It is a miracle, Dr. Cochran."

"Heather, how long did it take you to get better? How soon did you know something good was happening?"

"Within just an hour or so of taking the Ritalin. The first thing I noticed was that I was calm. I didn't feel anxious. I was astonished at how quickly it all happened. I am grateful to you, but I do have a question."

"Sure."

"You cured me overnight. How in the world did you know what to do?"

"Because I have learned how important narcolepsy is in people who suffer pain. It is really quite common, and I have learned that by treating the narcolepsy, I can relieve the pain."

As Heather and I concluded our visit, I found a Post-It note in the chart. It had been written by my nurse after Heather's phone call from six days before. She had written the words "Heather Johnson; called about Ritalin and dental sedation."

"Heather, I remember now, you tried to call me a few days ago. I returned your call and left a message, but I never heard back from you. I really did want to talk to you because I was interested in how you were doing. What is this Ritalin and dental sedation thing all about?"

"Oh, I hope you didn't spend too much time trying to reach me. I suppose I should have called you back, but it turned out there was really no problem at all."

"Tell me about it."

"Well, I have had an awful lot of dental work done, and it has been very painful for me. I developed a dentist phobia. I always have to take a sedative before I see a dentist, and I wanted to know if it was okay to do that while I was on the Ritalin."

"Well, it is okay to use the two together."

She smiled and said excitedly, "I have to tell you what happened. You are not going to believe this. I called you the day before my dental appointment, and when I didn't hear back from you right away, I decided I didn't need a sedative. For some reason I just wasn't worried or nervous about going to the dentist. I just marched in, sat down in the chair, and let him work on me, and it didn't bother me at all."

"Say that again, please."

"Going to the dentist didn't make me nervous. I didn't need a sedative. You didn't just cure my headaches and my nightmares, you cured my dentist phobia!"

Oh, my God, how I love this work!

I had cured a phobia, one sufficient in severity to require premedication with a sedative before this young woman sat down in a dentist chair.

There were few clues in her past history. She had none of those conditions that so often predict the appearance of pain.

And with Ritalin! Hardly a first-line drug for phobia—indeed, a last-line drug. We would reasonably anticipate that Ritalin (an energizing, activating brain drug) would make a phobia (characterized by anxiety) worse. How atypical and bizarre a response to pharmacy. You remember I have used those words before. Recall Joan of the 10 mg. Methadone on top of 300 mg. of morphine. I judged her response to be atypical and bizarre, but it was not. I have seen the effect duplicated in dozens, even perhaps hundreds of patients. So it was not really atypical and bizarre. It was merely unrecognized.

Manone was a buxom, dimpled, middle-school teacher with progressive migraine. She had the disease all her life, but in recent months the attacks had become much more frequent and of longer duration, sometimes lasting days on end. Triptan therapy was ineffective in relieving her pain, and trials of several different anticonvulsants to prevent the attacks were unhelpful.

"It is the stress. I know it is the stress. Being a schoolteacher was fun twenty years ago. It's not now. The demands on my time are more than I can really manage. I don't have time to prepare anymore, and that bothers me a lot. I am really unhappy with my job."

"I've heard that kind of complaint from many schoolteachers, Manone. I'm not sure I can do much about your job or your stress, but I suspect I can help your migraine."

"Please do. I am desperate."

I initiated my interview and learned that she had been happily married for many years and had two teenage daughters. There were few clues in her past history. She had none of those conditions that so often predict the appearance of pain. I did notice, however, on the intake history that she was taking the SSRI Luvox.

"Why are you taking Luvox, Manone? Do you have a problem with depression or did your doctor give you that for the migraines?"

"Neither. You see, I have obsessive-compulsive disorder. I've always been obsessive about doing things just so, but in the last few years it has become a real problem."

"Tell me about it."

"Well, this is really bizarre, but when I walk on a patterned surface such as a tile floor or a brick walkway, I feel compelled to step a certain way, avoiding every other one. If I am unable to do that and I misstep, I become very anxious. It is almost like panic, and it can be incapacitating. Sometimes I feel like I am going to fall when this happens to me. On a couple of occasions, I have actually fallen. I guess I was just so anxious I couldn't hold myself up."

"What has the Luvox done for you?"

"It helps the anxiety. I don't get as disturbed when I misstep now, but it is still quite a problem."

I concluded the interview with the now inevitable question, "Are you subject to vivid dreams?"

"Oh, very vivid dreams. They are frightening, and they are real—or at least they seem real to me."

"Do you ever awaken from a dream and feel that you are paralyzed and unable to move?"

"I certainly do. When it first started happening, it was very frightening to me, but now I know it will go away in just a few moments."

"How long have you had these dreams?"

"Well, I remember very vivid dreams, night terrors, when I was young, but they went away. The dreams that I have now began a few months ago. What does all this mean?"

"It may mean a lot. Let me ask you, do you ever get sleepy during the day? Do you have sleep attacks?"

"Yes, I am beginning to have attacks of sleepiness during the day. They don't happen much, but they do happen."

"Another question. Do you have episodes where your muscles seem to give out with you—when you suddenly feel weak and fall or at least have to grab something for support to keep from falling?"

"Yes, that is what I just told you about. When I become anxious about misstepping, I can fall."

Her descriptions were quite typical for cataplexy, and that disorder often manifests itself under the provocation of disturbed emotion.

"Well, Manone, you have migraine and obsessive-compulsive disorder. You also have narcolepsy. And as bad as all that might seem, it gives us a wonderful window of opportunity."

"You are moving along pretty fast."

"I know, but I am excited about treating you. I want you to be, too, because you have a good chance of getting well."

I first saw Manone a few months from my encounter with Heather, and the memory of that spectacular outcome (simultaneous cure of narcolepsy, migraine, and phobia) was very much with me. Could I possibly anticipate that the treatment of Manone's narcolepsy and migraine could relieve her obsessive-compulsive disorder? I prescribed Ritalin and scheduled a return appointment in two weeks. All my instincts, all that I had learned, told me that I just might see another clinical miracle.

She was beaming. "I can't believe it. I haven't had a migraine the past two weeks and—this is amazing—my obsessive-compulsive disorder is better. I don't get nearly as nervous when I misstep now. I am very excited about that, maybe even more than the migraine."

"How about the dreams?"

"They've gone."

"Manone, that's great! I am happy for you, and I think we are going to continue to get better, but there may be some bumps on the road yet, so I want you to be patient. Continue the Ritalin as before, and we will meet again in a month."

It wasn't going to be perfect, but it was awfully good.

A month later, Manone was back in my office.

"I am doing well, but I need to tell you that I did have another headache, and I had to take some Hydrocodone that my daughter had been given after a wisdom tooth extraction, but that was my only headache."

"That's okay, Manone. I don't expect you to never have another migraine. You had them for a long time, but I do think we are going to be able to control them. I am pleased with what you have told me. Let me ask you about some other things. How about the obsessions? How about misstepping on the tiles or the brick?"

"This is unbelievable. Most of the time I don't even look where I am walking. I don't need to. I am not worried about misstepping."

"No more anxiety? No more drop attacks?"

"No, none at all."

I will remind the reader that Ritalin is hardly first-line therapy for obsessive-compulsive disorder, which is a disease characterized by anxiety, but if the victim of obsessive-compulsive disorder (or in Heather's case, phobia) also suffers narcolepsy as a part of the bipolar spectrum, that which was formerly illogical, counterintuitive, atypical, and bizarre becomes quite the opposite. This raises an important question. Are there other phobics and obsessive-compulsives out there who carry some features of the bipolar spectrum who might be cured by the treatment of that underlying disease? Phobias and obsessive-compulsiveness are generally acknowledged to be two of the most pharmacy-resistant of the psychiatric disorders. And yet within a span of but a few months, I had cured one of each with the drugs administered seemingly counterintuitively and illogically. The possibility that there are other phobics and obsessive-compulsives out there whose symptoms represent an expression of bipolar disease and, therefore, would be amenable to pharmacy, absolutely boggles my mind.

I advise the reader that Heather and Manone were referred to me for the treatment of the disease migraine. I did not, however, choose to treat that disease. Rather, I chose to treat their narcolepsy, a disorder that I am sure neither referring physician was aware of. Whether the referring physicians were aware of their patient's phobia or obsessive-compulsive disorder, I do not know, but if they did, I am rather sure they considered it irrelevant to the issue of migraine. With this in mind, let's go back to the quotation of Sir William Osler in the front of this book. It dates back more than one hundred years ago. He was a great and wise man, arguably the greatest physician of the twentieth century. His sayings are still remembered. I will offer his again and alter it only slightly. "It is much more important to know what sort of patient [narcoleptic and phobic or narcoleptic and obsessive-compulsive] has a disease than what sort of a disease [migraine] a patient has."

Do you see it? Don't treat the pain—treat the patient.

Chuck dropped a hot cup of coffee on Christmas Day. It shattered on the floor, and a shard entered the side of his left foot. He removed it and applied a Band-Aid. The next day, he returned to work as a satellite-dish installer. Within a few hours, his left foot had become intensely painful and so swollen that he had difficulty removing it from his boot. It was dusky maroon in color, and it was cool to touch. He went to the emergency room and was treated appropriately with aggressive antibiotic therapy.

He did not improve, and within a few days, his physicians told him he had reflex sympathetic dystrophy (RSD). It is one of the most catastrophic forms of chronic pain. And nobody understands why it happens. It is almost always initiated by some injury, usually to an extremity. In response to that affront, the central nervous system (the brain and spinal cord) goes haywire, and there is no better description than that. Messages are sent down through the sympathetic nervous system (that which controls blood flow) causing the blood vessels within the damaged area to constrict. For want of blood supply, the bones become osteoporotic, the muscles wither and contract into deformity, and the skin becomes thin and atrophic. The pain can be intense. One of the defining features of RSD is allodynia. I have used that word before. It means the perception of pain in response to a sensory stimulus that should not be painful at all. Even touching the area with a tissue or blowing gently across it will incite pain.

A time-honored, but rarely truly effective, form of treatment for RSD is the blockade, with anesthetic, of the sympathetic nerves that arise from the spinal cord. Chuck had several of these procedures and, predictably, blood flow would increase, the skin would become warm, and the pain would diminish. When the anesthetic wore off, however, it all came back.

The protocol for the treatment of RSD with pharmacy is quite simple. It dictates that the physician treat with anything he can think of, forewarned that it is almost certainly not going to work. RSD is, without question, the most pharmacy resistant of the many states of chronic pain. Fortunately, Chuck got lucky. A few months into his illness, his doctor gave him Neurontin, and on that drug the swelling in the foot went away, the discoloration diminished, and the pain and sensitivity to touch diminished also. His foot, however, remained cool and quite uncomfortable. Nonetheless, a most unusual and favorable response!

The finger hurting when the foot pain is severe is . . . a new pain picking up an old pain and bringing it along for the ride.

Chuck became sleep disordered early on, and several times he would go three or four nights without sleeping at all. During these times, he would be extremely restless and anxious. He also became very depressed. Wellbutrin was prescribed, but it made him think about murdering people, and he stopped using it quickly. With time, his pain evolved into a curious pattern of behavior. It would appear in waves, seizing him in the left foot. When really severe, it would migrate over the left side of his body, especially to the fourth finger of the left hand (which had been fractured and satisfactorily healed some six months before his foot injury). I accepted his descriptions without reservation because I have heard similar things so many times. The finger hurting when the foot pain is severe is not an uncommon phenomenon. It is a new pain picking up an old pain and bringing it along for the ride—a form of remembered pain, as it were.

He told me that his sieges occurred almost invariably at night and lasted for several hours. A certain trigger for pain was inclement weather. With the approach of a storm, his pain could be agonizing. Considering the evident severity of his pain, his opiate use was modest, only 20 mg. of Hydrocodone a day.

He was two years into his illness when he came to me, almost exactly one year from the date of writing this chapter. It has been a year of incredible excitement and discovery for me as I have learned about the complexity and the many expressions of the bipolar spectrum, its frequent association with chronic pain, and its sometimes remarkable response to drugs that I would not have attempted to use before. I think I was anticipating all of this when I first saw Chuck, and I concluded my consultation letter to the referring rheumatologist with the words, "I do think this man is going to teach us something about the interface of psychiatric illness and chronic pain."

"Chuck, how would you grade your pain now? How severe is it?"

"I would put it at a four or five over ten. That is my baseline pain. When I have the sieges, though, it is a twelve or thirteen over ten."

"How often do they occur?"

"Oh, maybe once a week and whenever there is a storm."

"Does the Hydrocodone do a pretty good job?"

"It helps a little bit, but nothing helps the bad pain. My doctors really have made me feel kind of guilty about taking the Hydrocodone though, and I am reluctant to take stronger painkillers. I am still a young man, and I don't want to be taking painkilling drugs the rest of my life."

"Are you depressed?"

"Probably. I have been given Trazodone and Cymbalta, but neither one of them helped very much. I think that if I didn't have this pain, I wouldn't be depressed at all."

"Any thoughts of suicide?"

"No, never."

"Chuck, the way your pain comes in sieges is interesting to me. I hear that quite a lot from my patients. Walk me through one of those sieges. Tell me just what it is like. Tell me what happens to your mood and feelings also."

"I can tell when they are coming on because I begin to feel angry. I don't know why I am angry, but I am just overwhelmed with it. And then, and this is just a matter of a few minutes or so, I'll start feeling very nervous and anxious and sometimes I tremble a little bit. After maybe fifteen minutes of that, the intense pain will come over my leg and spread sometimes over the entire left side of my body."

"Do you have anger at other times? Is that a problem for you?"

"Yes, I guess so. I find myself getting angry at my mother, and I really shouldn't. I'll admit I do have a problem with road rage. That has been with me for a long time."

"And your sleep. How is your sleep now?"

"Really not very good. I am taking sleeping pills, but they don't work very well. My mind seems to stay too busy at night, and then the pain often strikes at night, and that will always keep me awake."

The interview complete, I began my examination of Chuck by noticing that he was wearing heavy boots on both feet. Unusual, I thought, for a foot-painful RSD victim to wear such heavy shoes. I asked him to remove them, and I examined the feet. The left had a faint, livid discoloration and was cool to touch. I performed that exercise very carefully, expecting him to complain bitterly of pain when I touched him. He expressed no discomfort at all. I gradually increased the pressure of my palpation, and it did not bother him.

"Chuck, I am holding your foot quite firmly now. I would expect that to give you pain, but it is not. Is that correct?"

"You are not hurting me at all."

"Chuck, I am sure you have researched RSD and know something about the disorder. You know it is very common for victims of the disease to be very sensitive to the touch, but you are not."

"No, ever since I have been on the Neurontin, it doesn't hurt to touch my feet. At night, though, I have to sleep with my foot out from under the bedcovers. Their weight hurts my feet. It just seems to happen at night."

I have written, reader, have I not, about pain worsening at night or appearing only at night. What a strange disease is chronic pain and its relationship to nighttime and attempts to sleep.

"One last question, Chuck. Do your moods shift? Do you go up and down?"

"Only when I have my sieges of pain. I feel very depressed when that happens."

I suspected that Chuck might be bipolar, chiefly on the basis of the periodicity of his pain and the change in his emotional state when it struck. I knew back then that bipolar disease was very common in the painful. I did not, however, know that anger was such an important and common expression of the disease. Nor did I appreciate that his four or five nights of sleeplessness and restlessness was almost certainly an expression of bipolar mania.

I told him to continue his Hydrocodone and Neurontin, and I prescribed Imipramine and Clonazepam. He developed urinary hesitancy, almost certainly due to the Imipramine. With the Clonazepam, he was sleeping better, but he experienced no change in his pain and its periodic flares. He did tell me that with the Clonazepam he was able to sleep at night with the bedcovers over his painful foot. Well, maybe some progress.

I knew back then that bipolar disease was very common in the painful. I did not, however, know that anger was such an important and common expression of the disease.

On the next visit I added Zoloft, and he said he felt somewhat more energized and focused on that drug, telling me it was like taking a couple of cups of coffee in the morning. I offered him a stronger opiate, perhaps Oxycontin, but he was reluctant. Along the way, this measuring over a few months, I added Seroquel, which helped his sleep a bit, and I increased his dose of Neurontin with some benefit. A trial of Lithium, however, only made him depressed.

Some four or five months into his treatment, I had my first really good idea. I prescribed the anticonvulsant Topamax. It can be analgesic and also mood stabilizing, but it has another singular attribute. It is derivative of the diuretic drug Diamox, which is used to treat mountain sickness. No need to go into just how it works, but Topamax (and Diamox) can be used to diminish the sensitivity of the painful to changes in barometric pressure.

Chuck felt that his pain was at least partially relieved by the Topamax, and he told me that storms didn't bother him quite as much. I was rather happy with what I had accomplished. No resurrection by any means, but at least he was back in school working for a degree in communications.

Chuck lived some two hundred miles away, and his visits to me were exhausting and quite uncomfortable because travel in any form is difficult for the painful. I wrote a six-month supply of medicines and told him to return for recheck then.

He came at the appointed time to see a doctor armed with far more knowledge than the one he had known before.

"Long time, Chuck. How are you doing?"

"I am doing pretty well. I would like to take more Topamax, though."

"How much are you taking now?"

"300 mg."

"Why do you need more?"

"Well, just today coming to see you, we drove up on the Cumberland Plateau, and my pain was becoming intense, so I took an extra Topamax. It went away almost immediately."

"Did anything else happen with the Topamax?"

"Yes, I usually get depressed and angry when I hurt, and that went away too."

"Chuck, you mean that driving up the Cumberland Plateau will make you painful, nervous, angry, and depressed, and you can make that go away with an extra Topamax?"

"Yes, exactly."

The reader is advised that the Cumberland Plateau is a landmass with an elevation of up to one thousand feet from its base. In my state of Tennessee, it lies between the cities of Knoxville and Nashville. Chuck lived near Knoxville, so each visit to me entailed ascending and then descending one thousand feet. In most of us, that would produce no perceptible change in the way we feel. But for Chuck, it incited severe pain, depression, and anger.

The sensitivity of pain to change in weather and barometric pressure has not received nearly the attention it deserves. It is real and it happens a lot. The notion, however, that change in atmospheric pressure influences our emotions and makes us (at least some of us) angry, is truly fascinating and a facet of bipolar disease that I don't believe anyone has ever explored.

"Chuck, is anger still a problem for you?"

"Yes, there was a man in your waiting room, and he was talking too much. I really wanted to pop him," he said calmly and smilingly.

"I'm glad you didn't."

"Well, I wanted to."

"Chuck, we will surely go up on your Topamax. Do you have anything else to report?"

"Yes." He handed me a report of a nerve conduction study done a couple of months before. "I was up late one night working on my computer, and I fell asleep in the chair. When I woke up, my right arm was paralyzed. I couldn't lift my hand. I went to the doctor, and he did these tests. He told me that I had a radial nerve palsy. When I fell asleep, my forearm was on the armrest of the chair, which was hard, and the nerve was compressed. He called the paralysis a wrist drop, and he told me it would slowly improve, but I should avoid sleeping in chairs again."

"That sounds like good advice. Have you recovered?"

"Yes, I've got full strength in my wrist now, but I need to tell you something that is really strange. When I started getting my strength back, when I was able to lift my hand and wrist again, my foot pain got a whole lot worse. It didn't happen when I was paralyzed. It happened when I started recovering my strength. Can you possibly explain that to me?"

"No, but that is the kind of thing I am used to hearing in the painful. I accept what you have told me, but I don't understand it."

As the arm started getting better, the foot got worse. How strange! How much we don't know. How fertile is the field for study. I can only surmise, and this represents the grandest of generalizations, that brain energy, normally directed toward controlling the pain in the foot, was diverted to other matters like the restoration of an injured nerve on the other side of the body. Perhaps the brain was too preoccupied with that task and was, therefore, unable to control an RSD-painful foot.

I know, reader, but it is the best I can do.

"Chuck, it has been a long time since we talked, so I want to review some things with you. How are you sleeping now?"

"The same. Thought-racing and still attacks of pain at night."

"Do you dream?"

"Oh boy, do I dream. They are really weird."

"Have you had weird dreams all your life, or have they come on just since your RSD?"

"Since the RSD."

"Vivid dreams, very vivid dreams?"

"Yes, sometimes extremely vivid. Sometimes I feel like they are real."

"Are they good dreams or bad dreams?"

"Usually bad. There is just a sense of evil in my dreams. Sometimes they really frighten me."

"Do you ever wake up from a dream paralyzed?"

"Yes, that happens a lot. What does that mean?"

"It may mean a lot."

"You are on to something, aren't you? You are really on to something."

"Maybe. I think you have narcolepsy, and I am prescribing Ritalin for you, one pill a day for the first week and then two. I want you to call me in a few days and let me know how you are doing. Will you do that?"

"Yes, I will. Do you think the Ritalin will help my pain?"

"I hope so, and I am writing another prescription for the Topamax. You can take up to five pills a day, and I want you to take an extra one before you start going up on the Cumberland Plateau, and when you call, I want you to tell me what happened."

It is my custom, when I see patients at infrequent intervals, to scan the chart and particularly the original consultation note to see if there was anything I was missing. As we have already seen, that exercise can lead to some interesting discoveries. I was taken with his descriptions of going four or five days without sleep during which time he would be very anxious and agitated.

"Chuck, we haven't talked about this in a while, but how about these sleepless spells and the nervousness. Do you still have those?"

"No, they went away when I got started on the Neurontin."

"Really?"

"Yes, really. The Neurontin has been the best drug I have taken. The Topamax has been helpful also, but when I started on the Neurontin, the swelling in my foot went down, the pain diminished, and I quit having my spells of insomnia."

Remarkable. The anticonvulsant Neurontin had terminated his attacks of mania and also diminished his swelling and pain. We already know, don't we, reader, that pain can be a presenting symptom of bipolar disease. Could that most strange form of pain we call reflex sympathetic dystrophy actually be an expression of bipolar disease? Maybe this young man, indeed, was going to teach us something about the interface of psychiatric illness and chronic pain.

Of all the states of chronic pain, reflex sympathetic dystrophy is certainly the most destructive and the least understood.

Exploring its relationship to bipolar disease seems . . . worth the effort.

I took his call ten days later.

"Dr. Cochran, I am taking four of the Topamax and two of the Ritalin. I made it up and down the Plateau without any pain, and I know you are interested in this, without anger. We had a storm the other day, and it didn't bother me as much as I expected. I think we are getting somewhere, and I think you are on to something."

It was not to last. He called two weeks later to report that the Ritalin was disagreeing with him. He said it caused "time loss," which I finally discovered was his curious way of describing amnesia. There were intervals in his everyday life that he was quite unable to remember. He also told me that he was procrastinating, putting off tasks that he normally performed diligently. I told him to stop the Ritalin, and I mailed him a prescription for Methadone, instructing him to return in three weeks.

"It's a miracle, Dr. Cochran. It is really a miracle. The past three weeks have been the best I have had in a long time. I think you have hit on the perfect combination."

"Tell me about it."

"It's the pain. The pain is almost gone. I still have some flares at night, but they are not near as bad as they used to be."

"I'm happy for you, Chuck. I am really happy. Let me ask you a few more questions. How is your mood? Do you still feel depressed?"

"No, the depression is a lot better. I don't know how to say this, but I just feel more even. Things that used to upset me and make me angry don't bother me anymore. My mother has noticed it. She says I am calmer—that I am not as irritable as I used to be."

"How about the dreams?"

"Gone, absolutely gone."

"Chuck, this is truly remarkable. Like you said, it's a miracle. I must tell you that I have never had an RSD patient do as well as you have. You know we were bucking pretty long odds, don't you?"

"Yes, I am aware of that, and I am grateful to you. Now I have a question."

"Sure."

"You are on to something, aren't you? You are really on to something."

"Yes, Chuck, I may be."

Let's go back to glutamine, the brain's excitatory and destructive neurotransmitter. We believe, almost certainly correctly, that mania, panic, and probably pain are types of glutamine storms. We know also, and I have already illustrated this, that migraine in the bipolar can be a particularly virulent form of the disease. We can at least theorize that migraine is also a glutamine storm, for I have described cases in which the bipolar migraineur was cured by the glutamine-fighting drug Methadone and also by stimulants, which are glutamine-fighting through their agency of the stimulation of dopamine. We also know that migraine can be controlled by anticonvulsants, which are, in their unique way, also glutamine-fighting.

Let's continue our derivations. Migraine is a disorder of the reactivity of blood vessels in the head. RSD is a disorder of the reactivity of blood vessels in an extremity. Could RSD be a type of glutamine storm? Could it be a disease that comes preferentially to the bipolar? Could we possibly cure RSD by treating bipolar disease?

The reader must be reminded that of all the states of chronic pain, reflex sympathetic dystrophy is certainly the most destructive and the least understood. Exploring its relationship to bipolar disease seems to me to be at least worth the effort. There is no certain evidence that the two are related, but I have a feeling. My instincts tell me that there may be a relationship, and I have learned to trust my instincts.

There is so much about chronic pain that we don't know, and I think that is because there are so many places where we haven't looked. Think about this chapter alone. Migraine, backache, reflex sympathetic dystrophy, hypnagogic hallucinations, sleep paralysis, cataplexy, daytime sleep attacks, nighttime pain attacks, anxiety, phobia, obsessive-compulsive disorder, anger, and changes in barometric pressure. Has anybody ever tried to put all that together? I can answer that one for you—no. But there is a relationship. There is meaning, and there is understanding to be had. There are so many places to go, places we haven't even thought about looking. Of this I am confident. There is an answer out there, and finding it may not be far ahead.

Epilogue

Primary care physicians constantly struggle with their role in the prescription of pain-relieving opiates over the long term, that is for the treatment of chronic pain. They fear that the act, however well-intentioned, will lead ultimately to addiction with all the unfortunate consequences that attend that disease. The conundrum is well expressed in this note from a very thoughtful internist.

Dear Bob:

RE: Ed Smith
DOB: 6/1/53

Mr. Smith brought up the idea of chronic pain therapy with me today. He had stones (renal) in the fall and noticed significant improvement in "quality of life" while he was on Hydrocodone. He said everything was better. He wonders about continuing. I told him I would like to get a consult from a pain specialist for the following reasons:

1. Euphoria versus pain relief.
2. His main pain now is from compression fractures, lumbar spine, sustained 1999.
3. He does have a history of drug use—periodic cannabis with a certain circle of friends.

Let me know what you think. I told him I would be happy to prescribe the drugs myself unless you thought it would be better for you to do it. Thanks.

Roger Watson, MD

Ed had suffered multiple compression fractures following a fall some eight years previous. He was hospitalized for a few days and then wore a back brace for several weeks. Painful though he was, Ed continued his contracting work, and in his spare time he farmed. Some four years later, his business partner died suddenly of a heart attack. There were unpleasant legal maneuverings, and Ed's farm was taken from him by his partner's family.

"I was really sad when I lost my buddy, but after what his family did, my grief turned into anger. I felt betrayed."

"I quite understand. What happened to your emotional health after that?"

"I started getting nervous. Dr. Watson gave me some Alprazolam. After a while, he referred me to a psychiatrist because I really was depressed. I couldn't sleep, I lost weight, and I was very forgetful and cross."

"And then?"

"He gave me Wellbutrin. I took it for a while and I did get better. I stopped the Wellbutrin a couple of years ago. I don't think I need it now."

"And what happened to your pain when you were depressed?"

"It got worse, a lot worse, but I was so used to my back hurting, I didn't pay too much attention to it. I didn't let it slow me down."

"Let's talk about your kidney stones and the Hydrocodone. You got started on that a few months ago?"

"Yes. I required treatment with litho-something. I can't pronounce that word."

"Lithotripsy."

"Yes, that is what it was. They shattered the kidney stones by sound waves. It was very painful. My doctor gave me Hydrocodone, and I just couldn't believe how much relief of pain I got—not just in the kidneys, but in my back. It made me realize just how much I had been hurting. I felt much better taking Hydrocodone. I didn't have nervous attacks anymore, and my wife tells me my disposition improved. I really want to stay on the Hydrocodone. Will you let me do that?"

We talked for quite some time, and I gradually sensed that Ed, over the course of a couple of years, had been in some kind of denial regarding his pain and his depression. He didn't realize how much he had been hurting until he actually got pain relief from Hydrocodone. I suspected that he would be reluctant to come to a kindred conclusion, that is, he didn't realize how depressed he was until he got on a medicine that relieved it. He did acknowledge that he suffered periodic anxiety and depressed moods. He volunteered that his sexual energy was also much diminished, and that it had improved when he was started on the Hydrocodone.

What to do? Deny him the use of a drug that gave him relief from both pain and depression because it was potentially addictive? Or use a lesser pain medicine, perhaps Darvocet or Tramadol (neither of which are totally free of the potential for addiction)? Or introduce a more conventional antidepressant such as Prozac, or even resume Wellbutrin? That drug had helped him before and relieved his depression, but would it relieve his pain? I suspect not. Darvocet, Ultram, Prozac, and others were of potential benefit, but only potential. Hydrocodone was of proven benefit.

I wrote a prescription for 10 mg. four times daily. He has maintained his improvement for several months now, and as best as I can tell has been quite compliant with his therapy. I hope I have done the right thing.

Go back to the referring physician's letter and note his use of the phrase "everything was better." Does that not tell us that we have the absolutely perfect drug? Note also his "euphoria versus pain relief." That word, euphoria, has come up before, hasn't it? Euphoria may not represent something that the patient doesn't deserve. It may represent something that the he does—recovery.

Jo was an attractive, but weight-gained thirty-four-year-old. She described childhood trauma. She was subject to frequent whippings with belts and, on one occasion, with baling wire. Following the birth of her child, she entered a postpartum depression. She became anxious and had trouble concentrating. She told me she lost her self-confidence and found it difficult to speak in front of people. She went into a sweet craving mode with forty-pound weight gain. She was treated with Alprazolam and Zoloft, and although her depression ameliorated, she began to experience painful joints and then widespread muscular pain. Fibromyalgia was diagnosed and she was given Hydrocodone. She found the drug extraordinarily helpful but had begun to overuse it.

She told me she was always subject to moodiness and had left college for a couple of weeks because of a severe depression. She acknowledged in response to my questions that although she and her husband had been quite economical and well-fixed, she had, following the birth of her child, started spending money foolishly. She had accumulated nearly twenty thousand dollars in credit card debt.

I told her to continue the Zoloft, Alprazolam, and Hydrocodone, and I added Imipramine and Clonazepam.

On her return, she said she was sleeping better on my medicine but admitted that she was taking six to eight Hydrocodone pills a day rather than the prescribed four. I elected to change her to Oxycodone, giving her the generous dose of 15 mg. five times daily.

Her next visit was earlier than scheduled. She came in to get another prescription for Oxycodone. She was clearly overusing it. Knowledgeable now and confident of the effects of Methadone in those whom I believe are bipolar, I prescribed that drug.

She called me a few days later to tell me that she felt sedated on the Methadone, and that her husband, fearful of that particular drug, had thrown it away. I elected to add Lamictal.

On her next visit, Jo told me that she had fallen and broken some ribs. On this account, her primary care physician wrote a prescription for extra Oxycodone, and it was giving her a measure of relief. She was on Zoloft, Alprazolam, Imipramine, Clonazepam, Lamictal, and way too much Oxycodone. I saw her drug addiction as the major issue with bipolarity a close second. Her pain was a low priority at that particular juncture. I admonished her to take her pain medicines as I prescribed and to receive them from no other physician.

She returned but a few days later in the company of her mother, telling me that she was increasingly craving the Oxycodone and using ever more of it. She was tearful and distraught, and I had to tell her that her opiate use was out of hand and that she must, if she was remain under my care, go to a drug abuse treatment center. She submitted to my request and spent several days there. With the drug Subutex, she experienced a relatively comfortable withdrawal from the Oxycodone.

I saw her shortly after her discharge from the treatment center, and she told me she had suffered a fall and hurt her wrist. Her primary care physician had prescribed Oxycodone, which she was taking—again in large quantities.

"You can take the Oxycodone if you want, Jo, but you are drug addicted, and you are in denial. I will be frank with you. I believe you have bipolar disease, and unfortunately drug addiction is very common with that disorder. I will continue to work with you and do the best I can, but I will never provide opiates for you, and I think your prognosis for recovery is very poor indeed unless you make some very big changes in your life."

A few weeks later, I received a phone call. "Dr. Cochran, I am sure you are right. I am getting more and more bipolarish. I am beginning to believe what you have been saying. I am spending money, lots of it. I am buying aquariums and tropical fish. I have spent thousands of dollars that I don't have. Now, I must tell you something important. I found some of the Methadone that you prescribed before. My husband told me he had thrown it away, but he hadn't. I took just a little bit of it, and I started feeling better. I feel calmer. I don't know how to say this, but I am more even."

I told her to come see me very soon, so we could talk.

"Dr. Cochran, it is amazing. I feel calm when I am on the Methadone, and I don't feel the need to buy fish."

"But you told me before that you had trouble with the Methadone. Now you tell me the Methadone is helping you. What is going on? I need to know, Jo. I really need to know."

"It was my husband. He didn't want me to take the Methadone. I think the sedation was from all the Oxycodone I was taking."

"You mean you are tolerating the Methadone now? It is not sedating or bothering you in any way?"

"No, it is the best drug I have ever had. I don't feel driven to spend money and I feel calm. I still hurt, and I am still taking Oxycodone but, and you may not believe this, I am not craving it like I did before. Since I have been on the Methadone, the Oxycodone seems to work better."

"Okay, Jo. Continue all the other medicines and take the Methadone three times daily. I want you to come back in two weeks."

"I understand. I think we are close to getting well."

How resolute I am! But a few weeks from the date when I told her I would never give her opiates, I was encouraging her to use them. Well, changing one's mind is not always bad. It can indicate that one has learned something.

Look, reader, where we are. Jo was a painful bipolar who was also opiate addicted. With Methadone, she was calmed, her pain was relieved, and her lust for buying fish was arrested. Could Methadone have also arrested her lust for Hydrocodone and Oxycodone? We have long known that Methadone relieves cravings for heroin. We also have learned that it relieves cravings for other opiates, and we are increasingly using it for that purpose. Astonishing, isn't it? Methadone, a drug that the user often takes less than prescribed to treat addiction to other opiates, drugs that, by definition, the user takes more than prescribed.

I was embarking on a new drug adventure, perhaps, just perhaps, the noblest of all. I was going to simultaneously treat her bipolar disease, her pain, and her drug addiction by the administration of Methadone. It seems counterintuitive and illogical. It seems like zebras, not horses, but I suspect it is going to work.

Before concluding this book, I must address once again the vexing and confusing issue of using addictive drugs for the treatment of chronic pain and its many and varied attendants. I want to go back four years when *Understanding Chronic Pain* was published. Many of the judgments I expressed in that book are, I believe, still appropriate. Those relating to the role of childhood abuse, particularly sexual abuse, substance abuse, and depression in the generation of pain are standing the test of time. In some regards, the book was prescient. It anticipated the possibility that bipolar disorder and attention deficit disorder might be kindred diseases, and that they might have something, perhaps a lot, to do with chronic pain. I made some big mistakes, however, the greatest of these being my bias against therapy with opiates. My views on this matter reflected those of the great majority of physicians of my age and experience and of many others quite younger. We have long believed that the addictive opiates are to be avoided and to be used only as a last resort. It was my view at that time that the use of opiates was an admission of failure—that I had been unable to cure my patient with antidepressants or anticonvulsants and, therefore, had to resort to the dangerous and destructive use of opiate painkillers.

The last four years have taught me much. Learning of the complexity of the bipolar spectrum, including narcolepsy, and the astonishing frequency with which it accompanies chronic pain has been revelatory. Revelatory also has been in the discovery, sometimes by accident, that the addictive stimulants and opiates can be antidepressant, mood-stabilizing, thought- and memory-restoring, nightmare-diminishing, and even phobia- and obsessive-compulsiveness curing. This has created a sea change in my thinking, and if this book can do anything, I will hope it will induce a sea change in the thinking of others.

The stimulants and opiates (particularly Methadone) have an enormous advantage over the antidepressants and anticonvulsants that we use in the treatment of pain: it is the suddenness and totality of their benefit. I have certainly given many examples of that. It is this quickness of response that makes them ideal for the employ of a therapeutic trial. If the trial is successful, the physician has cured the patient. If the trial is unsuccessful, the physician has really done no harm, for the drug can be immediately withdrawn.

There is a belief that the administration of addictive drugs renders everybody who receives them addicted. This is by no means the case. The ingestion of alcohol does not render all of its users alcoholic, and the same with Ritalin, Clonazepam, Methadone, and all the rest. However, the fear of addiction remains paramount in the minds of most physicians. It is this fear, I believe, that so often leads them to weigh the risk of addiction as greater than the probability of recovery. That was the way I felt four years ago, but it is not the way I feel now. I have learned that opiates and all the others can be miraculously curative, and I want to suggest that the risk of true addiction is virtually nil when the addictive drug is employed successfully in the treatment of disease. I have given many examples of miraculous cures with the use of addictive drugs, and there is little need to single out one as an example, but I cannot resist.

Think of Casey, she of the two years living-deathbed, painful bipolarity who was restored to health. She can now go to the mall, work on her computer, buy new dresses, read books and, by the way, become engaged to be married. We could not have achieved this incredible outcome had I been fearful of employing the potentially addictive Methadone. Will

Casey become an addict? Emphatically no. She achieved recovery with Methadone. She needs nothing more.

There are incredible drugs out there for the treatment of chronic pain. To use them effectively, however, we will have to disobey convention and change some of our thinking, but they are out there.

Index

A

abdominal pain,
4–14, 216
Abilify, 29
Actiq, 28, 264
Adderall/Adderall
XR. *See also*
stimulants
case studies
involving, 111,
218, 221, 232,
239–40, 244,
247, 297, 304
uses for, 31
adjustment disorder,
78, 193
agoraphobia, 92
alcohol, 25, 153,
155–56
alcoholism, 145–58,
173–78. *See also*
drug abuse;
marijuana
allodynia, 14, 18,
312–13
Alprazolam, 29, 156
Alzheimer's disease,
20, 126–28
Amerge, 30
Amitriptyline, 27,
184–86, 253

Amphetamine, 31
Anafranil, 26
analgesic rebound
headache, 187,
193, 195, 198,
202–4, 264
anger, 44, 74, 82,
107, 142, 144, 206,
252, 257, 261-62,
279–81, 286–87,
291–92, 294–95,
298, 300, 302,
315–18, 321
annual rhythms,
189
anticonvulsants,
23–24, 30–31
antipsychotic drugs,
29
anxiolytic drugs, 24,
29
Aripiprazole, 29
arm pain, 93–95
arthritis, 60–65
Ativan, 29
Atomoxetine, 31
attention deficit
disorder, 31, 158,
218, 242, 247,
284–85

B

back pain, 93–95,
98–109, 113–18,
138–50
benzodiazepines, 24,
29, 53
bipolar disease
anger and, 257,
279–80, 298,
302, 315
case studies in,
4–14, 60–65,
73–82, 93–102,
158–62, 178–81,
211–14, 223–27,
229–53, 255–62,
267–76,
280–321, 325–28
and childhood
abuse, 227–28
cyclothymia, 98
drugs for, 11,
28–32, 232,
295–96
identifiers of, 23
migraine and, 321
nature of, 9–11,
82, 226, 235, 273
reflex sympathetic
dystrophy and,
321–22

treating pain and,
238
use of Methdone
for, 276–78
Botox injection, 2
brain. *See also*
neurotransmitter
systems in
Alzheimer's
disease, 126–27
case studies in
damage to,
113–26
effect of opiates
on, 199
in Parkinson's
disease, 123–26
Buphrenorphine, 28
Bupropion, 28
Butorphanol, 28

C
Carbamazepine, 31
cataplexy, 235, 283
celestial rhythms,
188–89
Celexa, 26, 52
childhood abuse
and bipolar
disease, 227–28
and pain, 129, 135,
140–41, 205–27
as risk factor, 20,
157, 210–11, 228
chronic pain. *See*
pain, chronic
chronobiology,
188–89

circadian rhythms,
188
Citalopram, 26
Clomipramine, 26
Clonazepam
case studies
involving, 4, 9,
45, 53, 70, 118,
132, 142, 149,
157, 160, 190,
230, 238, 240,
302, 304
uses for, 24, 29
Clorazepate, 29
cocaine, 25, 159
comorbidity, 71
Concerta, 31
conversion reaction
case studies
involving,
129–44
pain behavior as
symptom of,
130–33
convulsive seizures,
258
cyclothymia, 98
Cymbalta, 23, 27,
40, 158

D
Darvocet, 29
Darvon, 28
delusion, 69–71,
118, 125
Demerol, 28
denial, 45, 55, 70,
90, 107, 109, 131,

150, 167–68, 170,
324, 327
Depakote, 30
depression
atypical, 60, 121–22
case studies in,
49–71, 138–44,
156–58
drugs for, 28, 52
and memory, 91
and pain, 53–54,
150
stigma of, 138–39,
143–44
Desipramine, 27
Desyrel, 27
Dexedrine, 31
Dexmethylphenidat,
31
Dextroamphetamin,
31
diabetes, 38–41
Diamox, 316
Diazepam, 24, 29
Dilantin, 31
Dilaudid, 28
Dolophine, 28, 32
dopamine, 24–25,
27–29, 31, 123–24,
155
dorsal column
stimulator, 80, 179
Doxepin, 27
drug abuse, 19,
158–71, 178–81,
325–28. *See also*
alcoholism;
marijuana

drug contract, 178
Duloxetine, 27
Duragesic, 28

E
Effexor, 23, 27, 211,
    240
Elavil, 27
Eletriptan, 30
Emsam, 27–28
epidural steroid
    injection, 1, 69,
    134, 150, 205
Equanil, 253
Escitalopram, 26
Eskalith, 31

F
fatigue, 18–19, 31,
    46, 51, 55, 83, 97,
    102, 104, 107–110,
    120–22, 197, 211,
    221, 231–33, 235,
    238–43, 248, 260,
    285, 294, 300–301
Fentanyl, 28, 266
Fentora, 28
fibromyalgia, 17,
    88–89, 120, 134,
    205, 209, 211,
    216–17, 223, 236,
    239, 245–46, 255,
    260–61, 279, 281,
    325
flashbacks, 91, 209,
    220, 256
Fleming, Alexander,
    277

Fluoxetine, 26
Fluvoxamine, 26
Focalin XR, 31
Frova, 30
Frovatriptan, 30

G
Gabapentin, 30–31
gamma-aminobu-
    tyric acid (GABA),
    24–25, 29, 155
genetic pleomor-
    phism, 33, 47
Geodon, 29
glutamine, 23–25,
    32, 127, 321

H
hallucinations, 24,
    67–68, 70–71, 75,
    82, 90, 110–11,
    117–18, 125, 128,
    153, 220–21, 235,
    273, 300, 322
head pain, 1–4, 14
hemorrhage, 54–55,
    57–58
Hydrocodone
    case studies
        involving use of,
        129, 150, 162,
        187, 205, 291
    case study in abuse
        of, 163–71
    for depression and
        pain, 323–25
    uses for, 28
Hydromorphone, 28

hypnagogic halluci-
    nations, 90, 300

I
Imipramine
    case studies
        involving, 53,
        132, 142, 149,
        160, 190
    in early pharmacy,
        253
    effects of, 26–27, 33
Imitrex, 30, 203
insouciance, 55
interstitial cystitis,
    148–49, 228, 245
irritable bowel
    syndrome, 4–14

J
jaw pain, 35–46

K
Kadian, 28
Keppra, 31
Ketalar, 32
Ketamine, 32
kindling, 92–95,
    98–102. *See also*
    memory
Klonopin, 29

L
Lamictal, 31, 33,
    227, 290
Lamotrigine, 31
leg pain, 93–95,
    138–44

Levetiracetam, 31
Lexapro, 26, 52, 230
Librium, 253
lingual nerve, 35–38, 41–42
Lithium, 30–31, 80–81, 161
Lithonate, 31
Lorazepam, 24, 29, 98, 214
Lorcet, 29
Lortab, 28
Luvox, 26
Lyrica, 30–31, 160

M
marijuana, 25, 155–56. *See also* alcoholism; drug abuse
Maxalt, 30
Memantine, 32
memory. See also kindling
  case studies in pain and, 93–111
  role in illness and pain, 40–42, 91–93, 111
menstrual cycle, 188–89
Meperidine, 28
Meprobamate, 253
mesencephalic subarachnoid hemorrhage, 57

Methadone
  for bipolar disease, 276–78
  case studies involving, 63, 154, 253, 259, 262, 264, 269–70, 275, 283, 286, 293, 299, 302, 304, 320, 326
  for opiate addiction, 254, 277–78
  uses for, 28, 32, 254–55
Methadose, 28, 32
Methylphenidate, 31
Metoprolol, 240
migraine
  and bipolar disease, 321
  case studies in, 54–60, 183–202, 262–67, 300–303, 305–11
  and depression, 194–95
  drugs for, 30–31
  nature of, 193–94, 321
  in pregnancy, 185
  transformed, 194–95
Miltown, 253
Modafinil, 31
Morphine, 24, 28, 160, 172–73, 251, 253

MS Contin, 28, 251, 259

N
Nalbuphine, 28
Naltrexone, 28, 155
Namenda, 32, 126–27
Naratriptan, 30
narcolepsy
  case studies in, 82–90, 102–11, 221, 240, 305–21
  drugs for, 31
  nature of, 235
  and pain, 112
neck pain, 1–4, 14, 93–95
Nefazodone, 27
neurologic disease, 20
Neurontin, 30–31, 214, 313
neurotransmitters, 21–22
neurotransmitter systems, 21–22
  dopamine, 24–25, 27–29, 31, 123–24, 155
  effect of childhood abuse on, 210–11
  GABA, 24–25, 29, 155
  glutamine, 23–25, 32, 127, 321

noradrenaline,
22–23, 26–27, 31
opioid, 24–25,
155–56
serotonin, 22–23,
26–27, 29–30
in youth, 210
non-steroidal anti-
inflammatory
drugs (NSAID), 28
noradrenaline,
22–23, 26–27, 31
Norpramine, 27
Nortriptyline, 4, 9,
27, 118, 142, 238,
246
Nubain, 28

O

obsessive-compulsive
disorder, 308–11
occipital nerve
block, 2
Olanzapine, 29
opiates. *See also*
individual drug
names addiction/
dependence,
165–66, 199
for bipolar disease,
295
case studies in
overuse of,
163–71, 178–81,
325–28
case studies in use
of, 249–76

effect on brain, 199
function of, 24–25
for mental illness,
253–55, 276
Methadone for
addiction to, 254,
277–78
use in treatment of
chronic pain,
328–30
uses for, 28–29
opioid hyperalgesia,
170–73
opioid transmitter
system, 24–25,
155–56
Osler, William, 312
osteonecrosis, 43
Oxazepam, 29, 151,
153
Oxycodone, 28,
173–78, 214, 326
Oxycontin, 28, 150,
157, 171, 178–81,
295

P

pain
migration beyond
origin, 36–38,
41–42, 50
nighttime, 1–4,
35–47, 312–21
pain, chronic
as disease of the
mind, 6, 41,
46–47

examples of, 17
identifiers of,
17–18, 107–8
nature of, 4–5, 9,
12, 15, 18–19,
52, 121
risk factors for,
19–20
use of pharmacy
for, 10–11,
20–21, 25–33,
70–71, 133, 210
pain behavior
case studies in,
129–44
with chronic versus
nonchronic
pain, 130
as symptom of
conversion,
130–33
Pamelor, 27
panic disorder,
91–92, 139, 205,
239, 248–49
Parkinson's disease
case studies in,
118–26
dopamine and, 24
nature of, 123–26
as risk factor, 20
Paroxetine, 26
Paxil, 26
penicillium mold,
277
Percocet, 29
Percodan, 28

periodic diseases,
189
personality disorder,
78
phantom limb
syndrome, 92
pharmacy
anticonvulsants,
23–24, 30–31
anti-migraine
drugs, 30
antipsychotic
drugs, 29
anxiolytics/
tranquilizers,
24, 29
dopamine anti-
depressants,
27–28
early advances in,
253
effect on neuro-
transmitter
systems, 21–25
glutamine
antagonists, 32
opioid analgesics,
28–29
psychostimulants,
31
selective serotonin
reuptake
inhibitors (SSRI),
22, 26, 52
serotonin and
noradrenaline
reuptake
inhibitors
(SNRI), 23, 27

tricyclic anti-
depressants, 11,
22–23, 26–27, 53
tricyclic-like anti-
depressants, 22,
27
use in chronic
pain, 10–11,
20–21, 25–33,
70–71, 133, 210
Phenytoin, 31
pleomorphism,
genetic, 33, 47
post-traumatic stress
disorder, 9, 14, 91,
178–81, 255–60
Pregabaline, 30–31
Propoxyphene, 28
Provigil, 31
Prozac, 22, 26
pruritis, 128
pseudoaddiction,
199
pseudoseizures, 258

Q
Quetiapine, 29

R
reflex sympathetic
dystrophy (RSD),
312–22
Relpax, 30
repression, 45, 91,
131, 258
Reserpine, 253
Restoril, 29
Riseridone, 29
Risperdal, 29

Ritalin, 31, 90, 306,
308, 310–11. *See
also* stimulants
Rizatriptan, 30

S
schizophrenia, 24, 29
selective serotonin
reuptake
inhibitors (SSRI),
22, 26, 52
Selegiline, 28
Serax, 29
Seroquel, 11, 29, 70
serotonin, 22–23,
26–27, 29–30
serotonin and
noradrenaline
reuptake inhibitors
(SNRI), 23, 27
Sertraline, 26
Serzone, 27
sexual abuse, 20. *See
also* childhood
abuse
Sinemet, 125
Sinequan, 27
sleep paralysis, 90,
110–11, 235, 301,
322
Soma, 129, 158
spinal fusion,
158–59, 173, 214,
216, 249
Stadol, 28
stimulants, 248, 329.
See also Adderall/
Adderall XR;
Ritalin

straight leg raising test, 129–30
Strattera, 31, 158
stroke, 20
Subutex, 28, 170, 200, 278, 326
Sumatriptan, 30
sundowning, 117

T
Tegretol, 31, 253
Temazepam, 29
Thorazine, 253
tongue pain, 35–42, 49–54
Topamax, 31, 100, 316
Topiramate, 31
Tramadol, 28
tranquilizers, 24–25, 29
transcutaneous electrical nerve stimulation (TENS), 80, 179

transference, 65, 131, 204
Tranxene, 29
trauma, emotional, 8, 14, 45
Trazadone, 27
tricyclic antidepressants (TCA), 11, 22–23, 26–27, 53
tricyclic-like anti-depressants, 22, 27
triptan, 30
Trofranil, 27
Tylox, 28

U
Ultracet, 29
Ultram, 28

V
vagus nerve stimulator, 179
Valium, 29

Valproate, 30
Venlafaxine, 27
Viagra, 177
Vicodin, 28

W
Wellbutrin, 28, 214
Wolff-Parkinson-White Syndrome (WPW), 102–9

X
Xanax, 29

Z
Ziprasidone, 29
Zolmitriptan, 30
Zoloft, 26, 68
Zomig, 30
Zonegran, 31
Zonisamide, 31
Zyprexa, 29

About the Author

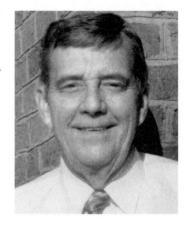

A graduate of Vanderbilt University Medical School, Robert T. Cochran Jr., MD, completed his residency in internal medicine and neurology at the University of Texas and Duke University. In 1963, he founded his private medical practice, and over the course of many years has treated thousands of patients with chronic pain.

This experience, in conjunction with that gained as co-director of the Pain Center at Centennial Hospital (Nashville) in the 1990s, led Dr. Cochran to make groundbreaking links between pain and various psychiatric disorders. His first book, *Understanding Chronic Pain* (Hillsboro Press, 2004), explored these relationships.

Curing Chronic Pain offers the thesis that chronic pain is actually a form of mental illness, one that with the imaginative use of pharmacy can be cured in many cases.

Dr. Cochran continues his active medical practice in Nashville, where he resides with his wife, Donna. They have three children and seven grandchildren.

For additional information about Dr. Cochran, a recognized leader in the field of chronic pain management and a national speaker on the subject, visit www.understandingpain.com.